Essential
Microbiology for
Dentistry

Commissioning Editor: Michael Parkinson
Project Development Manager: Janice Urquhart
Project Manager: Frances Affleck
Design direction: Erik Bigland
Illustrated by: Robert Britton

Essential Microbiology for Dentistry

L. P. Samaranayake
BDS, DDS, FRCPath, MIBiol, FHKAM (Pathology), FHKAM (Dental Surgery)

Chair Professor of Oral Microbiology, Faculty of Dentistry,
The University of Hong Kong, Hong Kong

With a section on Basic Immunology by

Brian M. Jones, BSc, PhD
Senior Hospital Immunologist, Department of Pathology, Faculty of Medicine,
The University of Hong Kong

Foreword by

Crispian Scully CBE
MD, PhD, MDS, MRCS, FDSRCS, FDSRCPS, FFDRCSI, FDSRCSE, FRCPath, FMedSci

Dean, Director of Studies and Research, Eastman Dental Institute for Oral Health Care Sciences,
University of London, UK

SECOND EDITION

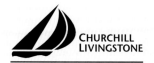

CHURCHILL
LIVINGSTONE

EDINBURGH LONDON NEW YORK OXFORD PHILADELPHIA ST LOUIS SYDNEY TORONTO 2002

CHURCHILL LIVINGSTONE
An imprint of Elsevier Limited

First published 1996
Second edition 2002
  Reprinted 2002 (twice), 2003, 2004

ISBN 0 443 06461 X

British Library Cataloguing in Publication Data
A catalogue record for this book is available from the British Library

Library of Congress Cataloging in Publication Data
A catalog record for this book is available from the Library of Congress

Note
Medical knowledge is constantly changing. As new information becomes available, changes in treatment, procedures, equipment and the use of drugs become necessary. The author and the publishers have taken care to ensure that the information given in this text is accurate and up to date. However, readers are strongly advised to confirm that the information, especially with regard to drug usage, complies with the latest legislation and standards of practice.

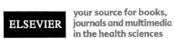

ELSEVIER your source for books,
journals and multimedia
in the health sciences

www.elsevierhealth.com

The
publisher's
policy is to use
paper manufactured
from sustainable forests

Printed in China
C/05

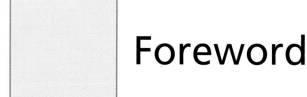

Foreword

I am delighted to see the second edition of this excellent text. The emergence of innumerable infectious diseases, the ever expanding HIV pandemic, mass migrations from the developing world and war zones, and the increase in global travel, soon to be escalated with a new generation of passenger aircraft, bring exotic diseases to all our doorsteps and increase the need for access to information on these areas. One has only to open any newspaper or watch the news, to be aware of the emerging problems of HIV, tuberculosis, ebola virus and transmissible spongiform encephalopathies. The changes in microbiology, not least due to the advances in DNA technology, also mean that students must keep abreast of advances. This book will no doubt assist them in that task.

Professor Crispian Scully CBE

Contents

1 Introduction

Microbiology, so called because it primarily deals with organisms too small for the naked eye to see, encompasses the study of organisms that cause disease, the host response to infection, and ways in which such infection may be prevented. For our purposes the subject can be broadly classified into **general**, **medical** and **oral microbiology**.

Dental students need both a basic understanding of general and medical microbiology and a detailed knowledge of clinical oral microbiology in order to diagnose oral microbial infections, which are intimately related to the overall treatment plan for their patients. Moreover, the two major oral disorders — **caries** and **periodontal disease** — that the dental practitioner is frequently called upon to treat are due to changes in the oral bacterial ecosystem, and a grasp of these disease processes is essential for their appropriate management.

The impact of these infections on the health and welfare of the community is simply astonishing. It has been estimated, for instance, that caries and periodontal disease are the most costly diseases that the majority of the population has to contend with during their lifetime, and the number of working hours lost due to these infections and the related cost of dental treatment worldwide amounts to billions of dollars per annum (e.g. 46 billion dollars in the USA in 1995).

The advent of the human immunodeficiency virus (HIV) infection in the early 1980s and the subsequent concerns about cross-infection via contaminated blood and instruments have resulted in an increased regimentation of **infection control** practices in dentistry. Furthermore, many patients are acutely concerned about possible infection transmission in clinical settings because of the intense, and sometimes unwarranted, publicity given to these matters by the media. The dental practitioner should therefore be conversant with all aspects of infection control in the clinical environment, not only to implement infection control measures but also to advise the dental team (dental hygienists and other dental ancillary personnel) and to allay patients' unfounded fears. For all these and many other reasons, which the student will discover in the text, the discipline of microbiology is intimately woven into the fabric of dentistry and comprises a crucial component of the dental curriculum.

About this book

This text is divided into six parts in order to highlight the different features of microbiology related to dentistry, but it should be remembered that such division is artificial and is merely an attempt to simplify the learning process.

The first few chapters in **Part 1** essentially describe general microbiological features of bacteria and viruses and how they cause human infections (i.e. **pathogenesis**). **Diagnostic microbiology**, by which clinical microbiologists ascertain the nature of agents causing various infections, is described in Chapter 6. The laboratory aspect of the latter fascinating subject is analogous to the work of a crime detection bureau! When a specimen (e.g. pus, urine) from a patient with an infectious disease is sent to the laboratory for identification of the offending agent, the clinical microbiologist has to resort to many methods and techniques, as well as a fair amount of thought, to identify the pathogenic organism or organisms lurking in the clinical sample. In many situations the organism may be dead, in which case other, indirect clues need to be pursued to incriminate the suspect pathogen. Once an offending pathogen is identified, antimicrobial chemotherapy is the mainstay of treatment; a description of chemotherapeutic agents and how they are chosen in the laboratory is given in Chapter 7.

The host responds to infection by mounting an immune response. A highly abbreviated account of **basic immunology** is given in **Part 2**; supplemental reading is essential to augment this material and the reader is referred to the lists of recommended texts for this purpose. Immunological nomenclature is complex and often difficult: a glossary of terms and abbreviations is therefore provided as an appendix.

Although there are thousands of offending pathogens, only some are of direct import to dental practice and to the comprehension of the **mechanisms of disease**; these are described in **Part 3**. Arguably this section may appear to be the most daunting part of the book because of the complex nomenclature of microbes; hence only the salient bacterial genera — some of which are more closely related to dental practice (e.g. streptococci) than others (e.g. legionellae) — are outlined. Similarly, the chapters on viruses and fungi are relatively brief, with thumbnail sketches of only the most relevant organisms.

The major **infections of each organ system** are discussed in **Part 4**, with emphasis on those that are most relevant to dentistry. The student is strongly advised to cross-refer to organisms and their characteristics (described in Part 3) when studying this section, as the microbial attributes and the diseases they cause form a single continuum.

Part 5 specifically outlines the **microbial interactions in the orofacial region**, in both health and disease. This 1 section should be particularly useful for the later years of the dental curriculum, to reinforce the studies in conservative dentistry, periodontics, oral and maxillofacial surgery and oral medicine.

Last but not least, the subject of **cross-infection and its control** in dentistry is encapsulated in **Part 6**. It provides a comprehensive summary of the routine infection-control regimens that must be implemented in every dental practice. The relevance of this information in routine clinical practice cannot be overemphasized and a thorough understanding of this material should pay rich dividends in years to come.

As the student will discover, the comprehensive nature of this text has made almost all the material significant. Thus the reader will be intellectually challenged to learn a new concept or terminology in almost every sentence or phrase. In addition, an attempt has been made to summarize the information as key facts, to serve as an aide-mémoire, at the end of each chapter. It is important, however, that the subject matter is augmented with additional reading and it is to this end that the list of recommended texts is given.

Finally, in most of the chapters the text is arranged under the following important features of microbiology, which the student must understand in order to deal with infectious diseases.

- **epidemiology**: spread, distribution and prevalence of infection in the community
- **pathogenesis**: the means by which microbes cause disease in humans, an understanding of which is critical for successful diagnosis and management of infections
- **diagnosis**: detection of an infection; depends on the collection of the correct specimen in the most appropriate manner, and subsequent interpretation of the laboratory results
- **treatment**: antibacterial, antifungal or antiviral therapy combined with supportive therapy leads to resolution of most infections
- **prevention** (prophylaxis): immunization is the most useful mode of preventing diseases such as tetanus and hepatitis B; however, increasing public awareness of diseases and their modes of spread significantly helps to curb the spread of infections in the community (e.g. HIV infection).

FURTHER READING

Coggan, D, Rose, G, and Barker, DJP (1997). *Epidemiology for the uninitiated* (4th edn). BMJ Publishing Group, London.

Morse, SS (1995). Factors in the emergence of infectious diseases. *Emerging Infectious Diseases* 1, 7–15.

General microbiology

The aim of this section is to present (1) the structural features of microbes and how they cause disease, and (2) a perspective of diagnostic laboratory methods to explain the relationship between the scientific basis of microbiology and its practical application in patient care.

- Bacterial structure and taxonomy
- Bacterial physiology and genetics
- Viruses and prions
- Pathogenesis of microbial disease
- Diagnostic microbiology and laboratory methods
- Antimicrobial chemotherapy

2 Bacterial structure and taxonomy

Microorganisms can be classified into major groups: algae, protozoa, fungi, bacteria, viruses and a number of organisms intermediate between bacteria and viruses (e.g. rickettsiae, chlamydiae). Bacteria, fungi and protozoa belong to the kingdom of **protists** and are differentiated from animals and plants by being unicellular or relatively simple multicellular organisms leading a parasitic existence. Viruses are unique, acellular, metabolically inert organisms and therefore can replicate only within living cells. Other differences between viruses and cellular organisms include:

- **Structure**. Cells possess a nucleus or, in the case of bacteria, a nucleoid with DNA. This is surrounded by the cytoplasm where energy is generated and proteins are synthesized. In viruses the inner core of genetic material is either DNA or RNA, but they have no cytoplasm and hence depend on the host for their energy and proteins (i.e. they are metabolically inert).
- **Reproduction**. Bacteria reproduce by **binary fission** (a parent cell divides into two similar cells), but viruses disassemble, produce copies of their nucleic acid and proteins, and then reassemble to produce another generation of viruses. As viruses are metabolically inert they must replicate within host cells. Bacteria, however, can replicate extracellularly (except rickettsiae and chlamydiae, which are bacteria that also require living cells for growth).

The major characteristics of bacteria, mycoplasmas, rickettsiae, chlamydiae and viruses are given in Table 2.1.

Eukaryotes and prokaryotes

Another way of classifying cellular organisms is to divide them into **prokaryotes** and **eukaryotes**. Fungi, protozoa and humans, for instance, are eukaryotic, whereas bacteria are prokaryotic. In prokaryotes the bacterial **genome**, or chromosome, is a single, circular molecule of double-stranded DNA, lacking a nuclear membrane (smaller, single or multiple, circular DNA molecules called plasmids may also be present in bacteria), whereas the eukaryotic cell has a true nucleus with multiple chromosomes surrounded by a nuclear membrane. The main differences between prokaryotes and eukaryotes are listed in Table 2.2.

Shape and size

The **shape** of a bacterium is determined by its rigid cell wall. Bacteria are classified by shape into three basic groups (Fig. 2.1):

- cocci (spherical)
- bacilli (rod-shaped)
- spirochaetes (helical).

Some bacteria with variable shapes, appearing both as coccal and bacillary forms, are called **pleomorphic** (*pleo* many, *morphic* shaped) in appearance.

The **size** of bacteria ranges from about 0.2 μm to 5 μm. The smallest bacteria approximate the size of the largest viruses (poxviruses), whereas the longest bacilli attain the same length as some yeasts and human red blood cells (7 μm).

Arrangement

Bacteria, whichever shape they may be, arrange themselves (usually according to the plane of successive cell division) as pairs (diplococci); chains (streptococci); grape-like clusters (staphylococci); or as angled pairs or palisades (corynebacteria).

Gram-staining characteristics

Bacteria can be classified into two major subgroups according to the staining characteristics of their cell walls. The stain used, called the **Gram stain** (first developed by a Danish physician, Christian Gram), divides the bacteria into **Gram-positive** (purple) and **Gram-negative** (pink) groups. The Gram-staining property of bacteria is useful both for their identification and in the therapy of bacterial infections because, in general, Gram-positive bacteria are more susceptible to penicillins than Gram-negative bacteria.

Structure

The structure of a typical bacterium is shown in Figure 2.2. Bacteria have a rigid cell wall protecting a fluid **protoplast** comprising a **cytoplasmic membrane** and a variety of other components (described below).

5

Table 2.1 Differential characteristics of major groups of organisms

	Bacteria	Mycoplasmas	Rickettsiae	Chlamydiae	Viruses*	Fungi
Visible with light microscope	+	+	+	+	−	+
Capable of free growth	+	+	−	−	−	+
Both DNA and RNA present	+	+	+	+	−	+
Muramic acid in cell wall	+	+	+	+	−	+
Rigid cell wall	+	−	+	Variable	−	+
Susceptible to penicillin	Variable	−	−	−	−	−
Susceptible to tetracycline	Variable	+	+	+	−	−
Reproduce essentially by binary fission	+	+	+	+	−	−

* Prions (agents responsible for Creutzfeldt–Jakob disease) are not included as their status is unclear.

Structures external to the cell wall

Flagella. Flagella are whip-like filaments which act as propellers and guide the bacteria toward nutritional and other sources (Fig. 2.3). The filaments are composed of many subunits of a single protein, **flagellin**. Flagella may be located at one end (monotrichous, a single flagellum; lophotrichous, many flagella) or all over the outer surface (peritrichous). Many bacilli (rods) have flagella, but most cocci do not and are therefore non-motile. Spirochaetes move by using a flagellum-like structure called the **axial filament**, which wraps around the cell to produce an undulating motion.

Fimbriae and pili. Fimbriae and pili are fine, hair-like filaments, shorter than flagella, that extend from the cell surface. Pili, found mainly on Gram-negative organisms, are composed of subunits of a protein, **pilin**, and mediate the adhesion of bacteria to receptors on the human cell surface — a necessary first step in the initiation of infection. A specialized type of pilus, the sex pilus, forms the attachment between the male (donor) and the female (recipient) bacteria during conjugation, when genes are transferred from one bacterium to another.

Glycocalyx (slime layer). The glycocalyx is a polysaccharide coating that covers the outer surfaces of many bacteria

Table 2.2 The major differences between prokaryote and eukaryote genetic and cellular organization

Prokaryotes	Eukaryotes
Organization of the genetic material and replication	
DNA free in the cytoplasm	DNA is contained within a membrane bound nucleus. A nucleolus is also present
Only one chromosome	More than one chromosome. Two copies of each chromosome may be present (diploid)
DNA associated with histone-like proteins	DNA complexed with histone proteins
May contain extrachromosomal elements called plasmids	Plasmids only found in yeast
Introns not found in mRNA	Introns found in all genes
Cell division by binary fission — asexual replication only	Cells divide by mitosis
Transfer of genetic information occurs by conjugation, transduction and transformation	Exchange of genetic information occurs during sexual reproduction. Meiosis leads to the production of haploid cells (gametes) which can fuse
Cellular organization	
Cytoplasmic membrane contains hopanoids	Cytoplasmic membrane contains sterols
Lipopolysaccharides and teichoic acids found	
Energy metabolism associated with the cytoplasmic membrane	Mitochondria present in most cases
Photosynthesis associated with membrane systems and vesicles in cytoplasm	Chloroplasts present in algal and plant cells
	Internal membranes, endoplasmic reticulum and Golgi apparatus present associated with protein synthesis and targeting
	Membrane vesicles such as lysosomes and peroxisomes present
	Cytoskeleton of microtubules present
Flagella consist of one protein, flagellin	Flagella have a complex structure with 9 + 2 microtubular arrangement
Ribosomes — 70S	Ribosomes — 80S (mitochondrial and chloroplast ribosomes are 70S)
Peptidoglycan cell walls (eubacteria only: different polymers in archaebacteria)	Polysaccharide cell walls, where present, are generally either cellulose or chitin

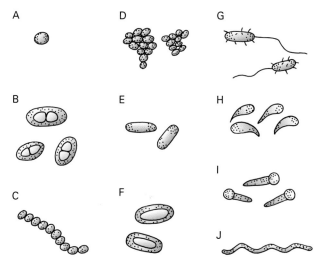

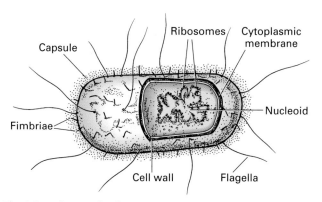

Fig. 2.1 Common bacterial forms. **A** coccus; **B** capsulated diplococci; **C, D** cocci in chains (e.g. streptococcus) and clusters (e.g. staphylococcus); **E** bacillus; **F, G** capsulated and flagellated bacillus (e.g. *Escherichia coli*); **H** curved bacilli (e.g. *Vibrio* sp.); **I** spore-bearing bacilli (e.g. *Clostridium tetani*); **J** spirochaete.

Fig. 2.2 A bacterial cell.

and allows the bacteria to adhere firmly to various structures, e.g. oral mucosa, teeth, heart valves and catheters. This is especially true in the case of *Streptococcus mutans*, a major cariogenic organism, which has the ability to produce vast quantities of extracellular polysaccharide in the presence of dietary sugars such as sucrose.

Capsule. An amorphous, gelatinous layer (usually more substantial than the glycocalyx) surrounds the entire bacterium; it is composed of polysaccharide, and sometimes protein (e.g. anthrax bacillus). The sugar components of the polysaccharide vary in different bacterial species and frequently determine the serological type within a species (e.g. 84 different serological types of *Streptococcus pneumoniae* can be distinguished by the antigenic differences of the sugars in the polysaccharide capsule). The capsule is important because:
- It mediates the **adhesion** of bacteria to human tissues — a prerequisite for colonization and infection.
- It hinders or inhibits **phagocytosis**; hence, the presence of a capsule correlates with virulence.
- It helps in laboratory **identification** of organisms (in the presence of antiserum against the capsular polysaccharide the capsule will swell greatly — a phenomenon called the **quellung reaction**).

- Its polysaccharides are used as antigens in certain vaccines because they elicit protective antibodies (e.g. polysaccharide vaccine of *S. pneumoniae*).

Cell wall

The cell wall confers rigidity upon the bacterial cell. It is a multilayered structure outside the cytoplasmic membrane. It is porous and permeable to substances of low molecular weight.

The inner layer of the cell wall is made of **peptidoglycan** and is covered by an outer membrane that varies in thickness and chemical composition, depending upon the Gram-staining property of the bacteria (Fig. 2.4). The term 'peptidoglycan' is derived from the peptides and the sugars (glycan) that make up the molecule. (Synonyms for peptidoglycan are murein and mucopeptide.)

The cell walls of Gram-positive and Gram-negative bacteria have important structural and chemical differences (Fig. 2.5):
- The peptidoglycan layer is common to both Gram-positive and Gram-negative bacteria but is much thicker in the Gram-positive bacteria.
- In contrast, the Gram-negative organisms have a complex outer membrane composed of lipopolysaccharide, lipoprotein and phospholipid. These form 'porins', through which hydrophilic molecules are transported in and out of the organism. The O antigen of the lipopolysaccharide and the lipid A component of the endotoxin are also embedded in the outer membrane. Lying between the outer membrane and the cytoplasmic membrane of Gram-negative bacteria is the **periplasmic space**. It is in this space that some bacterial species produce enzymes that destroy drugs such as penicillins (e.g. lactamases).
- The lipopolysaccharide of Gram-negative bacteria contains **endotoxin**. (Hence, by definition, endotoxins cannot be produced by Gram-positive bacteria as they do not have lipopolysaccharides in their cell walls.) It is responsible for many of the features of disease, such as fever and shock (see Ch. 5).

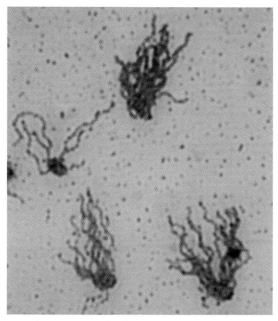

Fig. 2.3 Photomicrograph of a bacterium showing peritrichous flagella. Note the relative length of the flagella compared with the size of the organism.

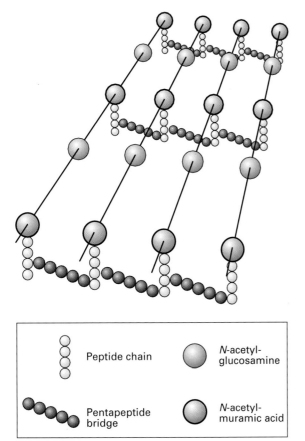

Fig. 2.4 Chemical structure of cross-linking peptidoglycan component of cell wall, common to both Gram-positive and Gram-negative bacteria (after Sharon N, The bacterial cell wall, *Scientific American* 1969;220: 92).

- The cell walls of some bacteria (e.g. *Mycobacterium tuberculosis*) contain lipids called mycolic acids which cannot be Gram-stained, and hence are called **acid-fast** (i.e. they resist decolorization with acid–alcohol after being stained with carbolfuchsin).

Bacteria with defective cell walls. Some bacteria can survive with defective cell walls. These include mycoplasmas, L-forms, spheroplasts and protoplasts.

Mycoplasmas do not possess a cell wall and do not need hypertonic media for their survival. They occur in nature and may cause human disease (e.g. pneumonia).

L-forms are usually produced in the laboratory and may totally or partially lack cell walls. They may be produced in patients treated with penicillin and, like mycoplasmas, can replicate on ordinary media.

Both **spheroplasts** (derived from Gram-negative bacteria) and **protoplasts** (derived from Gram-positive bacteria) lack cell walls, cannot replicate on laboratory media and are unstable and osmotically fragile. They require hypertonic conditions for maintenance and are produced in the laboratory by the action of enzymes or antibiotics.

Cytoplasmic membrane

The cytoplasmic membrane lies just inside the peptidoglycan layer of the cell wall and is a 'unit membrane' composed of a phospholipid bilayer similar in appearance to that of eukaryotic cells. However, eukaryotic membranes contain sterols, whereas prokaryotes generally do not (the only exception being mycoplasmas). The membrane has five major functions:

1. Active transport of molecules into the cell.
2. Passive diffusion of other nutrients through the semipermeable membrane.
3. Energy generation by oxidative phosphorylation.
4. Synthesis of cell wall precursors.
5. Secretion of enzymes and toxins.

Mesosome. This is a convoluted invagination of the cytoplasmic membrane which functions as the origin of the transverse septum that divides the cell in half during cell division. It is also the binding site of the DNA which will become the genetic material of each daughter cell.

Cytoplasm

The cytoplasm comprises an inner, nucleoid region (composed of DNA) which is surrounded by an amorphous matrix that contains ribosomes, nutrient granules, metabolites and various ions.

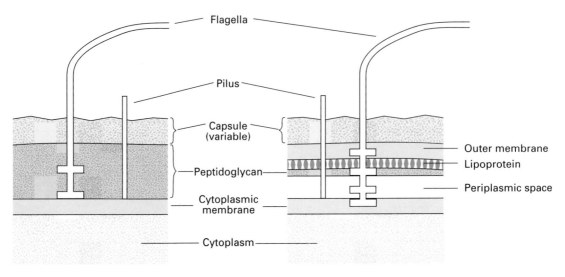

Fig. 2.5 Structural features of Gram-positive and Gram-negative cell walls.

Nuclear material or nucleoid. Bacterial DNA comprises a single, supercoiled, circular chromosome that contains about 2000 genes. During cell division it undergoes semiconservative replication bidirectionally from a fixed point.

Ribosomes. Ribosomes are the sites of protein synthesis. Bacterial ribosomes differ from those of eukaryotic cells in both size and chemical composition. Bacterial ribosomes are organized in units of 70S, compared with eukaryotic ribosomes of 80S. These differences are the basis of the selective action of some antibiotics that inhibit bacterial, but not human, protein β-synthesis.

Cytoplasmic inclusions. The cytoplasm contains different types of inclusions, which serve as sources of stored energy; examples include polymetaphosphate, polysaccharide and β-hydroxybutyrate.

Bacterial spores

Spores are formed in response to adverse conditions by the medically important bacteria that belong to the genus *Bacillus* (which includes the agent of anthrax) and the genus *Clostridium* (which includes the agents of tetanus and botulism). These bacteria **sporulate** (form spores) when nutrients, such as sources of carbon and nitrogen, are scarce (Fig. 2.6). The spore develops at the expense of the vegetative cell and contains bacterial DNA, a small amount of cytoplasm, cell membrane, peptidoglycan, very little water, and, most importantly, a thick, keratin-like coat. This coat, which contains a high concentration of calcium dipicolinate, is remarkably resistant to heat, dehydration, radiation and chemicals. Once formed, the spore is metabolically inert and can remain dormant for many years. Spores are called either 'terminal' or 'subterminal', depending on their position in relation to the cell wall of the bacillus from which they developed.

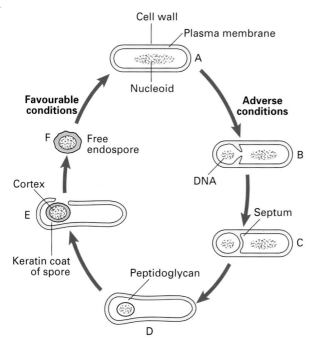

Fig. 2.6 The cycle of sporulation. **A** Vegetative cell; **B** ingrowth of cytoplasmic membrane; **C** developing forespore; **D** forespore completely cut off from the cell cytoplasm; **E** development of cortex and keratin spore coat; **F** liberation of spore and conversion to vegetative state under favourable conditions.

When appropriate conditions supervene (i.e. water, nutrients) there is enzymic degradation of the coat and the spore transforms itself into a metabolizing, reproducing bacterial cell once again (Fig. 2.6).

Clinical relevance of bacterial spores

The clinical importance of spores lies in their extraordinary resistance to heat and chemicals. Because of this, sterilization cannot be easily achieved by boiling; other, more efficacious methods of sterilization, such as steam under pressure (autoclaving), are required to ensure the sterility of products used for surgical purposes (Ch. 37). This property of bacterial spores is exploited when they are used for evaluating the sterilization efficacy of autoclaves; spores of *Bacillus stearothermophilus* and other species are used for this purpose.

TAXONOMY

Systematic classification and categorization of organisms into ordered groups is called 'taxonomy'. A working knowledge of taxonomy is useful for diagnostic microbiology and for studies in epidemiology and pathogenicity.

As mentioned at the beginning of this chapter, bacteria and fungi are protists. Although higher organisms are classified according to their evolutionary pathways (i.e. phylogenetically), bacteria cannot be similarly categorized because of the insufficiency of their morphological features. Bacterial classification is somewhat artificial in that they are categorized according to **phenotypic** features, which facilitate their laboratory identification. These comprise:

- **morphology** (cocci, bacilli, spirochaetes, etc.)
- **staining properties** (Gram-positive, Gram-negative, etc.)
- **cultural requirements** (aerobic, facultative anaerobic, anaerobic)
- **biochemical reactions** (saccharolytic and asaccharolytic, according to sugar fermentation reactions, etc.)
- **antigenic structure** (serotypes).

Most of the medically and dentally important bacteria are classified according to their morphology, Gram-staining characteristics and their atmospheric requirements. A simple classification of medically important bacteria is given in Figures 2.7 and 2.8.

Genotypic taxonomy

In contrast to the classical phenotypic classification methods outlined above, **genotypic** classification and speciation of organisms are becoming increasingly important and useful. Genotypic taxonomy exploits the genetic characteristics, which are more stable than the sometimes transient phenotypic features of organisms. These methods essentially evaluate the degree of DNA homology of organisms in order to speciate them, for example by assessing molecular guanine and cytosine (GC) content, ribotyping, randomly amplified polymorphic DNA (RAPD) analysis, and pulsed-field gel electrophoresis (PFGE). Further details of these methods are given in Chapter 3.

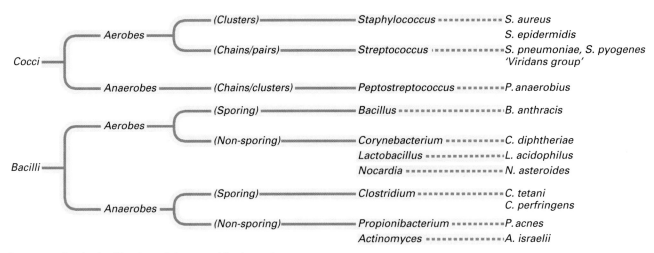

Fig. 2.7 A simple classification of Gram-positive bacteria.

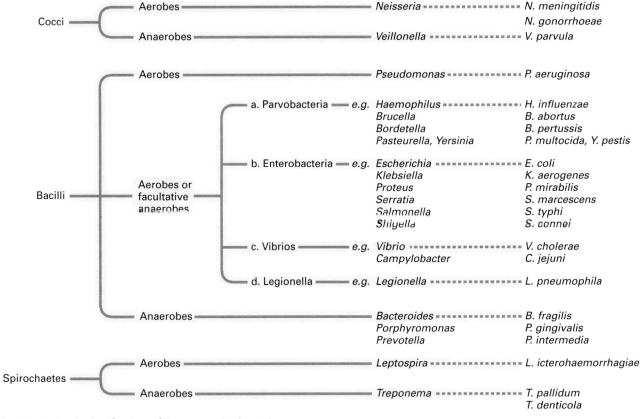

Fig. 2.8 A simple classification of Gram-negative bacteria.

How do organisms get their names?

Organisms are named according to a hierarchical system, beginning with the taxonomic rank **kingdom**, followed by **division, subdivision, order, family, genus** and **species** (Table 2.3). The scientific name of an organism is classically a binomial of the last two ranks, i.e. a combination of the generic name followed by the species name, e.g. *Streptococcus salivarius* (note that the species name does not begin with a capital letter). The name is usually written in italics with the generic name abbreviated (e.g. *S. salivarius*). When bacterial names are used adjectivally or collectively the names are not italicized and do not begin with a capital letter (e.g. staphylococcal enzymes, lactobacilli).

Table 2.3 Hierarchical ranks in classification of organisms

Taxonomic rank	Example
Kingdom	Procaryotae
Division	Firmicutes
Subdivision	Low GC content of DNA
Order	—
Family	Streptococcaceae
Genus	Streptococcus
Species	Streptococcus salivarius

KEY FACTS

Note: clinically relevant facts and practice points are *italicized*; key words are in **bold**

- The word 'microorganism' (microbe) is used to describe an organism that cannot be seen without the use of a microscope
- The main groups of microbes are **algae, protozoa, fungi, bacteria** and **viruses**; with progressively decreasing size
- All living cells are either **prokaryotic** or **eukaryotic**
- Prokaryotes such as **bacteria are simple cells** with no internal membranes or organelles
- **Eukaryotes have a nucleus, organelles** such as mitochondria, and complex **internal membranes** (e.g. fungi, human cells)
- Bacteria are divided into two major classes according to staining characteristics: **Gram-positive** (purple) and **Gram-negative** (pink)
- **Structures external** to the cell wall of bacteria are **flagella** (whip-like filaments), **fimbriae** or pili (fine, short, hair-like filaments), **glycocalyx** (slime layer) and **capsule**
- Flagella are used for movement, the fimbriae and pili for adhesion, and the glycocalyx for adhesion and protection

- Cell wall **peptidoglycan is common to both Gram-positive and Gram-negative bacteria**, but thicker in the former; it gives rigidity and shape to the organism
- Peptidoglycan comprises long chains of *N*-acetyl-muramic acid and *N*-acetyl-glucosamine cross-linked by peptide side-chains and cross-bridges
- *Lipopolysaccharides (LPS) are integral components of the outer membranes of Gram-negative (but not Gram-positive) bacteria; **LPS is the endotoxin** and therefore Gram-positive bacteria cannot produce endotoxin*
- Cell walls of some bacteria such as the **mycobacteria** contain lipids (mycolic acids) that are resistant to Gram staining; these bacteria are called **acid-fast organisms**
- **Bacterial cytoplasm contains** chromosomal nuclear material — **nucleoid, ribosomes,** inclusions/storage **granules**
- Spore formation or **sporulation** is a **response to adverse conditions** in *Bacillus* spp. and *Clostridium* spp.
- **Taxonomy (systematic classification of organisms** into groups) can be performed according to morphology, staining reactions, cultural requirements, biochemical reactions, antigenic structure and DNA composition

FURTHER READING

Mims, C, Playfair, J, Roitt, I, Wakelin, D, and Williams, R (1998). Microbes and parasites; and The host-parasite response. In *Medical microbiology* (2nd edn), Chs 1 and 2. Mosby, London.

Morello, JA, Mizer, HE, Wilson, ME, and Granato, PA (1998). Character of microorganisms. In *Microbiology in patient care* (6th edn), Chs 1 and 2. McGraw-Hill, Boston.

Murray, PR, Rosenthal, KS, Kobayashi, GS, and Pfaller, MA (1998). Bacterial morphology and cell wall structure and synthesis; and Bacterial metabolism and growth. In *Medical microbiology* (3rd edn), Chs 3 and 4. Mosby Year Book, St Louis.

3 Bacterial physiology and genetics

BACTERIAL PHYSIOLOGY

Growth

Bacteria, like all living organisms, require nutrients for metabolic purposes and for cell division, and grow best in an environment that satisfies these requirements. Chemically, bacteria are made up of polysaccharide, protein, lipid, nucleic acid and peptidoglycan, all of which must be manufactured for successful growth.

Nutritional requirements

Oxygen and hydrogen. Both oxygen and hydrogen are obtained from water; hence water is essential for bacterial growth. In addition, the correct oxygen tension is necessary for balanced growth. While the growth of aerobic bacteria is limited by availability of oxygen, anaerobic bacteria may be inhibited by low oxygen tension.

Carbon. Carbon is obtained by bacteria in two main ways:
- **Autotrophs**, which are free-living, non-parasitic bacteria, use carbon dioxide as the carbon source.
- **Heterotrophs**, which are parasitic bacteria, utilize complex organic substances such as sugars as their source of carbon dioxide and energy.

Inorganic ions. Nitrogen, sulphur, phosphate, magnesium, potassium and a number of trace elements are required for bacterial growth.

Organic nutrients. Organic nutrients are essential in different amounts, depending on the bacterial species.
- Carbohydrates are used as an energy source and as an initial substrate for biosynthesis of many substances.
- Amino acids are crucial for growth of some bacteria.
- Vitamins, purines and pyrimidines in trace amounts are needed for growth.

Reproduction

Bacteria reproduce by a process called **binary fission**, in which a parent cell divides to form a **progeny** of two cells. This results in a **logarithmic growth rate** — one bacterium will produce 16 bacteria after four generations. The **doubling** or **mean generation time** of bacteria may vary (e.g. 20 minutes for *Escherichia coli*, 24 hours for *Mycobacterium tuber-*

culosis); the shorter the doubling time, the faster the multiplication rate. Other factors that affect the doubling time include the amount of nutrients, the temperature and the pH of the environment.

Bacterial growth cycle

The growth cycle of a bacterium has four main phases (Fig. 3.1):
1. **Lag phase**: may last for a few minutes or for many hours as bacteria do not divide immediately but undergo a period of adaptation with vigorous metabolic activity.
2. **Log (logarithmic, exponential) phase**: rapid cell division occurs, determined by the environmental conditions.
3. **Stationary phase**: is reached when nutrient depletion or toxic products cause growth to slow until the number of new cells produced balances the number of cells that die. The bacteria have now achieved their **maximal cell density** or **yield**.
4. **Decline** or **death phase**: this is marked by a decline in the number of live bacteria.

Growth regulation

Bacterial growth is essentially regulated by the nutritional environment. However, both intracellular and extracellular regulatory events can modify the growth rate. Intracellular factors include:
- **End-product inhibition**: the first enzyme in a metabolic pathway is inhibited by the end-product of that pathway.
- **Catabolite repression**: enzyme synthesis is inhibited by catabolites.

Extracellular factors that modify bacterial growth are:
- **Temperature**: the optimum is required for efficient activity of many bacterial enzymes, although bacteria can grow in a wide range of temperatures. Accordingly bacteria can be classified as:
  - **mesophiles**, which grow well between 25°C and 40°C, comprising most medically important bacteria (that grow best at body temperature)
  - **thermophiles**, which grow between 55°C and 80°C (*Thermus aquaticus*, for instance, grows in hot springs and its enzymes such as *Taq* polymerase are therefore heat-resistant, a fact exploited by molecular biologists)
  - **psychrophiles**, which grow at temperatures below 20°C.

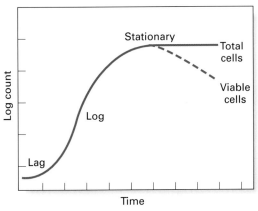

Fig. 3.1 Bacterial growth curve. Lag, lag phase of growth; Log, logarithmic phase of growth.

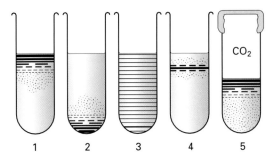

Fig. 3.2 Atmospheric requirements of bacteria, as demonstrated in agar shake cultures: **1**, obligate aerobe; **2**, obligate anaerobe; **3**, facultative anaerobe; **4**, microaerophile; **5**, capnophilic organism (growing in carbon dioxide-enriched atmosphere). (See also Table 3.1)

- **pH**: the hydrogen ion concentration of the environment should be around pH 7.2–7.4 (i.e. physiological pH) for optimal bacterial growth. However, some bacteria (for example lactobacilli) have evolved to exploit ecological niches, such as carious cavities where the pH may be as low as 5.0.

Aerobic and anaerobic growth

A good supply of oxygen enhances the metabolism and growth of most bacteria. The oxygen acts as the hydrogen acceptor in the final steps of energy production and generates two molecules, hydrogen peroxide (H_2O_2) and the free radical superoxide (O_2). Both of these are toxic and need to be destroyed. Two enzymes are used by bacteria to dispose of them: the first is **superoxide dismutase**, which catalyses the reaction

$$2O_2 + 2H^+ \rightarrow H_2O_2 + O_2$$

and the second is **catalase**, which converts hydrogen peroxide to water and oxygen:

$$2H_2O_2 \rightarrow 2H_2O + O_2.$$

Bacteria can therefore be classified according to their ability to live in an oxygen-replete or an oxygen-free environment (Fig. 3.2, Table 3.1). This has important practical implications, as clinical specimens must be incubated in the laboratory under appropriate gaseous conditions for the pathogenic bacteria to grow. Thus bacteria can be classified as follows:

- **Obligate (strict) aerobes**, which require oxygen to grow because their ATP-generating system is dependent on oxygen as the hydrogen acceptor (e.g. *Mycobacterium tuberculosis*).
- **Facultative anaerobes**, which use oxygen to generate energy by respiration if it is present, but can use the fermentation pathway to synthesize ATP in the absence of sufficient oxygen (e.g. oral bacteria such as mutans streptococci, *Escherichia coli*).
- **Obligate (strict) anaerobes**, which cannot grow in the presence of oxygen because they lack either superoxide dismutase or catalase, or both (e.g. *Porphyromonas gingivalis*).
- **Microaerophiles**, that grow best at a low oxygen concentration (e.g. *Campylobacter fetus*).

BACTERIAL GENETICS

Genetics is the study of inheritance and variation. All inherited characteristics are encoded in DNA, except in RNA viruses.

The bacterial chromosome

The bacterial chromosome contains the genetic information that defines all the characteristics of the organism. It is a single, continuous strand of DNA (Fig. 3.3) with a closed, circular structure attached to the cell membrane of the organism. The 'average' bacterial chromosome has a molecular weight of 2×10^9.

Replication

Chromosome replication is an accurate process that ensures that the progeny cells receive identical copies from the mother

Table 3.1 Effect of oxygen on the growth of bacteria

Degree of oxygenation	Term	Example
Oxygen essential for growth	Obligate aerobe	*Pseudomonas aeruginosa*
Grows well under low oxygen concentration (5%)	Microaerophile	*Campylobacter fetus*
Grows in presence or absence of oxygen	Facultative anaerobe[a]	*Streptococcus milleri*
Only grows in absence of oxygen	Obligate anaerobe	*Porphyromonas gingivalis*

[a] Facultative anaerobes may be subgrouped as capnophiles or capnophilic organisms if they grow well in the presence of 8–10% carbon dioxide (e.g. *Legionella pneumophila*).

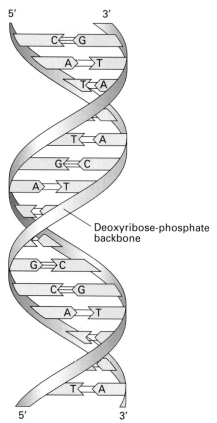

Fig. 3.3 The structure of DNA.

G, C, T, A = Bases $\equiv/\!=\!/$llllll = Hydrogen bonds

cell. The replication process is initiated at a specific site on the chromosome (*ori*C site) where the two DNA strands are locally denatured. A complex of proteins binds to this site, opens up the helix and initiates replication. Each strand then serves as a template for a complete round of DNA synthesis which occurs in both directions (bidirectional) and on both strands, creating a **replication bubble** (Fig. 3.4). The two sites at which the replication occurs are called the **replication forks**. As replication proceeds the replication forks move around the molecule in opposite directions opening up the DNA strands, synthesizing two new complementary strands until the two replication forks meet at a termination site. Of the four DNA strands now available, each daughter cell receives a parental strand and a newly synthesized strand. This process is called **semiconservative replication**. Such chromosomal replication is synchronous with cell division, so that each cell receives a full complement of DNA from the mother cell.

The main enzyme that mediates DNA replication is **DNA-dependent DNA polymerase**, although a number of others take part in this process. When errors occur during DNA replication, repair mechanisms excise incorrect nucleotide sequences with **nucleases**, replace them with the correct nucleotides and re-ligate the sequence.

Bacteria have evolved mechanisms to delete foreign nucleotides from their genomes. **Restriction enzymes** are mainly used for this purpose and they cleave double-stranded DNA at specific sequences. The DNA fragments produced by restriction enzymes vary in their molecular weight and can be demonstrated in the laboratory by gel electrophoresis. Hence these restriction enzymes are used in many clinical analytical techniques to cleave DNA and to characterize both bacteria and viruses (see below).

Genes

The genetic code of bacteria is contained in a series of units called **genes**. As the normal bacterial chromosome has only one copy of each gene, bacteria are called **haploid** organisms (as opposed to higher organisms, which contain two copies of the gene and hence are **diploid**).

A gene is a chain of **purine** and **pyrimidine** nucleotides. The genetic information is coded in triple nucleotide groups or **codons**. Each codon or triplet nucleotide codes for a specific amino acid or a regulatory sequence, e.g. start and stop codons. In this way the structural genes determine the sequence of amino acids that form the protein, which is the gene product.

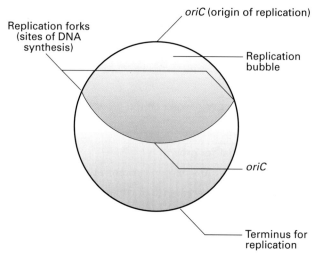

Fig. 3.4 Bidirectional replication of a circular bacterial chromosome.

No 631 — **RATING: MILD**

			7					3
6		8	3		1		9	
	3	2			4			
		4	8					
3	8	5				9	6	4
				6		3		
			9			1	5	
	9			4	3	7		6
2					7			

No 632 — **RATING: FIENDISH**

	3	8	6			1		4
1	4			8				2
	6							
			7	9	2			
		1			7			
		6	8	5				
6				4			2	5
	9	4			2	8	1	

KILLER No 133 — **RATING: TRICKY**

The genetic material of a typical bacterium (e.g. *E. coli*) comprises a single circular DNA with a molecular weight of about 2×10^9 and composed of approximately 5×10^6 base pairs, which in turn can code for about 2000 proteins.

Genetic variation in bacteria

Genetic variation can occur as a result of mutation or gene transfer.

Mutation

A mutation is a change in the base sequence of DNA, as a consequence of which different amino acids are incorporated into a protein, resulting in an altered phenotype. Mutations result from three types of molecular change, as follows.

Base substitution. This occurs during DNA replication when one base is inserted in place of another. When the base substitution results in a codon that instructs a different amino acid to be inserted, the mutation is called a **missense mutation**; when the base substitution generates a termination codon that stops protein synthesis prematurely, the mutation is called a **nonsense mutation**. The latter always destroys protein function.

Frame shift mutation. A frame shift mutation occurs when one or more base pairs are added or deleted, which shifts the reading frame on the ribosome and results in the incorporation of the wrong amino acids 'downstream' from the mutation and in the production of an inactive protein.

Insertion. The insertion of additional pieces of DNA (e.g. transposons) or an additional base can cause profound changes in the reading frames of the DNA and in adjacent genes (Fig. 3.5).

Mutations can be induced by chemicals, radiation or viruses.

Gene transfer

The transfer of genetic information can occur by:
- conjugation
- transduction
- transformation
- transposition.

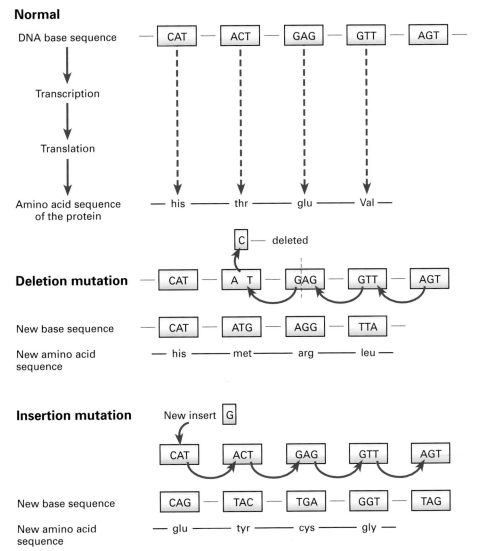

Fig. 3.5 Events that entail mutation: the effect of the deletion and insertion of a single base on the amino acid sequence (and the quality of the protein thus produced) is shown.

Clinically, the most important consequence of DNA transfer is that antibiotic resistance genes are spread from one bacterium to another.

Conjugation. This is the mating of two bacteria, during which DNA is transferred from the donor to the recipient cell (Fig. 3.6A). The mating process is controlled by an **F (fertility) plasmid**, which carries the genes for the proteins required for mating, including the protein pilin which forms the **sex pilus** (conjugation tube). During mating the pilus of the donor (male) bacterium carrying the F factor (F$^+$) attaches to a receptor on the surface of the recipient (female) bacterium. The latter is devoid of an F plasmid (F$^-$). The cells are then brought into direct contact with each other by 'reeling in' of the sex pilus. Then the F factor DNA is cleaved enzymatically and one strand is transferred across the bridge into the female cell. The process is completed by synthesis of the complementary strand to form a double-stranded F plasmid in both the donor and recipient cells. The recipient now becomes an F$^+$ male cell that has the ability to transmit the plasmid further. The new DNA can integrate into the recipient's DNA and become a stable component of its genetic material. It takes about 100 minutes for complete transfer of the bacterial DNA.

Transduction. Transduction is a process of DNA transfer by means of a bacterial virus – a **bacteriophage** (phage). During the replication of the phage, a piece of bacterial DNA is incorporated, accidentally, into the phage particle and is carried into the recipient cell at the time of infection (Fig. 3.6B). There are two types of transduction:

- Generalized transduction occurs when the phage carries a segment from any part of the bacterial chromosome. This may occur when the bacterial DNA is fragmented after

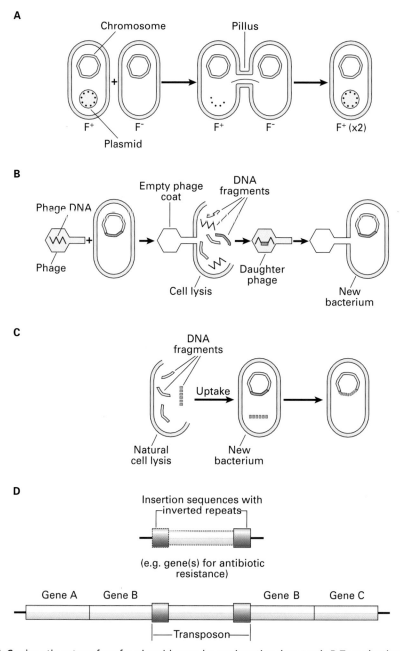

Fig. 3.6 Gene transfer. **A** Conjugation: transfer of a plasmid gene by conjugation (see text); **B** Transduction: phage-mediated gene transfer from one bacterium to another; **C** transformation: gene transfer by uptake of exogenous bacterial DNA by another bacterium in the vicinity (not mediated by plasmid or phage); **D** transposition: transposons (jumping genes) can move from one DNA site to another, thereby inactivating the recipient gene and conferring new traits such as drug resistance.

phage infection and pieces of bacterial DNA the same size as the phage DNA are incorporated into the latter.
- Specialized transduction occurs when the phage DNA that has been already integrated into the bacterial DNA is excised and carries with it an adjacent part of the bacterial DNA. Phage genes can cause changes in the phenotype of the host bacterium, for example toxin production in *Corynebacterium diphtheriae* is controlled by a phage gene. This property is lost as soon as the phage DNA is lost in succeeding reproductive cycles.

Plasmid DNA can also be transferred to another bacterium by transduction. However, the donated plasmid can function independently without recombining with bacterial DNA. The ability to produce an enzyme which destroys penicillin (β-lactamase) is mediated by plasmids that are transferred between staphylococci by transduction.

Transformation. This is the transfer of exogenous bacterial DNA from one cell to another. It occurs in nature when dying bacteria release their DNA, which is then taken up by recipient cells and **recombined** with the recipient cell DNA. This process appears to play an insignificant role in disease (Fig. 3.6C).

Transposition. This occurs when transposable elements (**transposons**; see below) move from one DNA site to another within the genome of the same organism (e.g. *E. coli*). The simplest transposable elements, called 'insertion sequences' are less than 2 kilobases in length and encode enzymes (*transposase*) required for 'jumping' from one site to another (Fig. 3.6D).

Recombination

When the DNA is transferred from the donor to the recipient cell by one of the above mechanisms, it is integrated into the host genome by a process called **recombination**. There are two types of recombination:
- **Homologous recombination**, in which two pieces of DNA that have extensive homologous regions pair up and exchange pieces by the processes of breakage and reunion.
- **Non-homologous recombination**, in which little homology is necessary for recombination to occur. A number of different enzymes (e.g. endonucleases, ligases) are involved in the recombination process.

Plasmids

Plasmids are extrachromosomal, double-stranded, circular DNA molecules within the size range 1–200 MDa. They are capable of replicating independently of the bacterial chromosome (i.e. they are replicons). Plasmids occur in both Gram-positive and Gram-negative bacteria, and several different plasmids can often coexist in one cell.

Transmissible plasmids can be transferred from cell to cell by conjugation. They contain about 10–12 genes responsible for synthesis of the sex pilus and for the enzymes required for transfer; because of their large size they are usually present in a few (1–3) copies per cell.

Non-transmissible plasmids are small and do not contain the transfer genes. However, they can be mobilized by coresident plasmids that do contain the transfer gene. Many copies (up to 60 per cell) of these small plasmids may be present.

Clinical relevance of plasmids

A number of medically important functions of bacteria are attributable to plasmids (i.e. are plasmid-coded). The plasmid-coded bacterial attributes include:
- antibiotic resistance (carried by R plasmids)
- the production of colicins (toxins that are produced by many species of enterobacteria and are lethal for other bacteria)
- resistance to heavy metals such as mercury (the active component of some antiseptics) and silver — mediated by a reductase enzyme
- pili (fimbriae), which mediate the adherence of bacteria to epithelial cells
- exotoxins, including several enterotoxins.

Transposons

Transposons, also called 'jumping genes', are pieces of DNA that move readily from one site to another, either within or between the DNAs of bacteria, plasmids and bacteriophages. In this manner plasmid genes can become part of the chromosomal complement of genes. Interestingly, when transposons transfer to a new site, it is usually a copy of the transposon that moves, the original remaining in situ (like photocopying). For their insertion transposons do not require extensive homology between the terminal repeat sequences of the transposon (which mediate integration) and the site of insertion in the recipient DNA.

Transposons can code for metabolic or drug resistance enzymes and toxins. They may also cause mutations in the gene into which they insert, or alter the expression of nearby genes.

In contrast to plasmids or bacterial viruses, transposons cannot replicate independently of the recipient DNA. More than one transposon can be located in the DNA; for example a plasmid can contain several transposons carrying drug resistance genes. Thus transposons can jump from:
- the host genomic DNA to a plasmid
- one plasmid to another
- a plasmid to genomic DNA.

RECOMBINANT DNA TECHNOLOGY IN MICROBIOLOGY

By definition, every classified species must have somewhere on its genome a unique DNA or RNA sequence that distinguishes it from another species. In diagnostic microbiology this attribute is used to identify microbes where the DNA sequence of the offending pathogen can be identified by means of a number of clever techniques, using clinical samples from the patient.

Gene cloning

Gene cloning is the artificial incorporation of one or more genes into the genome of a new host cell by various genetic recombination techniques.

The candidate DNA is first extracted from the source, purified, and cut or cleaved into small fragments by **restriction enzymes** — leaving 'sticky ends'. These are then inserted into a **vector DNA**, first by cutting the latter with the same enzyme so as to produce complementary sticky ends. The sticky ends of the vector and the candidate DNA are then tied or ligated together using enzymes called '**DNA ligases**' to produce a recombinant DNA molecule. This process can also be used for cloning RNA, when complementary copies of DNA are produced by reverse transcription using **reverse transcriptase** enzymes). The vector used for gene transfer is usually a plasmid or a virus.

The vector with the integrated DNA has to be inserted into a cell in order to obtain multiple copies of the organism that expresses the selected gene. This can be done by:

- **transformation** (see above) — very popular owing to its simplicity, but competent cells need to be found
- **electroporation** — here an electric current induces pores on the cell membrane for vector entry
- **gene gun** — tungsten or gold particles are coated with the vector and propelled into cells by a helium burst
- **microinjection** — direct manual injection of the vector into a cell by a glass micropipette.

The insertion of the vector containing the recombinant DNA does not necessarily mean that all the progeny bacteria will contain the inserted element, because the vector integration process is somewhat random. In order to select the clone of bacteria that expresses the recombinant gene, other devious manoeuvres have to be adopted. For instance, one can choose a plasmid vector that carries resistance to antibiotics A and B. If the foreign DNA is inserted in the middle of gene *A* which confers resistance to antibiotic A, then this gene will be inactivated as a consequence. In this manner bacteria with the cloned foreign DNA can be selected and are called the '**gene library**'.

Gene probes

DNA probes

Used extensively in diagnostic microbiology, gene probes are pieces of DNA that are labelled radioactively or with a chemiluminescent marker. The probes carry a single strand of DNA analogous to the pathogen that is sought in the clinical sample. There are different types of DNA probes:

- **Whole DNA probes** are derived from chromosomal DNA and are used to seek organisms where the genome is not well characterised. Owing to their relatively large size nonspecific reactions are common and the method is not very reliable.
- **Cloned DNA probes** are similar, but are smaller and the reaction is more specific. These are generally targeted at genes unique to the organism sought.

Oligonucleotide probes

Oligonucleotide probes are based on the variable region of the 16*S* ribosomal RNA genes. The nucleotide sequences of the latter gene of a number of microbes have been well characterized, and are known to be well preserved across species, except for several small variable regions. This property is helpful in the construction of specific oligonucleotide probes

of about 18–30 bases, which are much more specific than the DNA probes described above.

RNA probes

Cellular protein synthesis is dependent on ribosomal RNA (rRNA) and any mutation of the rRNA leads to cell death. Further, rRNA is highly species-specific and this property is exploited to produce RNA probes that are useful for both diagnostic microbiology and taxonomic studies. The most commonly used are the 5*S*, 16*S* and 23*S* probes.

DNA / RNA probes and oral microbiology

Cultivation of the complex mixture of bacteria residing in the oral cavity is fraught with problems, and it is now recognized that a number of bacterial genera are difficult or almost impossible to culture. The introduction of DNA and RNA probes has helped us to obtain a more complete picture of the oral flora. For example, commercially available probes can now be used in diagnostic laboratories not only to identify but also to quantify periodontopathic flora in subgingival plaque samples obtained from a periodontal pocket (Fig. 3.7). Further, the samples, say in paper points, could be simply sent by post to distant laboratories for identification without the fear of death of organisms and the associated cumbersome culture procedures.

Polymerase chain reaction

Gene cloning techniques revolutionized the molecular biological advances in the 1970s. The analogous event that took place in the late 1980s was the invention of the **polymerase chain reaction** (PCR). It is a simple technique in which a short region of a DNA molecule, a single gene for instance, is copied repetitiously by a DNA polymerase enzyme (Fig. 3.8).

Materials

The following materials are required:

- the region of the DNA molecule to be amplified
- *Taq* polymerase (a heat-stable enzyme from *Thermus aquaticus* (hence *Taq*), a bacterium that lives in hot springs)
- deoxyribonucleoside 5′-triphosphate (dNTP): adenine, guanine, cytosine, thymine
- primers (with a known DNA sequence).

Method

1. Choose a region of the DNA molecule where the nucleotide sequences of the borders are known. (The border sequence must be known because two short oligonucleotides must hybridize, one to each strand of the double helix of the DNA molecule for the PCR to begin.)
2. The double strand of the DNA molecule is first split into single strands by heating at 94°C (**denaturation** step).
3. The oligonucleotides now act as primers for the DNA synthesis and stick (or hybridize) to the region adjacent to the target DNA sequence, thus delimiting the region that is copied and amplified (**hybridization** step; around 55°C).
4. The DNA polymerase enzyme (*Taq* polymerase) and the nucleotides are added to the primed template DNA and incubated at 72°C for synthesis of new complementary strands (**synthesis** step).

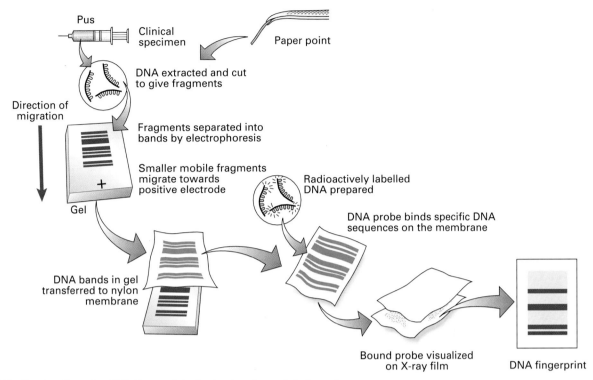

Fig. 3.7 Construction of a DNA fingerprint of microbes from clinical specimens.

5. The mixture is again heated to 94°C to detach the newly synthesized strands from the template.
6. The solution is cooled, enabling more primers to hybridize at their respective positions, including positions on the newly synthesized strands.
7. A second round of DNA synthesis occurs (this time on four strands) with the help of the *Taq* polymerase.
8. This three-step PCR cycle of **denaturation–hybridization–synthesis** can be repeated, usually 25–30 times (in a 'Thermocycler'), resulting in exponential accumulation of several million copies of the amplified fragment.
9. Finally, a sample of the reaction mixture is run through an agarose gel electrophoresis system in order to visualize the product, which manifests as a discrete band after staining with ethidium bromide (Fig. 3.8).

Why is PCR so widely used?

Some reasons why the use of PCR is so widespread:
- **To study minuscule quantities of DNA**, as a single DNA molecule is adequate for an amplification reaction (hence its use in forensic studies, archaeology, palaeontology).
- **Use in rapid clinical diagnostic procedures**. The sensitivity of the PCR has resulted in its use in rapid diagnosis of viral, bacterial and fungal and other diseases. For instance, amplification of viral DNA in a patient sample could be made within hours, and sometimes even before the onset of symptoms.
- **Amplification of RNA**. Here the RNA molecule has to be first converted to single-strand complementary DNA (cDNA) with an enzyme called reverse transcriptase (as it transcribes the RNA code into DNA in a reverse manner). Once this initial step is carried out the PCR primers and *Taq* polymerase are added; afterwards the experimental procedure is identical to the standard technique.

- **Comparison of different genomes**. Random amplification with short lengths of primers can be used in phylogenetics – the study of evolutionary history and lines of descent of species or groups of organisms. This technique is called **random amplification of polymorphic DNA (RAPD)**.

Other techniques for genetic typing of microorganisms

Restriction enzyme analysis

A genetic 'fingerprint' of the organism is obtained by extracting its DNA and cutting or cleaving the DNA at specific points by **restriction endonucleases**. The DNA fragments so generated are run on an agarose electrophoresis gel, and viewed under ultraviolet illumination after staining with ethidium bromide. The profiles of the bands produced on the gel (the 'fingerprints') can be compared or contrasted with those from other strains. This was the original molecular method used for genotyping organisms, but has been supplanted by newer methods that are more discriminatory.

Restriction fragment length polymorphism

In restriction fragment length polymorphism (RFLP), the DNA is first cleaved using restriction endonucleases and separated on the agarose gel. Afterwards the separated fragments are transferred by blotting on to a nitrocellulose or nylon membrane by a method called **Southern blotting**, and DNA probes constructed from genes of known organisms (species or strains) are then hybridized to the membrane; these will bind to complementary sequences in the DNA fragments on the membrane, revealing the species or strain identity.

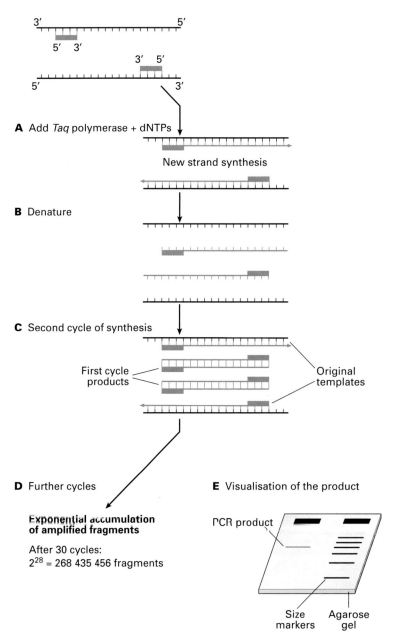

Fig. 3.8 The polymerase chain reaction.

Pulsed-field gel electrophoresis

Pulsed-field gel electrophoresis (PFGE) is similar to RFLP. Here the chromosomal DNA of an organism is cut into relatively large pieces by restriction enzymes and the resultant fragments are separated in an agarose gel with the help of a pulsed electric field, in which the polarity is regularly reversed. Large pieces of chromosomes usually do not separate in conventional agarose gels, hence the necessity of the pulsed/reversed electric field.

KEY FACTS

- **Bacteria**, like all living organisms, **require oxygen, hydrogen, carbon, inorganic ions** and organic **nutrients** for survival

- Other **factors that modify growth** are **end-product inhibition** and **catabolite repression**, and the **temperature** and **pH** of the medium

- Bacteria **reproduce** by **binary fission** leading to logarithmic growth of cell numbers; the doubling or mean generation time of bacteria can vary from minutes to hours or days

- Bacterial **growth** in laboratory media can be divided into a **lag** phase, **log** phase, **stationary** phase and **decline phase**

- Depending on their oxygen requirements, bacteria can be divided into **obligate aerobes, facultative anaerobes, obligate anaerobes** and **microaerophiles**

- Bacterial **chromosomes** comprise a single, **continuous strand of DNA** with a closed, **circular** structure **attached to the cell membrane**

- DNA replication is the synthesis of new strands of DNA using the original DNA strands as templates

- **DNA replicates** by a process called **semiconservative replication**; DNA-dependent DNA polymerase is the main enzyme that mediates DNA replication

- **Restriction enzymes** of bacteria **delete foreign nucleotides from their genomes**. These enzymes are therefore extremely useful in molecular biological techniques

- **Genetic variations** in bacteria can occur either by **mutation** or **gene transfer**

- **Mutation**, a change in the base sequence of the DNA, can be due to either **base substitution frame shifts** or **insertion** of additional pieces of DNA

- **Gene transfer** in bacteria may occur by **conjugation, transduction, transformation** or **transposition**

- **Plasmids** are **extrachromosomal, double-stranded circular DNA molecules** capable of **independent replication** within the bacterial host

- *The clinical relevance of plasmids lies in the fact that they code for antibiotic resistance, resistance to heavy metals, exotoxin production and pili formation*

- **Transposons** are '**jumping genes**' that move from one site to another either within or between the DNA molecules

- **Gene cloning** is the **introduction of foreign DNA into another cell** where it can replicate and express itself

- *Gene probes used in diagnostic microbiology are labelled (with chemicals or radioactively) pieces of DNA that can be used to detect specific sequences of DNA of the pathogen (in the clinical sample) by pairing with the complementary bases*

- *The polymerase chain reaction is a widely used technique that enables multiple copies of a DNA molecule to be generated by enzymatic amplification of the target DNA sequence*

FURTHER READING

Alberts, B, Bray, D, Lewis, J, Raff, M, Roberts, K, and Watson, JF (1994). *The molecular biology of the cell* (3rd edn). Garland, New York.

Beebee, T, and Burke, J (1992). *Gene structure and transcription* (2nd edn). IRL Press Oxford University Press, Oxford.

Collier, LH (ed.) (1998). *Topley and Wilson's Microbiology and microbial infections* (9th edn). Edward Arnold, London.

Moat, AG, and Foster, JW (1995). *Microbial physiology* (3rd edn). Wiley/Liss, New York.

4 Viruses and prions

Viruses are one of the smallest forms of microorganism and infect most other forms of life: animals, plants and bacteria. They can also cause severe acute oral and orofacial disease, produce oral signs of systemic infection, and be transmitted to patients and dental staff. The main features that characterize viruses are:

- **small size** (10–100 nm), averaging about one-tenth the size of a bacterium
- **genome** consisting of either DNA or RNA but never both; single- or double-stranded; linear or circular (the encoding of the whole of the genetic information as RNA in RNA viruses is a situation unique in biology)
- **metabolic inactivity** outside the cells of susceptible hosts; viruses lack ribosomes — the protein-synthesizing apparatus (the corollary of this is that viruses can multiply only inside living cells, i.e. they are obligate intracellular parasites).

STRUCTURE

Viruses consist of a nucleic acid core containing the viral genome, surrounded by a protein shell called a **capsid** (Figs 4.1 and 4.2). The entire structure is referred to as the **nucleocapsid**. This may be 'naked', or it may be 'enveloped' within a lipoprotein sheath derived from the host cell membrane. In many viruses (e.g. orthomyxoviruses, paramyxoviruses) the ensheathment begins by a budding process at the plasma membrane of the host cell, while others, such as herpesviruses, ensheath at the membrane of the nucleus or endoplasmic recticulum.

The protein shell or capsid consists of repeating units of one or more protein molecules; these protein units may go on to form structural units, which may be visualized by electron microscopy as morphological units called **capsomeres** (Fig. 4.1). Genetic economy dictates that the variety of viral proteins be kept to a minimum as viral genomes lack sufficient genetic information to code for a large array of different proteins. In enveloped viruses the protein units which comprise the envelopes and are visualized electron microscopically are called **peplomers** (loosely referred to as 'spikes').

Viral nucleic acid

Viral nucleic acid may be either DNA or RNA. The RNA, in turn, may be single-stranded (ss) or double-stranded (ds) and the genome may consist of one or several molecules of nucleic acid. If the genome consists of a single molecule, this may be linear or have a circular configuration. The DNA viruses all have genomes composed of a single molecule of nucleic acid, whereas the genomes of many RNA viruses consist of several different molecules or segments which are probably loosely linked together in the virion.

Viral protein

In terms of volume, the major bulk of the virion is protein, which offers a protective sheath for the nucleic acid. The viral protein is made up of two or three different polypeptide chains, although in some only one kind of polypeptide chain may be present. Virion surface proteins may have a special affinity for receptors on the surface of susceptible cells and may bear antigenic determinants.

Although most viral proteins have a structural function, some have enzymatic activity. For instance, many viruses such as the human immunodeficiency virus (HIV) contain a reverse transcriptase, whereas several enzymes (e.g. neuraminidase, lysozyme) are found in larger, more complex viruses.

Viral lipid and carbohydrate

In general, lipids and carbohydrates of viruses are found only in their envelopes and are mostly derived from the host cells. About 50–60% of the lipids are phospholipids; most of the remainder is cholesterol.

Virus symmetry

The nucleocapsids of viruses are arranged in a highly symmetrical fashion (symmetry refers to the way in which the protein units are arranged). Three kinds of symmetry are recognized (Fig. 4.3):

- **Icosahedral symmetry**. The protein molecules are symmetrically arranged in the shape of an icosahedron (i.e. a 20-sided solid, each face being an equilateral triangle). Herpesviruses are an example (Figs 4.1 and 4.2).
- **Helical symmetry**. The capsomeres surround the viral nucleic acid in the form of a helix or spiral to form a tubular nucleocapsid. Most mammalian RNA viruses have this symmetry, where the nucleocapsid is arranged in the form of a coil and enclosed within a lipoprotein envelope.
- **Complex symmetry**. This is exhibited by a few families of viruses — notably the retroviruses and poxviruses.

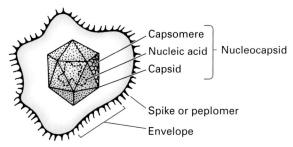

Fig. 4.1 Viral structure (schematic).

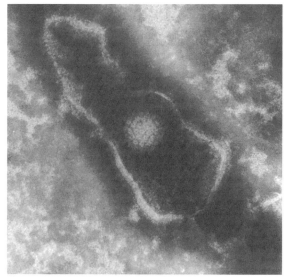

Fig. 4.2 Scanning electron micrograph of a herpesvirus. Note the extensive outer lipid envelope and the icosahedral nucleocapsid.

TAXONOMY

Vertebrate viruses are classified into families, genera and species. The attributes used in classification are their symmetry, the presence or absence of an envelope, nucleic acid composition (DNA or RNA), the number of nucleic acid strands, and their polarity. Classification of some of the recognized families of RNA and DNA viruses is given in Table 4.1. (*Note*: to memorize which viruses contain DNA, remember the acronym 'PHAD': P is for **pa**pova and **po**x, H for **h**erpes and AD for **ad**enoviruses. Most of the remainder are RNA viruses including the self-evident pi**corna**viruses.)

The following is a concise description of the families of mammalian viruses.

DNA viruses

Papovaviruses

Papovaviruses are small, icosahedral DNA viruses with a capacity to produce tumours in vivo and to transform cultured cell lines. The name 'papova' is an acronym derived from the **pa**pillomavirus, **po**lyomavirus and **va**cuolating agent SV40 virus, which make up this family.

Papillomavirus.
This genus contains human serotypes which cause benign skin tumours or warts and both oral and skin papillomas (e.g. hand and plantar warts). Although they were regarded as a cosmetic nuisance rather than a specific disease,

it is now known that the papillomaviruses may be involved in genital and oral cancers.

Polyomavirus.
This genus contains the polyomavirus of mice and simian virus 40 (SV40) of monkeys, which are used in experimental carcinogenesis in these animals.

Adenoviruses

Adenoviruses are icosahedral DNA viruses, commonly associated with respiratory and eye infections in humans. These viruses were so named because they were first isolated from cultured adenoid tissue eliciting cytopathic effects. Syndromes associated with adenoviruses include:
- acute febrile pharyngitis (primarily in infants and children), often indistinguishable from pharyngitis due to β-haemolytic streptococci
- acute adult respiratory disease, ranging from pharyngitis to pneumonia
- ocular infections.

Table 4.1 Classification of some of the viruses causing human disease

Morphology	Virus
DNA	
Enveloped, double-stranded nucleic acid	Herpesviruses
	Herpes simplex virus
	Varicella–zoster virus
	Epstein–Barr virus
	Cytomegalovirus
	Human herpesvirus 6
	Poxviruses
	Vaccinia
	Orf
Enveloped, single-stranded	Parvoviruses
Non-enveloped, double-stranded	Adenoviruses
	Papovaviruses
	Polyomaviruses
	Papillomaviruses
	Hepadnaviruses
	Hepatitis B virus
RNA	
Enveloped, single-stranded	Orthomyxoviruses
	Influenza virus
	Paramyxoviruses
	Parainfluenza
	Respiratory syncytial
	Mumps
	Measles
	Togaviruses
	Rubella
	Retroviruses
	Human immunodeficiency viruses HTLV-I, -III
	Rhabdoviruses
	Rabies
Non-enveloped, double-stranded	Reoviruses
	Rotavirus
Non-enveloped, single-stranded	Picornaviruses
	Rhinovirus
	Enterovirus
	Coxsackievirus
	Echovirus
	Poliovirus

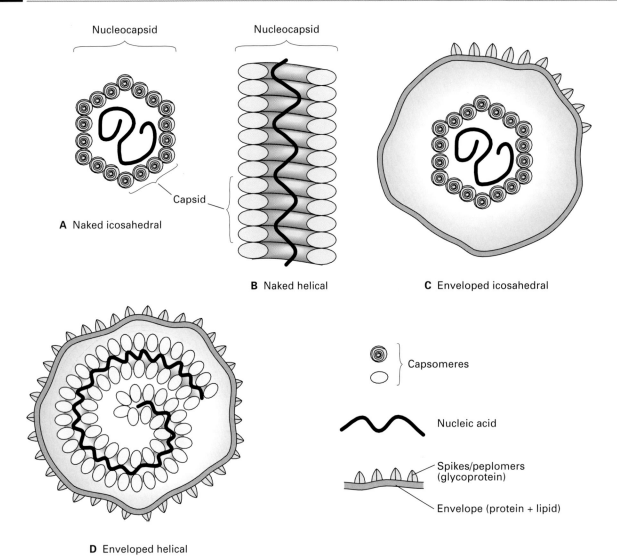

Fig. 4.3   Structural components and symmetry of different viruses.

Herpesviruses

Herpesviruses are the predominant viral cause of oral infections in humans; often the infections are recurrent, and latent.

Structure. These enveloped, icosahedral viruses are 180–200 nm in diameter and contain a linear, double-stranded DNA molecule. The *Herpesviridae* family has over 100 members spread widely among vertebrates and invertebrates and new species are continuously being added. Herpesviruses are unstable at room temperature, and are rapidly inactivated by lipid solvents such as alcohol and other common disinfectants owing to the disruption of the outer lipid envelope.

During reproduction maturation of the progeny begins in the nucleus of the host cell, which buds through the nuclear membrane and acquires the viral envelope. Typical and highly pathognomonic **intranuclear inclusions** are therefore found in cells that have undergone active virus replication. As many herpesviruses can fuse with the cells they infect, **polykaryocytes** or **giant cells** readily appear in tissue lesions. Such cells, e.g. Tzanck cells or nuclear inclusions (Lipschütz bodies), are hallmarks of herpetic infections.

Different herpesviruses cause a variety of infectious diseases, some localized and some generalized, often with a vesicular rash. Herpesviruses establish latent infection, which can be readily reactivated by immunosuppression (Table 4.2).

The nomenclature of herpesviruses is contentious; there is thus a historical or a traditional (trivial) nomenclature and an official name for each virus (Table 4.3). The herpesviruses that commonly infect humans can be distinguished by their antigenic and genomic profiles, although they cannot be differentiated by electron microscopy owing to identical capsid morphology. They also have a universal ability to establish latent infection in the host in which they reside, and manifest a number of common epidemiological features. Herpes simplex virus, herpes zoster virus, Epstein–Barr virus, human

Table 4.2   Latent viruses relevant to dentistry

Virus	Site of latency
Herpex simplex virus	Trigeminal ganglion
Varicella–zoster virus	Sensory ganglia
Epstein–Barr virus	Epithelial cells Blymphocytes
Cytomegalovirus	Salivary gland cells
Papillomaviruses	Epithelial cells
Human immunodeficiency viruses	Lymphocytes and other CD4+ cells (see Ch. 30)

Table 4.3 Official and trivial nomenclature of human herpesviruses (family *Herpesviridae*)

	Official name	Trivial name	Acronym
Subfamily	*Alphaherpesvirinae*		
Species	Human herpesvirus 1	Herpes simplex virus 1	HSV-1
	Human herpesvirus 2	Herpes simplex virus 2	HSV-2
	Human herpesvirus 3	Varicella–zoster virus	VZV
Subfamily	*Betaherpesvirinae*		
Species	Human herpesvirus 5	Cytomegalovirus	HCMV[a]
	Human herpesvirus 6	—	HHV-6
Subfamily	*Gammaherpesvirinae*		
Species	Human herpesvirus 4	Epstein–Barr virus	EBV
	Human herpesvirus 7	—	HHV-7
	Human herpesvirus 8	Kaposi's sarcoma herpesvirus	HHV-8

[a] HCMV, human cytomegalovirus.

cytomegalovirus and herpesviruses 6 and 8 can all cause infections in oral and perioral tissues (Fig. 4.4); see Ch. 35 for details.

Poxviruses

The poxviruses are the largest viruses to infect humans or animals. Molluscum contagiosum in humans is caused by a poxvirus, as is smallpox, which is now a disease of only historical interest. Humans occasionally acquire infection by animal poxviruses, e.g. cowpox.

Parvoviruses

Parvoviruses are icosahedral viruses with single-stranded DNA. Three serologically distinct types of autonomous parvoviruses are recognized in human disease. The first group is found in stool specimens, the second (the B19 virus) in the serum of asymptomatic blood donors, while the third has been recovered from synovial tissues of rheumatoid arthritis patients. The B19 virus is responsible for a febrile illness, particularly in children, manifesting as a maculopapular rash. The exanthem is characterized by a fiery-red rash on the cheeks — the 'slapped cheek' syndrome (also termed fifth disease).

Hepadnaviruses

Hepadnaviruses are small, spherical DNA viruses causing hepatitis, chronic liver infections and possibly liver cancer. They are of particular interest in dentistry because of their mode of transmission via blood and saliva (see Ch. 29).

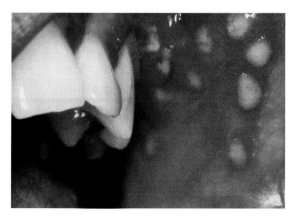

Fig. 4.4 Primary herpes simplex infection of the oral mucosa.

RNA viruses

Picornaviruses

Picornaviruses are the smallest family of RNA viruses, but incorporate a very large group of viruses, including the genus *Enterovirus*. Human enteroviruses have been further subdivided into three major subgroups:
- **polioviruses**
- **echoviruses** (acronym: enteric cytopathogenic, human, orphan)
- **coxsackieviruses** (Coxsackie, a town in the USA) types A and B.

The enteroviruses reside and multiply asymptomatically in the gut, but may cause a spectrum of disease ranging from mild undifferentiated rashes, respiratory infections and pharyngitis (coxsackie A) to more serious diseases, including carditis (coxsackie B) which may be lethal in the newborn (see Chs 21 and 35).

Orthomyxoviruses

The orthomyxoviruses are RNA viruses with a tubular nucleocapsid and a lipoprotein envelope. Influenza A viruses of birds, mammals and humans are in this category. Some of these viruses, for example Asian influenza viruses, may cause severe generalized infections.

Paramyxoviruses

Paramyxoviruses are large, pleomorphic enveloped RNA viruses. The family contains four common and important human pathogens: measles, mumps, parainfluenza and respiratory syncytial viruses. Paramyxoviruses are a common cause of croup (laryngotracheobronchitis), while respiratory syncytial viruses cause regular winter epidemics of bronchiolitis/pneumonitis in infants.

Retroviruses

Retroviruses are large, spherical enveloped RNA tumour viruses characterized by a unique genome, a unique enzyme and a unique mode of replication. The viral genome RNA is first transcribed into DNA by a virus-specific enzyme, reverse transcriptase. This DNA can then serve as a template for messenger RNA (mRNA) synthesis. The RNA viruses infecting humans comprise a single taxonomic group with three sub-families:

- **lentiviruses** cause slowly progressive disease and include HIV types 1 and 2 (see Ch. 30)
- **oncoviruses** include those that cause tumours: human T-cell leukaemia virus (HTLV-I), the agent of adult T-cell leukaemia–lymphoma (ATLL), and HTLV-II, associated with hairy cell leukaemia
- **spumaviruses** are not recognized human pathogens.

Other RNA viruses

Other RNA viruses that are important but are not known to cause oral disease include togaviruses, coronaviruses, arenaviruses, rhabdoviruses and filoviruses.

Viroids

As a result of advances in molecular biology, two new classes of infectious agents, prions and viroids, have been discovered. These are the smallest known agents of disease. Viroids cause diseases in plants and comprise naked, covalently linked, closed circles of single-stranded RNA, less than 300–400 nucleotides in length. Despite their minute size they replicate using host cell enzymes. Viroids are not associated with human disease, thus far. Prions are discussed at the end of this chapter.

VIRAL REPLICATION

Viral replication (Fig. 4.5) is a highly complex process and only a brief summary is given here. There are a number of general steps in the replication cycle of all viruses: **adsorption, penetration, uncoating and eclipse, transcription, synthesis of viral components, assembly** and **release of virions**. In some viruses, however, these steps may not be clearly defined and may overlap, e.g. penetration and uncoating. It is noteworthy that in some families (e.g. *Herpesviridae*) many of the critical events occur in the cell nucleus, while others (e.g. *Picornaviridae*) multiply exclusively within the cytoplasm. The period between infection and the production of the new virion (**eclipse** or **latent period**) could be as short as 3 hours (e.g. *Orthomyxoviridae*) or as long as several months or years (e.g. HIV).

Figure 4.5 depicts the steps in the replication of a DNA virus. However, this picture has to be somewhat modified when RNA viruses are considered, as the basic unit of information is now RNA instead of DNA. The strategies of viral replication become more complex when double-stranded (ds) rather than single-stranded (ss) viruses and those with RNA of positive polarity and negative polarity are considered. The basic steps in replication are:

1. **Adsorption** or **attachment** of the virus particle to the specific receptors of the host cell plasma membrane. Firm attachment requires the presence of receptors for the virus on the plasma membrane (e.g. orthomyxoviruses and paramyxoviruses bind via an envelope protein, known as haemagglutinin, to certain glycoproteins or glycolipids on the host cell).

2. **Penetration** or **uptake**. The process by which the virus or its genome enters the host cell cytoplasm. Penetration can be achieved by three separate mechanisms:
   - **endocytosis**: most of the virions taken up by endocytosis appear to be degraded by lysosomal enzymes

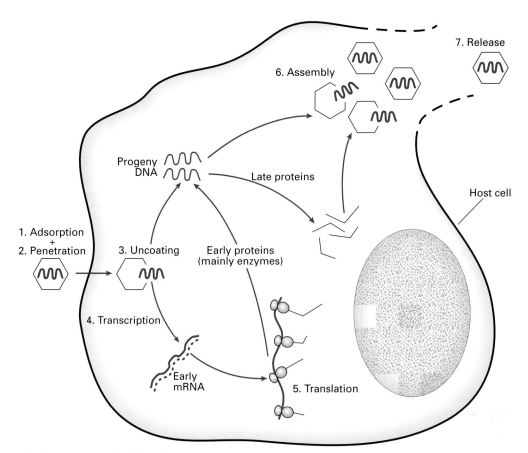

Fig. 4.5 Steps in the replication of a DNA virus.

and therefore fail to initiate infection, but this is the normal route to successful infection by many viruses
- **fusion**: direct fusion of the viral envelope with the plasma membrane of cells allows the nucleocapsid of some viruses to be released directly into the cytoplasm without an intervening phagocytic process
- **translocation**: some non-enveloped viruses have the capacity to pass directly through the plasma membrane.

3. **Uncoating** and **eclipse**. After penetration there is a period during which no intact infectious virus can be detected. This 'eclipse phase' begins with uncoating of the lipid membrane and protein capsid surrounding the nucleic acid viral core. As uncoating proceeds, the viral nucleic acid becomes free to act as a template for the synthesis of virus mRNA.

4. **Transcription**. The virus mRNA codes for the synthesis of enzymes necessary to complete the process of uncoating itself and also to initiate early steps in viral replication. When the virus initiates the reproductive cycle within the host cell the synthesis of host cell RNA is halted and host ribosomes are free to receive viral mRNA and provide a focus for transcription and synthesis of viral proteins.

5. **Synthesis of viral components**. Viral proteins are of two types:
- structural (the proteins that make up the virus particle)
- non-structural (enzymes required for virus genome replication).

Structural viral proteins are synthesized on cellular polyribosomes. There is a simultaneous synthesis of progeny viral nucleic acid, using newly synthesized nucleic acid polymerases.

6. **Assembly**. Viral assembly is accomplished by incorporation of viral nucleic acid into putative capsomeres — **procapsids**. Assembly may occur in the cell nucleus, cytoplasm or (with enveloped viruses) at the plasma membrane.

7. **Release** may occur either through gradual budding, in the case of enveloped viruses, or by sudden rupture.

The foregoing is a brief, composite picture of processes involved in viral multiplication. It should be noted that the replication cycle of each family of viruses has unique characteristics which differ from other viruses.

PATHOGENESIS OF VIRAL INFECTIONS

See Chapter 5.

CELLULAR ANTIVIRAL RESPONSE

The antiviral response is mostly mediated immunologically and is described in Part 2.

PRIONS AND PRION-INDUCED DISEASES

Prions (proteinaceous infectious particles) are unique elements in nature and they are the agents of a group of chronic diseases with extremely long incubation periods lasting up to decades. The major features of prions are given below.
- They are neither viruses nor viroids
- Prions do not have either DNA or RNA

- The native form of the prion protein is designated PrP^C, while the disease related isoform derived from the latter is designated PrP^{Sc}
- The abnormal form, PrP^{Sc} is derived from the native precursor by a post-translational process leading to a conformational change from an α-helical structure to an insoluble β-sheet structure
- They have the ability to self replicate but with a very long incubation period (up to 20 years in humans)
- The prototype prion agent caused **scrapie**, a CNS disease in sheep
- As the organism is highly resistant to heat, chemical agents and irradiation, either special autoclaving procedures are required to sterilise contaminated instruments or disposable instruments/material have to be used for surgical procedures on infected/suspect patients
- The prion agent can be transmitted to cows, mink, cats and mice for instance, when fed with infected material
- Iatrogenic transmission of prion disease by neurosurgical instruments has been reported.

Prion-induced diseases or transmissible spongiform encephalopathies (TSEs)

Kuru

Kuru is the fatal neurologic disease first described in societies in Papua New Guinea who consumed human brain. It is no longer prevalent owing to the cessation of this practice.

Creutzfeldt–Jakob disease

Creutzfeldt–Jakob disease (CJD) is a globally prevalent, rare, chronic encephalopathy; 10% of cases are **familial** and carry the mutated prion gene; the remainder are either **acquired** and **sporadic**. Onset is in middle to late life (40–60 years); the clinical course lasts for about 7–18 months.

Variant Creutzfeldt–Jakob disease. A variant form (vCJD) is localized to Europe, especially the UK; it almost always affects teenagers or young adults, with a mean age of onset of 24 years.

Fatal familial insomnia

Characterized by progressive insomnia, disruption of circadian rhythms and motor dysfunction, fatal familial insomnia has a late onset (40–60 years) and a clinical course that lasts for about 7 months.

Gerstmann–Straussler–Scheinker syndrome

Symptoms include profound chronic cerebellar ataxia and slow-onset dementia; early onset (20–30 years), clinical course about 5 years.

Pathogenesis

Prions appear to replicate incessantly, first in lymphoid tissue, and then in brain cells where they produce intracellular vacuoles and deposition of altered host prion protein. These vacuoles give rise to the sponge-like appearance of the brain on microscopic examination, hence the name 'spongiform encephalopathy'. The disease is uniformly fatal.

Transmission

Kuru is transmitted in infected human brain by cannibalism.

The mode of transmission of CJD is mostly unknown. There are a few reports of iatrogenic transmission by medical and surgical procedures; hereditary acquisition occurs in familial cases; contaminated food (beef from cattle with 'mad cow' disease, bovine spongiform encephalopathy) is thought to cause acquired disease.

Prevention and dental implications

- There is no treatment or vaccine against prion induced disease

- Hence the only preventive measure is not consuming suspect food (especially those containing neural tissues)
- The level of infectivity in oral and dental tissues is unknown, but in vCJD there is extensive lymphoreticular involvement
- For patients with highly suspected or confirmed CJD or vCJD, all instruments used in dental procedures must be incinerated after use
- For patients at risk (recipients of dura mater grafts; pituitary hormone injections before the mid 1980s; those with close family members with a history of CJD), either use disposable instruments or clean instruments thoroughly and sterilize for 18 minutes at 134°C in a vacuum autoclave (see Chapter 37).

KEY FACTS

- **Viruses** are **obligate intracellular parasites**, which are **metabolically inert**, and can replicate only within living cells
- The virus **genome** has either **DNA or RNA** but **never both**
- The genome is protected by an **outer protein coat (capsid)** composed of **capsomeres**; the **nucleocapsid** is the term given to the **protein and the viral genome** complex
- The nucleocapsid of viruses is arranged in one of three spatial configurations: **icosahedral, helical or complex symmetry**
- When a lipoprotein surrounds the virus it is called an envelope. **Non-enveloped viruses** are called **naked viruses**
- **Peplomers (spikes)** are **glycoprotein extensions** from the envelope, and play a role in the attachment of the virus to the target host cells
- Viruses are classified into families, genera and species. The attributes used in classification are their symmetry, the

presence or absence of envelope, nucleic acid composition (DNA or RNA), the number of nucleic acid strands and their polarity. In practice 'common names' are routinely used when describing viruses

- The stages of **viral replication** are **adsorption, penetration, uncoating, transcription and translation of the genome, assembly** of the virus particles, and **release**
- **Prions** are unique as they are **devoid of nucleic acids** and are **made of self-replicating, low-molecular-weight proteins (PrP)**; their mode of replication is unclear as yet
- *The human transmissible spongiform encephalopathies (e.g. kuru, Creutzfeldt–Jakob disease) are caused by prions*
- *In view of the difficulty of inactivating prions, either special autoclaving procedures are required to sterilize contaminated instruments or disposable instruments and materials have to be used for surgical procedures on infected or suspect patients*

FURTHER READING

Collier, L, and Oxford, J (1993). *Human virology: a text for students of medicine, dentistry and microbiology*. Oxford University Press, Oxford.

Evans, AS, and Kaslow, RA (eds) (1997). Epidemiologic concepts and methods. In *Viral infections of humans. Epidemiology and control* (4th edn), Ch. 1. Plenum, New York.

Field, DN, Knipe, DM, and Howlley, PM (eds) (1996). *Virology* (3rd edn). Lippincott-Raven, Philadelphia.

Samaranayake, LP, Peiris, JSM, and Scully, C (1996). Ebola virus infection: an overview. *British Dental Journal* 180, 264–266.

Scully, C, and Samaranayake, LP (1992). *Clinical virology in oral medicine and dentistry*, Chs 1 and 2. Cambridge University Press, Cambridge.

Taussig, MJ (1984). Infection: viruses. In *Processes in pathology and microbiology* (2nd edn), sect. 3. Blackwell, Oxford.

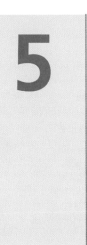

5 Pathogenesis of microbial disease

If a microorganism is capable of causing disease it is called a **pathogen**. Fortunately, only a minority of the vast multitude of microorganisms in nature are pathogenic. Whereas some organisms are highly virulent and cause disease in healthy individuals, even with a small inoculum, others cause disease only in compromised individuals when their defences are weak. The latter are called **opportunistic** organisms, as they take the opportunity offered by reduced host defences to cause disease. These opportunists are frequently members of the body's normal flora.

GENERAL ASPECTS OF INFECTION

Virulence

Virulence is a quantitative measure of pathogenicity and is related to an organism's **toxigenic potential** and **invasiveness**. Virulence can be measured by the number of organisms required to cause disease and is designated as LD_{50} or ID_{50}: the LD_{50} (50% lethal dose) is the number of organisms needed to kill half the hosts, and ID_{50} (50% infectious dose) is the number needed to cause infection in half the hosts. These values are determined by inoculation of laboratory animals.

Communicable diseases

Infections are called 'communicable diseases' if they are spread from host to host. Many, but not all, infections are communicable; for example, tuberculosis is communicable, as it is spread by airborne droplets produced by coughing, but staphylococcal food poisoning is not, as the exotoxin produced by the organism and present in the contaminated food affects only those eating that food. If a disease is highly communicable it is called a 'contagious disease' (e.g. chickenpox).

Depending on the degree of incidence and prevalence of an infectious disease in a community, it may be called an endemic, an epidemic or a pandemic infection.
- an **endemic** infection is constantly present at a low level in a specific population (e.g. endemic malaria in some African countries)
- an infection is an **epidemic** if it occurs much more frequently than usual (e.g. an epidemic of influenza in the winter)
- an infection is a **pandemic** if it has a worldwide distribution (e.g. HIV infection).

Natural history of infectious disease

An acute infection generally progresses through four stages:
1. The **incubation period**: time between the acquisition of the organism or the toxin and the commencement of symptoms (this may vary from hours to days to weeks).
2. The **prodromal period**: non-specific symptoms such as fever, malaise and loss of appetite appear during this period.
3. The **acute specific illness**: the characteristic signs and symptoms of the disease are evident during this period.
4. The **recovery period**: the illness subsides and the patient returns to health during this final phase.

A number of organisms may elicit an **inapparent** or **subclinical** infection, without overt symptoms, where the individual remains asymptomatic although infected with the organism. On the other hand, once infected, the body may not completely eliminate the pathogen after recovery and some individuals may become **chronic carriers** of the organism (e.g. *Salmonella typhi*, hepatitis B virus); they may shed the organism while remaining healthy. Some infections result in a **latent** state, after which reactivation of the growth of the organism and recurrence of symptoms may occur at a later stage (e.g. after primary herpes infection the virus may reside in a latent state in the trigeminal ganglion, causing recurrent herpes labialis from time to time). All the above groups may unknowingly shed pathogenic organisms and spread disease.

PATHOGENESIS OF BACTERIAL DISEASE

Determinants of bacterial pathogenicity

Bacterial pathogenicity is a vast subject. The following is a brief outline of the ways and means by which bacteria cause disease. The major steps are transmission, adherence to host surfaces, invasiveness, and toxigenicity.

Transmission

Most infections are acquired by transmission from external sources, i.e. they are **exogenous** in origin. Others are caused by members of the normal flora behaving as opportunist pathogens, i.e. they are **endogenous** in origin. Transmission can be by:
- inhalation — the airborne route
- ingestion — faecal contamination of food and water

29

Table 5.1 Portals of entry of some common pathogens

Portal of entry	Pathogen	Disease
Skin	*Clostridium tetani*	Tetanus
	Hepatitis B virus	Hepatitis B
Respiratory tract	*Streptococcus pneumoniae*	Pneumonia
	Neisseria meningitidis	Meningitis
	Haemophilus influenzae	Meningitis
	Mycobacterium tuberculosis	Tuberculosis
	Influenza virus	Influenza
	Rhinovirus	Common cold
	Epstein–Barr virus	Infectious mononucleosis
Gastrointestinal tract	*Shigella dysenteriae*	Dysentery
	Salmonella typhi	Typhoid fever
	Vibrio cholerae	Cholera
	Hepatitis A virus	Infectious hepatitis
	Poliovirus	Poliomyelitis
Genital tract	*Neisseria gonorrhoeae*	Gonorrhoea
	Treponema pallidum	Syphilis
	Human immunodeficiency virus	AIDS
	Candida albicans (fungus)	Vaginitis

- inoculation — by sexual contact, contaminated needles, skin contact, blood transfusions or biting insects.

There are four important portals (or gates) of entry of pathogens (Table 5.1):
- skin
- respiratory tract
- gastrointestinal tract
- genitourinary tract.

Adherence to host surfaces

This is the first step in the infection. Unless organisms have the ability to stick or adhere to host surfaces they will be unable to cause infection. Some bacteria and fungi have specialized structures or produce substances that facilitate their attachment to the surface of human cells or prostheses (e.g. dentures, artificial heart valves), thereby enhancing their ability to colonize and cause disease. These adherence mechanisms are critical for organisms that attach to mucous membranes; mutants that lack these mechanisms are often non-pathogenic (e.g. the hair-like pili of *Neisseria gonorrhoeae* and *Escherichia coli* mediate their attachment to the urinary tract epithelium; the extracellular polysaccharides of *Streptococcus mutans* helps it adhere to enamel surfaces).

Invasiveness

Invasiveness of bacteria plays a critical role in pathogenesis; this property is dependent upon secreted bacterial enzymes. A few examples are:
- **Collagenase** and **hyaluronidase** degrade their respective intercellular substances, allowing easy spread of bacteria through tissues, and are especially important in skin infections caused by *Streptococcus pyogenes*.
- **Coagulase**, produced by *Staphylococcus aureus*, accelerates the formation of a fibrin clot (from fibrinogen). It helps protect the organisms from phagocytosis by walling off the infected area and by coating the organisms with a fibrin layer.

- **Immunoglobulin A (IgA) protease** degrades protective IgA on mucosal surfaces, allowing organisms such as *N. gonorrhoeae*, *Haemophilus influenzae* and *Streptococcus pneumoniae* to adhere to mucous membranes.
- **Leucocidins** can destroy both neutrophilic leucocytes and macrophages; the periodontopathic organism *Actinobacillus actinomycetemcomitans* possesses this enzyme. The mutants that do not secrete the enzyme are less virulent.

Other factors also contribute to invasiveness by interfering with the host defence mechanisms, especially phagocytosis.
- The polysaccharide **capsule** of several common pathogens, such as *S. pneumoniae* and *Neisseria meningitidis*, prevents the phagocyte from adhering to the bacteria. (This can be verified by the introduction of anticapsular antibodies which allow more effective phagocytosis or opsonization to occur. Thus the vaccines against *S. pneumoniae* and *N. meningitidis* contain capsular polysaccharides that induce protective anticapsular antibodies.)
- The **cell wall proteins** of the Gram-positive cocci, such as the M protein of the group A streptococci and protein A of the staphylococci, are also antiphagocytic (Table 5.2).

Bacterial infection may lead to two categories of inflammation: pyogenic (pus-producing) and granulomatous (granuloma-forming).

Pyogenic inflammation. The neutrophils are the predominant cells in this type of inflammation. *Streptococcus pyogenes*, *Staphylococcus aureus* and *Streptococcus pneumoniae* are the common pyogenic bacteria.

Granulomatous inflammation. Macrophages and T cells predominate in this type of inflammation. The most notable organism in this category is *Mycobacterium tuberculosis*. Here, the bacterial antigens stimulate the cell-mediated immune system, resulting in sensitized T-lymphocyte and macrophage activity. Although the phagocytic activity of macrophages kills most of the tubercle bacilli, some survive and grow within

Table 5.2 Examples of surface virulence factors which interfere with host defences

Organism	Virulence factor	Used in vaccine
Bacteria		
Streptococcus pneumoniae	Polysaccharide capsule	Yes
Streptococcus pyogenes	M protein	No
Staphylococcus aureus	Protein A	No
Neisseria meningitidis	Polysaccharide capsule	Yes
Haemophilus influenzae	Polysaccharide capsule	Yes
Klebsiella pneumoniae	Polysaccharide capsule	No
Escherichia coli	Protein pili	No
Salmonella typhi	Polysaccharide capsule	No
Mycobacterium tuberculosis	Mycolic acid cell wall	No
Fungi		
Cryptococcus neoformans	Capsule	No

these cells, leading to granuloma formation. The organisms reside within phagosomes, which are unable to fuse with lysosomes, resulting in protection from degradative enzymes therein. Many fungal diseases are also characterized by granulomatous lesions.

Toxigenicity

Toxin production or toxigenicity is another major mediator of bacterial disease. Toxins are of two categories: **endotoxins** and **exotoxins**. Their main features are shown in Table 5.3.

Toxin production

Endotoxins

Endotoxins are the cell wall lipopolysaccharides of Gram-negative bacteria (both cocci and bacilli) and are not actively released from the cell. (*Note*: thus by definition Gram-positive organisms do not possess endotoxins.) Endotoxins cause fever, shock and other generalized symptoms.

A number of biological effects of endotoxin are described below. These are due mainly to the production of host factors such as **interleukin 1** (IL-1) and **tumour necrosis factor** (TNF) from macrophages.

1. **Fever** is due to the release of endogenous pyrogens (IL-1) by macrophages; these act on the hypothalamic temperature regulatory centre and reset the 'thermostat' at a higher temperature.
2. **Hypotension**, shock and reduced perfusion of major organs due to vasodilatation, is brought about by bradykinin release, increased vascular permeability and decreased peripheral resistance.
3. Activation of the **alternative pathway of the complement cascade** results in inflammation and tissue damage.
4. Generalized **activation of the coagulation system** (via factor XII) leads to disseminated intravascular coagulation, thrombosis and tissue ischaemia.
5. There is **increased phagocytic activity** of macrophages, polyclonal B-cell activation (but not T lymphocytes).
6. **Increased antibody production**.

Endotoxin-like effects may also occur in Gram-positive bacteraemic infections. However, as endotoxin is absent in Gram-positive bacteria, other cell wall components, such as teichoic acid or peptidoglycan, are thought to trigger the release of TNF and IL-1 from macrophages.

Exotoxins

Both Gram-positive and Gram-negative bacteria (Table 5.4) secrete exotoxins, whereas endotoxin is an integral component of the cell wall of Gram-negative organisms. Exotoxins in

Table 5.3 Comparison of main features of exotoxins and endotoxins

Property	Exotoxin	Endotoxin
Source	Some species of some Gram-positive and Gram-negative bacteria	Cell walls of Gram-negative bacteria
Origin	Secreted from cell	Cell wall constituent
Chemistry	Polypeptide	Lipopolysaccharide
Toxicity	High (fatal dose of the order of 1 μg)	Low (fatal dose in the order of hundreds of micrograms)
Clinical effects	Variable	Fever, shock
Antigenicity	Induces high-titre antibodies called antitoxins	Poorly antigenic
Vaccines	Toxoids used as vaccines	No toxoids formed and no vaccine available
Heat stability	Most are thermolabile (destroyed rapidly at 60°C)	Thermostable at 100°C for 1 hour
Typical diseases	Cholera, tetanus, diphtheria	Sepsis by Gram-negative rods, endotoxic shock

Table 5.4 Some important bacterial exotoxins and their mode of action

Organism	Disease	Mode of action	Toxoid vaccine
Gram-positive			
Corynebacterium diphtheriae	Diphtheria	Elongation factor inactivated by ADP-ribosylation	Yes
Clostridium tetani	Tetanus	Tetanospasmin blocks release of the inhibitory neurotransmitter glycine at motor nerve ends	Yes
Clostridium perfringens	Gas gangrene	Alpha-toxin — a lecithinase destroys eukaryotic cell membranes	No
Staphylococcus aureus	Toxic shock	Binds to class II MHC protein; induces IL-1 and IL-2	No
Gram-negative			
Escherichia coli	Diarrhoea	Labile toxin stimulates adenylate cyclase by ADP-ribosylation; stable toxin stimulates guanylate cyclase	No
Vibrio cholerae	Cholera	Stimulates adenylate cyclase by ADP-ribosylation	No
Bordetella pertussis	Whooping cough	Stimulates adenylate cyclase by ADP-ribosylation	No

particular can cause disease in distant parts of the body as a result of diffusion or carriage of the toxin via systemic routes (e.g. tetanus bacillus infecting a lesion in the foot produces an exotoxin which causes 'lockjaw' or spasm of masseter muscles on the face).

Exotoxins are polypeptides whose genes are frequently located on plasmids or lysogenic bacterial viruses. Essentially, these polypeptides consist of two domains or subunits: one for binding to the cell membrane and entry into the cell, and the other possessing the toxic activity.

Exotoxins are highly toxic (e.g. the fatal dose of tetanus toxin for a human can be less than 1 µg). Fortunately, exotoxin polypeptides are good antigens and induce the synthesis of protective antibodies called antitoxins, useful in prevention or treatment of diseases such as tetanus. The toxicity of the polypeptides can be neutralized when treated with formaldehyde (or acid or heat) and these **toxoids** are used in protective vaccines because they retain their antigenicity.

Bacterial exotoxins can be broadly categorized as:

● neurotoxins
● enterotoxins
● miscellaneous exotoxins.

Neurotoxins. Tetanus toxin, diphtheria toxin and botulinum toxin are all neurotoxins and their action is mediated via neuronal pathways.

Tetanus toxin, produced by *Clostridium tetani*, is a neurotoxin that prevents release of the inhibitory neurotransmitter glycine, thus causing muscle spasms (see Fig. 13.4). Tetanus toxin (tetanospasmin) comprises two polypeptide subunits: a heavy chain and a light chain. The former binds to the gangliosides in the membrane of the neuron, while the latter is the toxic component. The toxin is liberated at the peripheral wound site but is transmitted to the neurons of the spinal cord either by retrograde axonal transport or in the bloodstream. There it blocks the release of the inhibitory transmitter, which leads to sustained and convulsive contractions of the voluntary muscles (e.g. risus sardonicus, contraction of the facial muscles; lockjaw, contraction of the masseter muscles).

Diphtheria toxin, produced by *Corynebacterium diphtheriae*, is synthesized as a single polypeptide with two functional domains. Once secreted, one domain mediates the binding of the toxin to cell membrane receptors; the other domain pos-

sesses enzymatic activity and inhibits protein synthesis in all eukaryotic cells. The enzyme activity is highly potent: a single molecule can kill a cell within a few hours. *Escherichia coli*, *Vibrio cholerae* and *Bordetella pertussis* also possess exotoxins that act in a similar manner.

Botulinum toxin, produced by *Clostridium botulinum*, is one of the most toxic compounds known (1 µg will kill a man). The toxin blocks the release of acetylcholine at the synapse, producing paralysis of both voluntary and involuntary muscles. The toxin, encoded by the genes of a bacteriophage, comprises two polypeptide subunits.

Enterotoxins. These toxins act on the gut mucosa and cause gastrointestinal disturbances.

Escherichia coli enterotoxin is of two types: one heat-labile and one heat-stable. The heat-labile toxin (inactivated at 65°C in 30 minutes) is composed of two domains: one binds to a ganglioside in the cell membrane, while the other is the active component and mediates synthesis of cyclic adenosine monophosphate (cAMP) in the mucosal cells of the small intestine. This leads to an increase in the concentration of cAMP, which promotes cellular chloride ion excretion and inhibition of sodium ion absorption. The net result is fluid and electrolyte loss into the lumen of the gut (diarrhoea).

The heat-stable toxin of *E. coli* (not inactivated by boiling for 30 minutes) stimulates guanylate cyclase and thus increases the concentration of cyclic guanosine monophosphate (cGMP), which inhibits the reabsorption of sodium ions and causes diarrhoea (compare with heat-labile toxin). The genes for both toxins are carried on a plasmid.

The enterotoxins produced by the diarrhoea-causing organisms *V. cholerae* and *Bacillus cereus* act in a manner similar to that of the heat-labile toxin of *E. coli*.

Miscellaneous exotoxins. An array of exotoxins are produced by *Clostridium perfringens* and other species of clostridia that cause gas gangrene. These include the α-toxin (a phospholipase that hydrolyses lecithin, present in all eukaryotic cell membranes), collagenase, protease, hyaluronidase and deoxyribonuclease (DNAase). As the names imply, they destroy the cells and the connective tissue by a multiplicity of actions. In addition, a heterogeneous group of toxins with a haemolytic and necrotizing activity have been identified in clostridia.

PATHOGENESIS OF VIRAL DISEASE

Viral pathogenesis can be defined as the methods by which viruses produce disease in the host. The vast majority of viral infections are subclinical (symptomless) and go almost unrecognized. One individual may succumb to disease with an infection by a virus, while another may be entirely asymptomatic when infected by the identical strain of virus; genetic factors, immunity, nutrition and other factors influence the results of infection. The study of viral pathogenesis can be considered at two levels. First, at the level of the virus (parasite) and, second, at the level of the host.

Entry of viral infections

As in bacterial infections, viruses gain entry into the host by:
- inoculation (via the skin and mucosa)
- inhalation (via the respiratory tract)
- ingestion (via the gastrointestinal tract).

See Figure 5.1. (*Note*: although in this section viruses are considered separately, very similar host defence mechanisms operate to prevent the entry of all other pathogens through these portals.)

Skin and mucosa

The skin is an effective barrier against viral infection as the dead cells of the stratum corneum cannot support viral replication. Breach of skin integrity occurs:
- during accidental abrasions or needlestick injuries (during vaccination, virus is inoculated into the skin deliberately)
- via the bites of arthropod vectors, e.g. mosquitoes and ticks (these infect the host either because their saliva is infected as a result of viral multiplication within the arthropod, e.g. yellow fever virus in mosquitoes, or because their mouthparts are contaminated with the virus)
- as a result of deep inoculation into the subcutaneous tissue and muscle, which can follow hypodermic needle injections, tattooing, acupuncture, ear-piercing or animal bites. Once a virus has reached the dermis it has access to blood and lymphatic vessels as well as to macrophages, so the infection may spread readily (Fig. 5.2).

Oropharynx and intestinal tract

Natural defence mechanisms of the mouth and the gastrointestinal tract that prevent viral entry are:
- continuous desquamation of the epithelium
- the presence of saliva, the mucous layer of the intestine, gastric acid, bile and proteolytic enzymes, all of which nonspecifically inhibit viral entry
- mechanical movements of the tongue, cheek, peristalsis, etc.
- immune mechanisms (see Ch. 10).

Respiratory tract

A number of defence mechanisms operate to prevent viral entry through the respiratory tract. These include:
- secretion of mucus by goblet cells; this, propelled by the action of ciliated epithelial cells, clears inhaled foreign material (the mucociliary escalator)
- IgA present in respiratory secretions
- alveolar phagocytic cells.

To gain access to the respiratory tract, viruses need to be primarily in the form of aerosol particles or droplets. Other factors that affect viral respiratory infection include the humidity and air temperature (e.g. influenza is more common in the winter months) and the physical and chemical properties and structure of the virus particle.

Genitourinary tract

The vagina and urethra can be portals for entry of viral infection. The host factors that can influence viral entry via these routes include:
- natural mucosal desquamation
- vaginal secretions and cervical mucus, which contain both specific and non-specific defence factors
- intermittent flushing action of urine.

Sexual activity may cause tears or abrasions of the vaginal epithelium or trauma to the urethra, allowing viral ingress. Sexually transmitted viruses in humans include HIV, herpesviruses, human papillomaviruses and most hepatitis viruses.

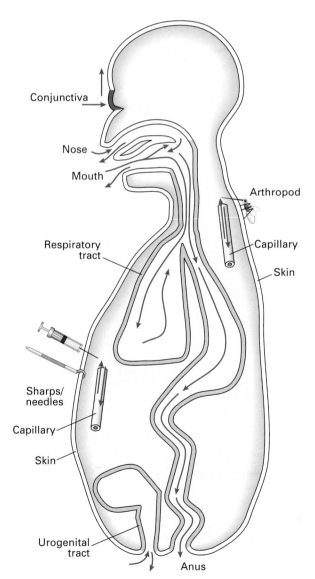

Fig. 5.1 Sites of the body where viral infections may ensue and subsequent shedding may occur.

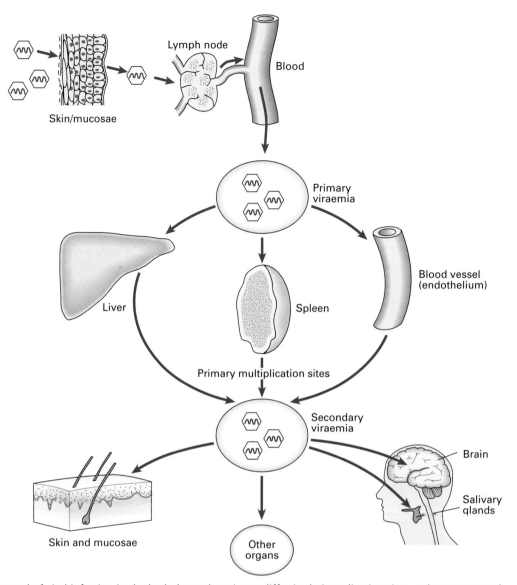

Fig. 5.2   The spread of viral infection in the body (note that viruses differ in their replicating sites and target organs).

Mechanisms of viral spread in the body

Viruses, unlike some bacteria, are completely devoid of organelles of transport, and they spread throughout the body by a number of routes. These include:
- direct local spread on epithelial and subepithelial surfaces
- lymphatic spread
- viraemic spread
- central nervous system and peripheral nerve spread.

Local spread on body surfaces

A number of viruses cause disease on epithelial surfaces without systemic spread. Such infections are characterized by:
- their localized nature
- direct viral shedding into the exterior or lumen (e.g. respiratory tract and alimentary tract infections with rhinoviruses and rotaviruses, respectively).

Once an invading virus overcomes the epithelial barrier it is exposed to the second line of body defences in the form of **phagocytic cells**, predominantly histiocytes of the macrophage series. When the virus is phagocytosed it will be destroyed not only by the low pH conditions in the phagocytic vesicle but also by enzymes in the **phagolysosome**.

Some viruses have developed mechanisms to evade this type of defence and, indeed, replicate within the macrophages.

Lymphatic spread

The phagocytosed and free viral particles lurking beneath the epithelium rapidly enter the subepithelial/mucosal network of lymphatic capillaries and are carried to regional lymph nodes (Fig. 5.2). Lymph nodes serve two main functions:
- they act as filters of extraneous microbes that gain access to the lymphatic system
- they are the sites where immune responses are generated.

Soon after entering the lymph node, viruses are exposed to the macrophages lining the marginal sinus. If the virus is phagocytosed, antigens are presented to the underlying lymphoid cells to evoke an immune response, on the success of which depends the outcome of the infection. If the virus is inactivated the infection resolves. However, the organism may infect macrophages and lymphocytes if the immune response at this stage is inadequate (e.g. herpesviruses, measles). The virus particles that escape the 'nodal filter' can then enter the bloodstream via the efferent lymphatics and the thoracic duct (Fig. 5.2).

There is a constant bidirectional movement of macrophages and lymphocytes from the blood into lymph nodes and vice versa. Thus if a virus infects cells in lymph nodes without damaging them, these cells can act as vehicles of virus dissemination. Sometimes the virus infects and multiplies in lymphatic endothelium, further increasing the virus load reaching the node and hence the lymphatic system. Viruses do not appear to enter the local blood vessels directly, except perhaps when these are damaged mechanically by trauma (e.g. needlestick injury, bites).

These events are closely followed by a local inflammatory response which alters the eventual outcome of the viral infection, as described below.

Viraemia and spread to organs

The entry of virus into the blood and its subsequent spread is called viraemia. Once a virus reaches the bloodstream, it is effectively disseminated within minutes. The first episode of viral entry into the blood is called a **primary viraemia** (Fig. 5.2). The virus may then be seeded in various distant organs, after which there is further replication at these sites and a second wave of viral entry into the bloodstream — a **secondary viraemia**. This is usually larger than the primary viraemia and the virus is more easily detected in blood samples. The secondary viraemia often leads to infection of other organs.

Viruses may be free in the plasma, in blood cells, or in both (Fig. 5.3). Those in the plasma can be relatively easily cleared, but viruses in leucocytes are not easily destroyed. If the infected leucocyte remains healthy it may disseminate infection to distant body sites. Once a virus reaches an organ, its localization depends on its ability to attach to and grow in vascular endothelial cells, and on phagocytosis by reticuloendothelial cells.

Central nervous system and peripheral nerve spread

During a viraemia, circulating viruses invade the central nervous system by localizing in blood vessels of:

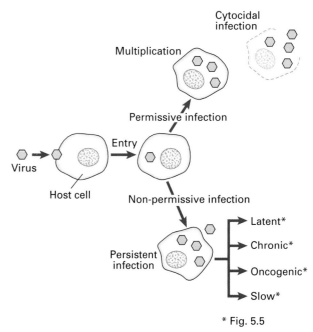

Fig. 5.4 The possible effects of viruses on host cells.

- the meninges and choroid plexus, with subsequent passage via cerebrospinal fluid into the neural tissues (e.g. mumps virus)
- the spinal cord or brain, with subsequent direct infection (e.g. poliovirus).

The process of localization is enhanced when there is an associated inflammatory focus. Peripheral nerves act as an effective path of transmission for some viruses, such as herpes simplex virus. Viral passage can be either **centripetal** (from body surface inwards) as in rabies, or **centrifugal** as in reactivation of herpes simplex (herpes labialis) or varicella–zoster. This mode of transport is a slow process (mm/h) compared with viraemic spread. Four possible routes of viral transmission in peripheral nerves are known:
- axon
- endoneural cell (e.g. Schwann cell)
- connective tissue space between nerves
- perineural lymphatics.

Virus and host cell interactions

Once the virus enters the host cell it can interact with the latter in two main ways:
1. **Permissive infection**, in which there is synthesis of viral components, their assembly and release.
2. **Non-permissive infection**, in which the infection can result in cell transformation, often with the integration of viral DNA into the host genome.

Permissive infection

The infection of a cell by a virus may have one or more sequelae (Fig. 5.4). The most common sequel is for the virus to replicate in a lytic or cytocidal infection, causing the cells to die and producing an acute illness. A virus-infected cell may die as a result of:
- 'shut–down' of host cell protein and nucleic acid synthesis
- cell lysis, by the release of progeny virions

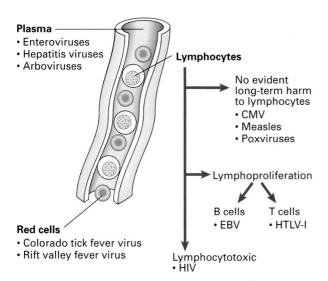

Fig. 5.3 Carriage of some important viruses in different compartments of blood. CMV, cytomegalovirus; EBV, Epstein–Barr virus; HIV, human immunodeficiency virus; HTLV-I, human T-cell leukaemia virus type I.

- intracellular release of lysosomal enzymes
- damage to cell membranes.

The adverse cellular consequence of viral infection, particularly that observed in virus-infected cells in tissue culture, is termed the **cytopathic effect** (see Ch. 7). During the early phase of infection, before cell death, characteristic alterations in the infected cell membrane may occur. Haemadsorption and giant cell formation are two examples.

Haemadsorption. In viruses that leave the cell by budding through the plasma membrane, viral glycoproteins (destined for the envelope) are first inserted into the membrane. A common envelope protein is haemagglutinin; this protein enables an infected cell to attract red cells at its surface, a phenomenon called haemadsorption. Haemadsorption can be used in the laboratory to detect cells infected with certain viruses (e.g. orthoviruses and paramyxoviruses).

Giant cell formation. Some viruses, such as herpes simplex and HIV, promote cell fusion in which membranes of adjacent cells coalesce to produce multinucleated giant cells (polykaryons, syncytia). Other markers of viral infection include intranuclear or cytoplasmic inclusion bodies.

Non-permissive infection

Cell death is not an inevitable accompaniment of viral replication. Sometimes a **persistent infection** may ensue in which there may be viral replication within the cell but the cell remains alive. Many viruses can produce persistent infections. Some relevant examples are hepatitis B virus, papillomaviruses, herpesviruses and retroviruses. Factors that favour persistence include:

- low pathogenicity of the virus
- ineffective or no antibody-mediated or cell-mediated host immune responses
- defective or no interferon production
- infection of lymphocytes and macrophages by the virus.

There are four categories of persistent infection: latent, chronic, oncogenic and slow (Fig. 5.5).

Latent viral infections. These occur when viral nucleic acids persist in the cell, usually integrated into the host DNA as a **provirus** (e.g. HIV, herpes simplex, varicella–zoster). As herpes simplex infection can be considered as the classic example of latent infection, the mechanism of its persistence is described. After an acute infection the herpes simplex virus travels along sensory nerve fibres (intra-axonal transport) to the appropriate dorsal root ganglion (e.g. in oral herpes the virus travels to the trigeminal ganglion). During latency, infectious virus is undetectable, but virus may be recovered by growing ganglion fragments in tissue culture. The re-emergence of virus is prevented, possibly due to host cell-mediated immunity but, when this wanes, there may be recrudescence and shedding of the virus in secretions from the area. Similarly, varicella–zoster virus remains latent for many years and may spontaneously recur as zoster (shingles) on dermatomes supplied by the specific sensory ganglion in which the virus is latent. Latent viral infections are reactivated particularly in immunocompromised patients, who subsequently suffer from infection and excrete the virus (see Ch. 30).

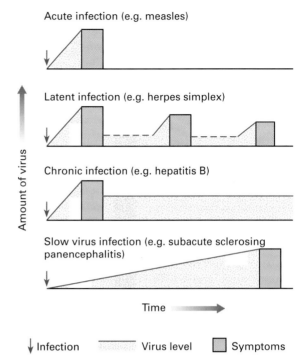

Fig. 5.5 Modes of viral infection, as a function of time (oncogenic infection not shown).

Chronic infections. These occur when viruses persist in quantity in the body over a prolonged period, with or without a history of disease. These chronically infected individuals, who are often asymptomatic, are called 'carriers' and are an important potential source of infection for others. Carriers make up a significant but unknown proportion of patients treated by dental health-care workers (see Ch. 36). The main difference between chronic and latent infections is that the virus is **continuously detectable** in the former but not in the latter.

Oncogenic infections. Persistent infections in which genetic and developmental factors are important in determining whether a particular virus is oncogenic in a given host (e.g. Epstein–Barr virus causing nasopharyngeal carcinoma and Burkitt's lymphoma).

Slow virus infections. These are rare, with incubations lasting months or years, leading to severe disability and eventual death (e.g. subacute sclerosing panencephalitis, a late consequence of measles).

Transmission of viral infections and infection control

See Chapter 36.

Host determinants of viral infection

The outcome of viral infection in a host depends not only on the type and virulence of the virus but also on host factors, including:

- **Immune status** — see Chapter 10.
- **Genetic constitution.** Genetic factors are now known to influence susceptibility to infection by herpesviruses, myxoviruses and poxviruses. Susceptibility may also be

associated with the presence of the appropriate host cell receptors on target cells.

- **Age.** Some viruses (such as mumps, polio, EBV or hepatitis) tend to produce less severe infection in infants, whereas others (such as respiratory syncytial virus and rotavirus) are more severe in children. The basis for this type of age dependence of viral infection is not clear.
- **Miscellaneous factors.** Hormonal and nutritional status may influence the outcome of viral infections, as shown by the fact that a number of viral infections (e.g. polio, hepatitis A and B) are often more severe during pregnancy, and protein malnutrition dramatically exacerbates the severity of measles infection. Personal habits (e.g. cigarette smoking) may influence the outcome of viral infections such as influenza — possibly due to impaired mucociliary clearance in the respiratory tract. Further, it is known that preceding vigorous exercise may accentuate the severity of a subsequent bout of poliomyelitis.

PATHOGENESIS OF FUNGAL DISEASE

See Chapter 22.

KOCH'S POSTULATES

A wide spectrum of microbes inhabit the human body. Some are permanent residents living as commensals, others are transient organisms and still others are commensals that behave as pathogens under suitable conditions (opportunistic pathogens). Hence when infection supervenes it is important to differentiate a commensal from a pathogen in order to identify and eliminate the latter. This problem was encountered by Robert Koch, a German general practitioner, in 1877 when he tried to determine the cause of an infection called anthrax in cattle and tuberculosis in humans. Koch defined the criteria for attributing an organism as the cause of specific disease. These criteria, called **Koch's postulates**, are as follows:

1. The organism must be isolated from every patient with the disease and its distribution in the body correspond to that of the lesions observed.
2. The organism must be isolated and cultured outside the body (in vitro) in pure culture.
3. The pure organism must cause the disease in healthy, susceptible animals.
4. The organism must be recovered from the inoculated animal.

Currently these four postulates are complemented with another:

5. The antibody to the organism should be detected in the patient's serum.

Clearly, these are ideal criteria and are not *always* attainable in practice (e.g. *M. leprae*, the leprosy bacillus, cannot be cultured in vitro), but they provide a framework for establishing an aetiological role of organisms in infectious diseases.

KEY FACTS

- The **virulence** of an organism can be measured by its **toxigenic potential** and **invasiveness**
- **Infections are either endogenous or exogenous** depending on whether the pathogen is derived from the patient's own flora or from an external source
- *Transmission of a pathogen to an infective focus can occur via inhalation, ingestion or inoculation*
- The **ability** of an organism to **adhere to host surfaces** is a **prerequisite** for initiating infection
- *Bacterial infection leads to pyogenic and granulomatous inflammation*
- **Toxins** of bacteria are classified as **endotoxins** or **exotoxins**
- **Endotoxins** are the lipopolysaccharide (LPS) components of cell walls of Gram-negative bacteria and hence, by definition, Gram-positive bacteria do not have endotoxins

- **Exotoxins** can be **produced by both Gram-positive and Gram-negative bacteria**; they are polypeptides whose genes are frequently located on plasmids or lysogenic bacterial viruses
- *Biological effects of endotoxins include fever, hypotension, activation of complement cascade, disseminated intravascular coagulation and increased phagocytic activity of macrophages*
- *Attenuated exotoxins of bacteria are called toxoids; they are not toxic but are antigenic and hence used in protective vaccines*
- **Viruses**, once they gain entry, **spread** throughout the body **by direct local spread, lymphatics, blood (viraemia)**, and the **central and peripheral nervous system**
- *Virus entry into a host cell may result in abortive, cytocidal, latent, chronic oncogenic (transforming) or slow infection*

FURTHER READING

Inglewski, BH, and Clark, LV (eds) (1990). *The bacteria. Molecular basis of bacterial pathogenesis*, vol. xi. Academic Press, London.

Mims, C, Dimmock, N, Nash, A, and Stephen, J (1995). *Mims' Pathogenesis of infectious disease* (4th edn). Academic Press, London.

Mims, C, Playfair, J, Roitt, I, Wakelin, D, and Williams, R (1998). Pathologic consequences of infection. In *Medical microbiology* (2nd edn), Ch. 12. Mosby, London.

Scully, C, and Samaranayake, LP (1992). *Clinical virology in oral medicine and dentistry*, Ch. 3. Cambridge University Press, Cambridge.

Taussig, MJ (1984). Infection: bacteria. In *Processes in pathology and microbiology* (2nd edn), sect. 4. Blackwell, Oxford.

6 Diagnostic microbiology and laboratory methods

DIAGNOSTIC MICROBIOLOGY

Diagnostic microbiology involves the study of specimens taken from patients suspected of having infections. The end result is a report, which should assist the clinician in reaching a **definitive diagnosis** and a **decision on antimicrobial therapy**. Hence clinicians should be acquainted with the techniques of taking specimens, and understand the principles and techniques behind laboratory analysis.

The diagnosis of an infectious disease entails a number of decisions and actions by many people. The diagnostic cycle begins when the clinician takes a microbiological sample and ends when the clinician receives the laboratory report and uses the information to manage the condition (Fig. 6.1). The steps in the diagnostic cycle are:
1. Clinical request and provision of clinical information.
2. Collection and transport of appropriate specimen(s).
3. Laboratory analysis.
4. Interpretation of the microbiology report and use of the information.

Clinical request

The first stage in the diagnostic cycle comprises the specimen and the accompanying request form. The following, which influence the quality of the specimen, should be noted:
- The clinical condition of the patient: if the patient is not suffering from a microbial infection then sampling for pathogens would be futile (e.g. tumours, trauma).
- Antibiotic therapy will alter the quality and quantity of the organisms. Hence specimens should be collected before antibiotic therapy, if possible; exceptions are where the patient is seriously ill, immunologically compromised, or not responding to a specific antibiotic, in which case the necessity of obtaining an interim report as a guide to further management justifies such action.

Provision of clinical information

The appropriate tests for each specimen have to be selected by the microbiologist according to clinical information given in the accompanying request form. Hence information such as age, main clinical condition, date of onset of illness, recent/current antibiotic therapy, antibiotic allergies and history of previous specimens are all important for the rationalization of investigations and should be supplied with the specimen.

Collection and transport of specimens

Always collect appropriate specimens.

Specimens should be as fresh as possible: many organisms (e.g. anaerobes, most viruses) do not survive for long in specimens at room temperature. Others, such as coliforms and staphylococci, may multiply at room temperature and subsequent analysis of such specimens will give misleading results.

Transport specimens in an appropriate medium (see below), otherwise dehydration and/or exposure of organisms to aerobic conditions occurs, with the resultant death and reduction in their numbers. The transport medium should be compatible with the organisms that are believed to be present in the clinical sample (e.g. virus specimens should be transported in viral transport medium, which is not suitable for bacteriological samples). Transport specimens in safe, robust containers to avoid contamination.

Laboratory analysis

A wide array of specimens are received and analysed by a number of methods in diagnostic microbiology laboratories. The analytical process of a pus specimen from a dental abscess is given below, as an illustration (Fig. 6.2).
1. Make a **smear** of the specimen, Gram **stain** and examine by **microscopy**. (A smear is made by spreading a small quantity of pus on a clean glass slide and heat fixing.)
2. **Inoculate** the specimen on two blood agar plates for **culture** under aerobic and anaerobic conditions (these plates are referred to as the **primary plates**).
3. **Incubate** the blood agar plates for 2–3 days at 37°C (because most oral pathogens are slow-growing anaerobes; for isolating aerobes an 18-hour incubation period is adequate).
4. **Inspect** plates for growth. Note the shapes and size of different colony types for subculture. Infections can be due to one organism (monomicrobial) or more than one organism (polymicrobial), as in the case of the majority of dentoalveolar infections, where samples usually yield a mixture of two or three organisms.

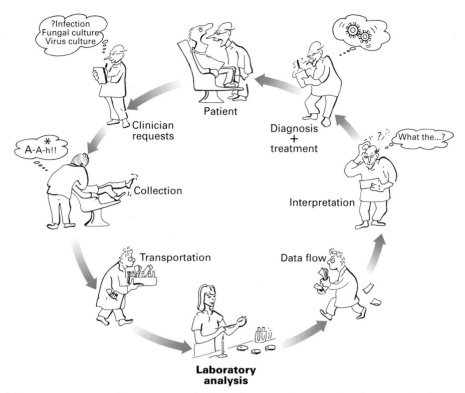

Fig. 6.1 The cycle of important events in diagnostic microbiology, depicting the interaction between the clinician and the microbiology laboratory.

5. **Isolate** the putative pathogen(s) by **subculturing** on to fresh blood agar plate(s) (single organism cultures) and incubating at 37°C for 24–48 hours.
6. **Harvest a pure culture** of the pathogen and identify using biochemical reactions, selective media or specific antibody reactions (see below).
7. **Antibiotic sensitivity tests** can be performed on the mixed growth obtained from pus (primary antibiotic tests) or on the pure organism(s) obtained in step 6 (secondary antibiotic tests) (see below).

Finally, it should be noted that the microbiologist can issue a provisional report after 2 days but the final report may take longer (Fig. 6.2).

Interpretation of the microbiology report and use of information

While interpretation of most microbiology reports may be straightforward, there are situations in which the clinician should contact the microbiologist, e.g. for guidance in relation to antibiotic therapy and the necessity for further sampling. Good collaboration between the clinician and the microbiologist is essential to achieve optimal therapy.

LABORATORY METHODS

A number of methods and techniques are used in the laboratory diagnosis of infection; they can be broadly categorized into:
- **Non-cultural methods**. These are many and varied, and include
  - microscopic methods (light microscopy, electron microscopy)
  - detection of microbes by probing for their genes.

- **Cultural methods**. Classic methods of diagnosis, in which
  - solid or liquid media are used for bacterial and fungal growth
  - cultured cells derived from animals and humans are used for viral growth.
- **Immunological methods**. These are used to
  - identify organisms
  - detect antibodies in a patient's body fluids (e.g. serum, saliva), especially when the organism cannot be cultured in laboratory media.

Microscopic methods

Light microscopy

Bright-field or standard microscopy. Routinely used in diagnostic microbiology, stained smears from lesions are examined with the oil immersion objective (×100) using the ×10 eyepiece, yielding a magnification of ×1000. **Wet films** are examined with a dry objective (×40) (e.g. to demonstrate motility of bacteria).

Dark-ground microscopy. The specimen is illuminated obliquely by a special condenser so that the light rays do not enter the objective directly. Instead the organisms appear bright, as the light rays hit them, against the dark background.

Phase-contrast microscopy. Although rarely employed in diagnostic microbiology, this technique may be used to define the detailed structure of unstained microbes.

Fluorescence microscopy. Fluorescence techniques are widely used, especially in immunology. This method employs the principle of emission of a different wavelength of light when

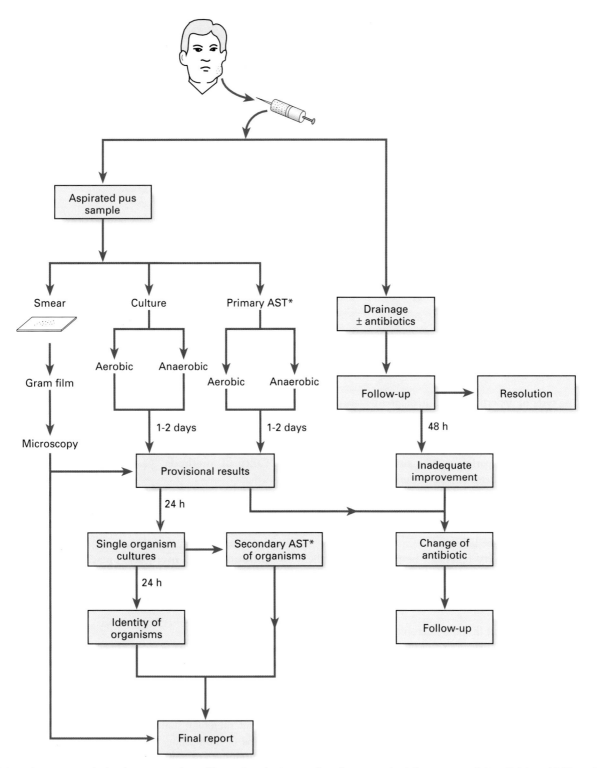

Fig. 6.2 Laboratory analysis of a pus specimen illustrating the interactions between the laboratory and the clinician. *AST, antibiotic sensitivity test.

light of one wavelength strikes a fluorescent object. Ultraviolet light is normally used, and the bacteria or cells are stained with fluorescent dyes such as auramine; for example, to detect microbial antigens in a specimen the latter is 'stained' with specific antibodies tagged with fluorescent dyes (immunofluorescence, see below).

Electron microscopy

In electron microscopy light waves are replaced by a beam of electrons, which allows resolution of extremely small organisms such as virions, e.g. 0.001 μm. Electron microscopy can

be used in diagnostic virology, for instance for direct examination of specimens (e.g. rotavirus, hepatitis A virus). Approximately one million virus particles are needed for such visualization. Clumps of such viral particles can be obtained by reacting the sample with antiviral antibody — **immunoelectron microscopy**.

Light microscopy and stains

In light microscopy bacterial stains are used:
- to visualize bacteria clearly
- to categorize them according to staining properties.

The most commonly used stain in diagnostic microbiology is the Gram stain.

Gram stain technique

1. After heat-fixing the dry film (by gently passing through a flame), flood with crystal violet for 15 seconds. Then wash the excess.
2. Flood with Lugol's iodine for 30 seconds (to fix the stain), wash the excess.
3. **Critical step**. Decolorize with acetone or alcohol for about 5 seconds. When no blue colour comes off the smear, wash immediately with water.
4. Counterstain with dilute carbolfuchsin for 30 seconds (or neutral red for 2 minutes).
5. Wash with water, and blot dry.

Staining characteristics. According to the results of Gram staining, bacteria may be either Gram-positive or Gram-negative:

- Gram-positive bacteria retain the violet stain by resisting decolorization and are stained deep **blue-black**.
- Gram-negative bacteria lose the violet stain during decolorization and are therefore counterstained with **pink**, the colour of carbolfuchsin.

Ziehl–Neelsen technique

Some bacteria, such as tubercle bacilli, are difficult to stain by the Gram method because they possess a thick, waxy outer cell wall. Instead, the Ziehl–Neelsen technique is used. The organisms are exposed to hot, concentrated carbolfuchsin for about 5 minutes, decolorized with acid and alcohol (hence the term acid- and alcohol-fast bacilli), and finally counterstained with methylene blue or malachite green. The bacilli will stain **red against a blue background**.

Other stains

A number of other stains are used in microbiology to demonstrate flagella, capsules and granules, and for staining bacteria in tissue sections.

Detection of microbes by probing for their genes

Polymerase chain reaction

Very small bacterial numbers (10–100) in patient specimens can be detected using the standard polymerase chain reaction (PCR) techniques (Ch. 3), while more sophisticated techniques can detect one HIV proviral DNA sequence in 10^6 cells. The main advantage of this method is its rapidity (a few hours compared with many days for conventional cultural techniques). However, PCR reactions may yield non-specific data and hence judicial selection of primers and careful conduct of the assays (to prevent contaminants giving rise to false positive results) are important. For these reasons PCR techniques are not common in the diagnostic laboratory, but with new developments such as microarray technology and nested PCR it is only a matter of time before this technique becomes more popular.

Nucleic acid probes

In this technique, a labelled, single-stranded nucleic acid molecule is used to detect a complementary sequence of DNA of the pathogen in the patient sample, by hybridizing to it.

The probes are obtained in the first instance from naturally occurring DNA by cloning DNA fragments into appropriate plasmid vectors and then isolating the cloned DNA. However, if the sequence of the target gene (in the pathogen) is known, oligonucleotide probes can be synthesized and labelled with a radioactive isotope or with compounds that give colour reactions under appropriate conditions.

This technique is not sensitive for detecting small numbers of organisms (i.e. few copy numbers of the gene) in clinical samples. However, a combination of the PCR technique (to produce high copy numbers) and hybridization with an oligonucleotide probe is likely to be the method of choice in identifying organisms that are slow or difficult to grow in the laboratory.

Cultural methods

Bacteria grow well on artificial media, unlike viruses which require live cells for growth. **Blood agar** is the most widely used bacterial culture medium. It is an example of a **non-selective** medium as many organisms can grow on it. However, when chemicals are incorporated into media to prevent the growth of certain bacterial species and to promote the growth of others, **selective** media can be developed (e.g. the addition of bile salts helps the isolation of enterobacteria from a stool sample by suppressing the growth of most gut commensals). Some examples of selective media and their use are given in Table 6.1.

Bacteriological media

The main constituents of bacteriological media are:
- water
- agar: a carbohydrate obtained from seaweed (as agar melts at 90°C and solidifies at 40°C, heat-sensitive nutrients can be added to the agar base before the medium solidifies)
- growth-enriching constituents: e.g. yeast extract, meat extract (these contain carbohydrates, proteins, inorganic salts and growth factors for bacterial growth)
- blood: defibrinated horse blood or sheep blood.

Preparation of solid media and inoculation procedure

When all the necessary ingredients have been added to the molten agar, it is dispensed, while still warm, into plastic or glass petri dishes. The agar will gradually cool and set at room temperature, yielding a plate ready for inoculation of the specimen.

The objective of inoculating the specimen or a culture of bacteria on to a solid medium is to obtain discrete colonies of organisms after appropriate incubation. Hence a standard technique (Fig. 6.3) should be used. Solid media are more useful than liquid media as they facilitate:

- Discrete colony formation, allowing single, pure colonies to be picked from the primary plate for subculture on a secondary plate. The pure growth from the secondary culture can then be used for identification of the organism using biochemical tests, etc.
- Observation of colonial characteristics helpful in identification of organisms.
- Quantification of organisms as **colony forming units** (CFU). This is valuable both in research and in diagnostic microbiology (e.g. if a urine specimen yields more than

Table 6.1   Some selective media used in routine microbiology

Medium	Selective agents	Differential substrate (indicator)	COLONIAL TYPES Selected organisms		Major organisms inhibited
			I	II	
MacConkey	Bile salts	Lactose (neutral red)	FERMENTER/RED *Escherichia coli* *Klebsiella*	NON-FERMENTER *Salmonella* *Pseudomonas*	Most cocci
Mitis salivarius	Tellurite, crystal violet	Sucrose (trypan blue)	BIG > 2 mm *Streptococcus salivarius*	SMALL < 1 mm *Streptococcus mitis* Other streptococci	Staphylococci enteric bacilli
Mannitol salt	7.5% NaCl	Mannitol (phenol red)	BIG/YELLOW *Staphylococcus aureus*	SMALL/PINK *Staphylococcus epidermidis*	Streptococci enteric bacilli
Löwenstein–Jensen	Malachite green	—	ROUGH *Mycobacterium tuberculosis*	SMOOTH/ PIGMENTED Atypical mycobacteria	Cocci
TCBS	Thiosulphate, citrate, bile salts, high pH (8.4)	Sucrose (bromothymol blue)	FERMENTER (YELLOW) *Vibrio cholerae* *Aeromonas*	NON-FERMENTER *Vibrio para-haemolyticus*	Cocci, enteric bacilli
Thayer–Martin	Antibiotics	—	GREY COLONIES *Neisseria gonorrhoeae* *Neisseria meningitidis*		Gram-positive cocci
Charcoal yeast extract	Cysteine, ferric sulphate	—	CUTGLASS COLONIES *Legionella* spp.		Gram-positive cocci
Sabouraud	Low pH (5.6) ± antibiotics	—	CREAM COLONIES Fungi		Most bacteria

10^5 CFU/ml the patient is deemed to have a urinary tract infection; a mixed saliva sample with more than 10^6 CFU/ml of *Streptococcus mutans* indicates high cariogenic activity).

Liquid media

Liquid media are used in microbiology to:
- Promote growth of small numbers of bacteria present in specimens contaminated with antibiotics. The antibiotic is diluted in the fluid medium, thereby promoting growth of the organism.

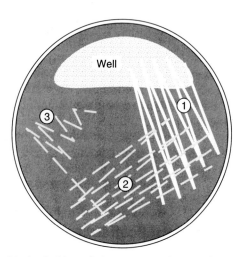

Fig. 6.3   Method of inoculating an agar plate to obtain discrete colonies of bacteria (after overnight incubation).

- Preferentially promote the growth of a specific bacterium while suppressing other bacterial commensals present in the sample. These are called **enrichment media** (e.g. selenite F broth used for stool cultures).
- Test the biochemical activities of bacteria for identification purposes.

Some examples of solid and liquid media are given in Table 6.2.

Media for blood culture

When the infectious agent is circulating in blood (e.g. in septicaemia, endocarditis, pneumonia) the latter has to be aseptically withdrawn by venepuncture and cultured. Blood culture has to be performed on special liquid media, both under aerobic and anaerobic conditions. The blood is aseptically transferred to a rich growth medium (e.g. brain–heart infusion broth) containing anticoagulants (Fig. 6.4). Cultures are checked for turbidity and gas production daily, up to a week (in many laboratories this process is now automated and machines are used to detect bacterial growth). Positive cultures are sampled and the organism(s) isolated and identified.

Transport media

Specimens are transported from the clinic to the laboratory in a transport medium, which helps to maintain the viability of the organisms in transit.

Bacteriological transport media.   A semisolid, non-nutrient agar such as the Stuart transport medium is widely used. It

Table 6.2 Constituents and uses of some commonly used solid and liquid media

Medium	Major ingredients	Use
Solid media		
Nutrient agar	Nutrient broth, agar	General purpose
Blood agar	Nutrient agar, 5–10% horse or sheep blood	Very popular, general use
Chocolate agar	Heated blood agar	Isolation of *Haemophilus* and *Neisseria* spp.
CLED agar	Peptone, L-cystine, lactose, etc.	Culture of coliforms
Antibiotic sensitivity	Peptone and a semisynthetic medium	Antibiotic sensitivity tests
Liqid media		
Peptone	Peptone, NaCl, water	General use; base for sugar fermentation tests
Nutrient broth	Peptone water, meat extract	General culture
Robertson's meat medium	Nutrient broth, minced meat	Mainly to culture anaerobes
Selenite F broth	Peptone water, sodium selenite	Enrichment medium for *Salmonella* and *Shigella* spp.

also contains thioglycolic acid as a reducing agent, and electrolytes.

Viral transport medium. This is a general term describing a solution containing proteins and balanced salts which stabilizes the virus during transportation. Antimicrobial agents are also added to kill any bacteria present in the sample.

Atmospheric requirements and incubation

Once inoculated the agar plates may be incubated:
- **Aerobically**: but addition of 10% carbon dioxide enhances the growth of most human pathogens.
- **Anaerobically**: most bacteria, especially the oral pathogens, are strict anaerobes and grow only in the absence of oxygen. Anaerobic conditions can be produced in a sealed jar or in large anaerobic incubators. In either case the environmental oxygen is replaced by nitrogen, hydrogen and carbon dioxide.
- **At body temperature**: 37°C (a few bacteria grow well at a higher or a lower temperature; fungi usually grow at ambient temperature).

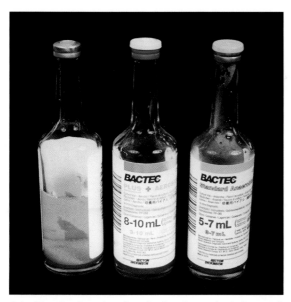

Fig. 6.4 Blood culture bottles: the bottle on the left contains the uninoculated medium.

BACTERIAL IDENTIFICATION

When the putative pathogen from the clinical specimen is isolated as a **pure culture** it is important to identify the organism(s). Bacterial identification (Fig. 6.5) initially entails:
1. Inspection of the **colonial characteristics**: size, shape, elevation (flat, convex, umbonate), margin (entire, undulate, filamentous), colour, smell and texture; effect on blood (α-, β-, or non-haemolytic).
2. Examination of **microscopic morphology** and **staining characteristics**: a stained film of the colony helps identification.
3. Identification of **growth conditions**: aerobic, anaerobic, capnophilic (i.e. grows well in carbon dioxide excess); growth on selective and enrichment media.

The foregoing will indicate the major group to which the organism belongs (e.g. streptococci, enterobacteria, clostridia). However, definitive identification to species level requires biochemical tests.

Biochemical tests

Each bacterial species has a characteristic biochemical profile valuable for its identification. These include:
- **Sugar fermentation and assimilation profile**. The pure culture is incubated with specific sugars and checked for the production of acid and gas or both.
- **Enzyme profile**. The organism is incubated with an appropriate enzyme substrate. If the enzyme is secreted by the organism this will react with the substrate and cause a colour change. In addition, some bacteria can be identified primarily by production of a characteristic enzyme. Thus, coagulase produced by *Staphylococcus aureus* clots (or coagulates) plasma and is a specific enzyme for this organism. Another example is lecithinase produced by *Clostridium perfringens* (see Ch. 13).

Commercial identification kits

Definitive identification of an organism requires testing for a spectrum of enzymes as well as its ability to ferment (anaerobic breakdown) or assimilate (aerobic breakdown) a number of carbohydrates. This is facilitated by commercially

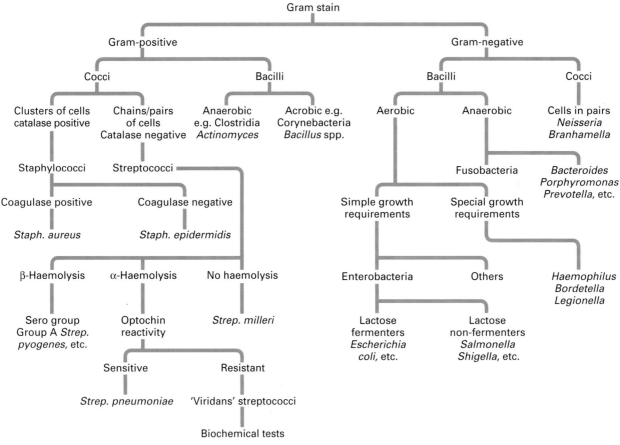

Fig. 6.5 A 'decision tree' used in the laboratory identification of organisms.

available kits, such as the API and AnIdent systems, which incorporate a wide range of the foregoing tests (usually 20) in a single kit system (Fig. 6.6).

Method

A pure culture of the test organism is inoculated into each small well (**cupule**) containing the appropriate carbohydrate or the chemical and incubated overnight. The resultant colour or turbidity change for each test is then compared with a standard colour chart (provided by the manufacturers) and scored. The numerical profile thus obtained for the organism is compared with a profile compiled from type cultures, and the

degree of concordance between the profiles of the two organisms enables identification of the test bacterium.

Sometimes the process of identifying an organism has to be extended further than **speciation** (i.e. identifying the bacteria beyond the species level) described above; this is called **bacterial typing**.

Typing of bacteria

It is important to realize that bacteria of the same species may have different characteristics (just as individual members of the species *Homo sapiens* vary in characteristics such as skin colour, stature, etc.). This is especially important when tracing

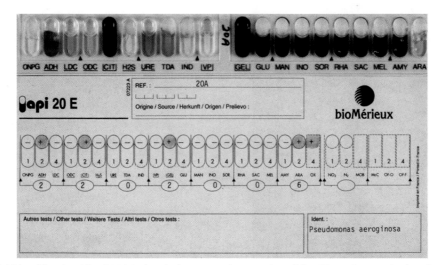

Fig. 6.6 A commercial identification kit of 20 biochemical tests used to speciate (identify to the species level) enterobacteria. Similar kits are used to speciate other genera of bacteria.

the epidemic spread of an organism either in the community or in a hospital ward (like tracing a criminal in a vast population). Tracing such an organism can be performed by strain differentiation using the following typing procedures:

- **serotyping**: differentiates bacteria according to antigenic structure
- **biotyping**: differentiates bacteria according to the biochemical reactivity
- **phagetyping**: differentiates bacteria on the basis of susceptibility to a panel of known bacteriophages (viruses that kill bacteria)
- **bacteriocin typing**: bacteriocins are potent proteins of bacteria which inhibit the growth of other members of the same class species; a panel of bacteriocins can be used to test the susceptibility of a test organism, and the profile thus obtained used for typing
- **genetic typing**: a number of novel genetic typing methods such as those described in Chapter 3 are now available and these produce very accurate 'fingerprints' of bacteria.

IMMUNOLOGICAL METHODS

Immunological methods are useful in diagnostic microbiology to identify organisms and to detect antibodies in a patient's body fluids (e.g. serum, saliva), especially when the organism cannot be cultured in laboratory media.

Identification of organisms using immunological techniques

Agglutination

Slide agglutination. Antibodies against the specific serotypes of the organism (e.g. *Salmonella* and *Shigella* species) can be used in identification. When a suspension of the organisms and a few drops of the specific antibody are mixed on a glass slide, visible agglutination (clumping) of the organism indicates a positive reaction.

Latex agglutination. Here the agglutination of latex beads coated with the specific antibody directed against the unknown organism is used, as above (e.g. *Neisseria meningitidis*, *Haemophilus influenzae*, the yeast *Cryptococcus neoformans*) (Fig. 6.7).

Immunofluorescence

If an organism is exposed to the specific antibody tagged with a fluorescent dye, then the organism binds to the antibody and can be visualized through an ultraviolet microscope. Principles of direct (one-step) and indirect (two-step) immunofluorescence techniques are shown in Figure 6.8.

Enzyme-linked immunosorbent assay

The enzyme-linked immunosorbent assay (ELISA) is a modification of the above test in which the fluorescent dye tagged to the antibody is replaced by an enzyme. The organism binds to the antibody and the tagged enzyme, and the amount of bound enzyme can then be demonstrated by reaction with the enzyme substrate. This is a highly popular test.

Detection of antibodies in a patient's serum

An example of this technique is the serological tests for syphilis. The agent of syphilis, *Treponema pallidum*, does not grow in laboratory media. Hence serological tests are useful. These are:

- The VDRL (non-treponemal) test, in which a cardiolipin, lecithin and cholesterol mixture is used as an antigen. Clumping of the cardiolipin occurs in the presence of antibody to *T. pallidum*. (*Note*: this is a non-specific test, and, if positive, confirmatory tests must be done.)
- The treponemal test, in which non-viable *T. pallidum* is used as the antigen (e.g. fluorescent treponemal antibody absorbed test, FTA-ABS) (see Ch. 18).

LABORATORY INVESTIGATIONS RELATED TO ANTIMICROBIAL THERAPY

Once the putative pathogen has been identified from a specimen its antimicrobial sensitivity can be predicted with some degree of accuracy, based on previous experience and avail-

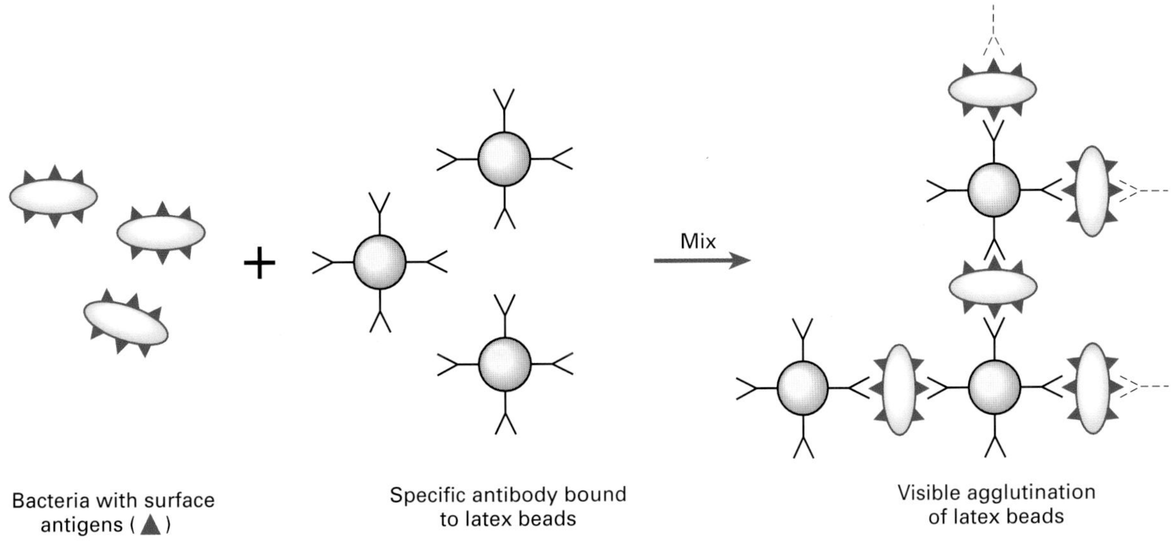

| Bacteria with surface antigens (▲) | Specific antibody bound to latex beads | | Visible agglutination of latex beads |

Fig. 6.7 Latex agglutination test: latex beads coated with a known, specific antibody (e.g. *Haemophilus influenzae*) is mixed with a suspension of the unknown organisms; visible agglutination of the beads occurs instantaneously if the identity is positive.

Direct immunofluorescence

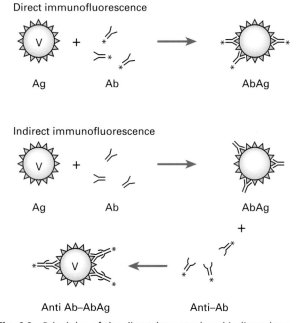

Indirect immunofluorescence

Fig. 6.8 Principles of the direct (one-step) and indirect (two-step) immunofluorescence techniques. This example illustrates the detection of a viral antigen (e.g. herpes simplex).
*, Immunofluorescence label; V, viral antigen; Ag, antigen; Ab, antibody.

able data. Prescribing in this manner is called **empirical therapy** (e.g. based on the sensitivity of staphylococci to flucloxacillin). However, it is essential to base **rational therapy** on the results of laboratory antibiotic tests performed on the isolated pathogen.

Susceptibility of organisms to antimicrobial agents

In clinical microbiology a microbe is considered **sensitive** (or **susceptible**) to an antimicrobial agent if it is inhibited by a concentration of the drug normally obtained in human tissues after a standard therapeutic dose. The reverse is true for a **resistant** organism. Organisms are considered **intermediate** in susceptibility if the inhibiting concentration of the antimicrobial agent is slightly higher than that obtained with a therapeutic dose.

Laboratory testing for antimicrobial sensitivity

The action of an antimicrobial drug against an organism can be measured:
- **qualitatively** (disc diffusion tests)
- **quantitatively** (minimum inhibitory concentration or minimum bactericidal concentration tests).

A semiquantitative technique called the break–point test is not described here. These in vitro tests indicate whether the expected therapeutic concentration of the drug given in standard dosage inhibits the growth of a given organism in vivo. Laboratory results can only give an indication of the activity of the drug in vitro, and its effect in vivo depends on factors such as the ability of the drug to reach the site of infection and the immune status of the host. A strong host defence response may give the impression of 'successful' drug therapy, even though the infecting organism was 'resistant' to a specific drug when laboratory tests were used.

Disc diffusion test

The disc diffusion test is the most commonly used method of testing the sensitivity of a microorganism to an antimicrobial agent. Here, the isolate to be tested is seeded over the entire surface of an agar plate and drug-impregnated filter paper discs are applied. After overnight incubation at 37°C, zones of growth inhibition are observed around each disc, depending on the sensitivity of a particular organism to a given agent (Figs 6.9 and 6.10).

Antimicrobial sensitivity tests of this type can be divided into **primary sensitivity** (direct) and **secondary sensitivity** (indirect). A primary test is carried out by inoculating the clinical sample, say pus, directly on to the test zone of the plate. The advantage of this is that the overall

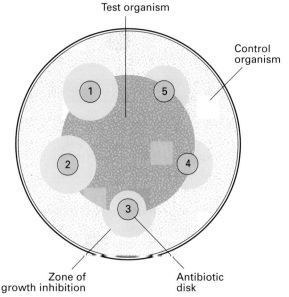

Fig. 6.9 The antibiotic susceptibility of an organism can be tested by an application of filter-paper discs impregnated with different antibiotics on to a lawn of the organism seeded on an agar plate. After overnight incubation, zones of growth inhibition around discs indicate sensitivity to the antibiotic, whereas growth of the organism up to the disc indicates resistance. In this example the test organism is sensitive to antibiotics 1 and 2, moderately sensitive to antibiotic 3, and resistant to antibiotics 4 and 5.

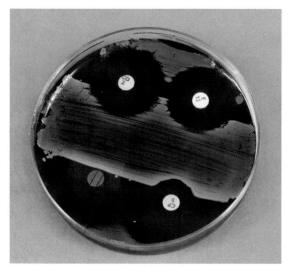

Fig. 6.10 Another example of an antibiotic sensitivity test; here the control organism is inoculated on the polar aspects of the plate and the test organism is inoculated in the middle. In this example the organism is resistant to ampicillin (AM disc, bottom left) and sensitive to the other three antibiotics.

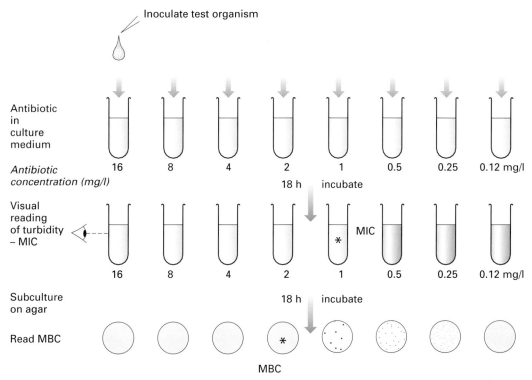

Fig. 6.11 Determination of the minimum inhibitory concentration (MIC) and minimum bactericidal concentration (MBC) of an antibiotic required to inhibit or kill a specific organism. This gives a quantitative estimate of the antibiotic sensitivity of the organism, compared with the disc diffusion method described in Figure 6.9. (In this example, MIC = 1 mg/l, MBC = 2 mg/l.)

sensitivity results for the organisms present in pus will be available after 24–48 hours' incubation (see Fig. 6.2). This is particularly useful when treating debilitated patients with acute infections such as dentoalveolar abscesses. However, because this is a rough estimate, secondary sensitivity tests are therefore performed on a pure culture of the organism isolated, but the results are not available for at least 2–4 days after sampling.

Assessment of MIC and MBC

Determining the minimum inhibitory concentration (MIC) and the minimum bactericidal concentration (MBC) gives a quantitative assessment of the potency of an antibiotic (Fig. 6.11).

Method. A range of twofold dilutions of an antimicrobial agent can be incorporated into a suitable broth in a series of tubes (tube dilution technique). The broth is inoculated with a standardized suspension of the test organism and incubated for 18 hours. The minimum concentration of the drug that inhibits the growth of the test organism in the tube is recorded as the MIC, i.e. the lowest concentration that will inhibit the visible growth in vitro. Subsequently, a standard inoculum from each of the tubes in which no growth occurred may be subcultured on blood agar to determine the minimum concentration of the drug required to kill the organism (MBC). The MBC is defined as the minimum concentration of drug that kills 99.9% of the test microorganisms in the original inoculum.

These tests are not routinely performed but are useful in patients with serious infections where optimal antimicrobial therapy is essential, for example to establish sensitivity of streptococci isolated from blood cultures from patients with infective endocarditis, and of bacteria causing septicaemia in immunosuppressed patients.

APPROPRIATE SPECIMENS IN MEDICAL MICROBIOLOGY

See Table 6.3.

Appropriate specimens for oral infections

Sampling for pathogens within the oral environment poses many problems due to the multitude of indigenous commensal flora that thrive in the oral cavity. Further, many of the pathogens are endogenous in origin and cause disease when an opportunity arises (opportunistic pathogens). In addition, obtaining an uncontaminated sample from sites such as the depths of periodontal pockets where disease activity and hence the numbers of periodontopathogens are likely to be high is extremely difficult. For these reasons, judicial and appropriate sampling techniques should be used when diagnosing oral infections (Table 6.4).

The specimens submitted to an oral microbiology laboratory can be categorized as those useful for the management of purulent infections, mucosal infections, and periodontal infections and caries.

Purulent infections

The appropriate specimen is an aspirated sample of pus, if possible. Take care to avoid needlestick injuries when re-sheathing the needle cap; drainage of residual pus by incision, after aspiration sampling, is obligatory. The laboratory steps in the diagnosis of a purulent infection are shown in Figure 6.2.

Mucosal infections

A common oral mucosal infection is oral candidiasis. Here, the lesion is sampled with a dry swab, and a smear taken

Table 6.3 Some appropriate specimens for microbiological investigations

Tissue or system	Specimen	Comments
Skin	Swab	Examine for bacteria and yeasts
	Scrapings	Examine for fungi
	Vesicle fluid	Examine for viruses (electron microscopy and culture)
	Serum	Viral serology
Blood (bacteraemia and septicaemia)	Blood culture	Sterile precautions necessary. Multiple specimens required
Gastrointestinal tract	Faeces	Culture for bacteria and viruses; toxin detection for *Clostridium difficile*; light microscopy for parasites and protozoa; electron microscopy for viruses
	Serum	Serological tests for enteric fevers
Urinary tract	Midstream specimen of urine/ suprapubic aspirate/catheter specimen of urine (not from a collecting bag)	For quantitative and qualitative bacteriology
Upper respiratory tract	Pernasal, throat and nose swabs; saliva	Culture for *Bordetella pertussis*. Culture for β-haemolytic streptococci, other bacteria and viruses
	Throat washings or nose and throat aspirates	Culture and immunofluorescence for viruses
Lower respiratory tract	Sputum	Culture for bacteria, viruses and fungi; fluorescent microscopy for many viruses, *Mycobacterium tuberculosis* and *Legionella* spp.
	Serum	Viral and fungal serology
Meninges	Cerebrospinal fluid	Cell count, microscopy and culture
	Serum	Viral serology
Genital tract	Swab in Amies' or Stuart's transport medium	For bacterial and yeast culture and microscopy for gonococci and *Trichomonas* spp. (wet film)
	Swabs in chlamydia and viral transport medium	Culture of chlamydia and viruses
	Smear of discharge	For detection of gonococci
	Serum	Serological test for syphilis
Abscess	Pus	Aspirates for culture and identification
Wounds	Pus or swab	Avoid contamination from skin; pus preferred
	Tissue	Send small samples in dry sterile containers for homogenization, culture and microscopy
Mucosal lesions	Swab	Avoid contamination with normal flora. Use transport medium if necessary; culture for bacteria, fungi and viruses
	Smear	Fluorescent microscopy; useful for gonococci and yeasts
	Serum	Serological tests for staphylococcal and streptococcal infection and viruses

Modified from Ross PW, Hollbrook WP. Clinical and oral microbiology. Oxford: Blackwell; 1984.

immediately thereafter (see the section on candidal infections below).

When evaluating the oral carriage of yeasts (or other organisms such as Enterobacteriaceae) then an **oral rinse** should be collected. This entails requesting the patient to rinse the mouth for 60 seconds with 10 ml of phosphate-buffered saline and then expectorating the rinse into a container, which is transported to the laboratory for quantification of yeast growth (in terms of CFUs).

Diagnosis of viral infections of the oral mucosa is described below.

Periodontal infections and caries

The value of microbiological sampling for the diagnosis of caries and periodontal diseases is limited. In the case of dental caries salivary counts of lactobacilli and *Streptococcus mutans*

could be used, and for this purpose saliva samples should be collected (Ch. 32).

The diagnosis of periodontal disease by microbiologic means is problematic. A deep gingival smear is useful for the diagnosis of acute necrotizing ulcerative gingivitis, while paper point samples appear useful for DNA analysis of periodontopathic bacteria. However, the latter is not a conclusive test.

LABORATORY ISOLATION AND IDENTIFICATION OF VIRUSES

The techniques for isolation and identification of viruses are significantly different from bacteriological techniques. Laboratory procedures for the diagnosis of viral infections are of four main types:

Table 6.4 Appropriate specimens for microbiological examination of oral infections

Lesion or site of lesion	Specimen	Comments
Lips and perioral skin	Moistened swab Vesicle fluid, swab Aspirate of abscess Serum	Culture for yeasts and bacteria Virus culture and electron microscopy Microscopy and culture (see Fig. 6.2) Serological tests for viruses and syphilis
Tongue and oral mucosa	Swab Smear of scraping (heat fixed) Vesicle fluid Biopsy tissue Serum	Culture for bacteria, yeasts and viruses Microscopy for yeasts and bacteria As above Culture for bacteria and viruses: microscopy for yeasts and suspected tuberculosis As above
Dental abscess or suspected infected cyst	Aspirate	Smear and culture (see Fig. 6.2)
Infected root canal	Paper point or barbed broach	Aseptic collection; use semisolid transport medium; semi-quantitative culture
Dental plaque	Scraping	A variety of sampling tools and procedures available
Gingivae and gingival crevice	Scraping on a sterile scaler	Smear can be diagnostic for fusospirochaetal infection; viral culture possible, DNA tests, BANA tests for periodontopathogens
Severe caries	Saliva	Lactobacillus/*Streptococcus mutans* counts
Prosthesis (dentures)	Swab and smear	In suspected denture stomatitis examine for yeasts

BANA, N-benzoyl-DL-arginine-2-naphthylamide.

- direct microscopic examination of host tissues for characteristic cytopathological changes and/or for the presence of viral antigens
- isolation and identification of virus from tissues, secretions or exudates
- detection of virus-specific antibodies or antigens in patients' sera
- molecular amplification methods for rapid viral diagnosis.

Direct microscopy of clinical material

Direct microscopy is the quickest method of diagnosis. Virus or virus antigen may be detected in tissues from lesions, aspirated fluid samples or excretions from the patient. The common techniques used are:

- **Electron microscopy**: a common diagnostic tool used in provisional identification of the virus on a morphological basis, although other tests need to be performed to confirm the virus type (e.g. widely used in the examination of stool specimens in infantile diarrhoea).
- **Serology**: tests include immunofluorescence and immunoperoxidase techniques, which commonly employ monoclonal antiviral antibody.

Isolation and identification from tissues

Viruses do not grow on inanimate media and they must be cultivated in living cells. Since no single type of host cell will support the growth of all viruses, a number of different methods of culturing viruses have been developed:

- tissue culture cells — the cheapest and most popular system (e.g. monkey kidney cells, baby hamster kidney cells)
- embryonated eggs — outdated

- laboratory animals (e.g. suckling mice) — expensive, rarely used.

Tissue culture

After the inoculation of a **monolayer** of tissue culture with a clinical sample it is examined daily for microscopic evidence of viral growth, for about 10 days. Viruses produce different kinds of degenerative changes or **cytopathic effects**, such as rounding of cells and net or syncytial formation, in susceptible cells (Fig. 6.12). The cell type supporting virus growth and the nature of the cytopathic effect help identification of individual viruses (e.g. herpesviruses growing in monkey kidney cells produce fused cells in which nuclei aggregate to form multinucleate giant cells). The time required for the cytopathic effect to be seen can vary from 24 hours up to several days, depending on the virus strain and the concentration of the inoculum. Once the virus is cultured it can be identified by:

- electron microscopy
- haemadsorption: added erythrocytes adhere to the surface of infected cells
- growth neutralization assays using virus-specific antiserum
- immunofluorescence: with standard or monoclonal antibody.

Serodiagnosis of viral infections

Many virus infections produce a short period of acute illness in which viral shedding occurs, and thereafter it is difficult to culture viral samples from clinical specimens. Hence diagnosis of viral infections by serology is widely used. A diagnosis of a recent viral infection depends on:

1. **Demonstration of IgM antibodies.** These are the earliest antibodies to appear after infection and, if present,

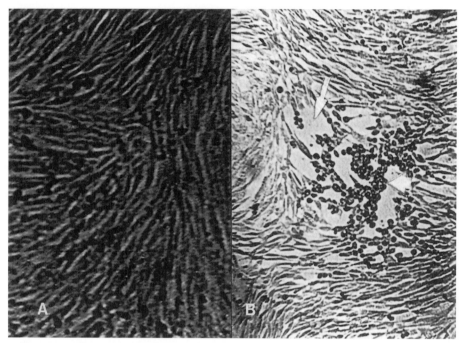

Fig. 6.12 Cytopathic effects caused by herpes simplex virus in baby hamster kidney fibroblasts. **A** Confluent monolayer of cells (control); **B** cytopathic effect with rounded cells and areas with detached cells (arrow).

indicate unequivocal recent disease. A number of tests are available and include detection of antihuman IgM using ELISA and immunofluorescence techniques.

2. **Demonstration of a rising titre of antibody.** For this, the timely collection of a pair of blood samples, one in the **acute** and the other in the **convalescent** phase of the disease, is essential. Acute-phase serum should be collected as early as possible when illness is suspected, while convalescent-phase serum is collected when the patient has recovered, usually some 10–20 days after the first specimen has been collected.

Serological test results are interpreted by comparing the antibody titres of the acute and convalescent sera. **Antibody titre** is defined as the reciprocal of the highest serum dilution that shows antibody activity, in a given test (e.g. if the patient's serum shows antibody activity when diluted by 1 in 64, then the antibody titre is 64.) A greater than fourfold rise in titre between the acute and convalescent samples is considered to be a positive result, indicating the patient has had an acute illness due to the specific virus.

Serological tests

A wide array of serological tests are used in virology. The classic and oldest technique of complement fixation is now being supplanted by a number of other tests. These include immunofluorescence, ELISA and radioimmunoassay (see Fig. 6.8). The advantages of the latter methods over the comparison of viral titre in paired sera, described above, are that only a single serum sample is needed and results are available quickly. Immunological and tissue culture detection methods have been successfully combined to shorten the time required to identify viral infections. Other methods frequently used in serodiagnosis of viral infections include haemagglutination.

Serodiagnosis using multiple antigen systems. Some viruses, such as mumps virus and hepatitis B virus, present with

more than a single antigen (and hence antibody), which appear at different periods of the illness. This feature can be exploited to detect the state of illness by using a single sample of serum without waiting for convalescence. A variety of antigens and antibodies used in the detection of various phases of hepatitis B virus infection is described in some detail in Chapter 29.

Molecular amplification methods for rapid viral diagnosis

Molecular methods are increasingly useful and should gradually supplant conventional methods of viral detection, as has already been discussed in Chapter 4. For example the polymerase chain reaction technique can detect even a few DNA molecules of a specific virus in a sample. Also, radioactive virus DNA can detect virus genome or mRNA in tissues by molecular hybridization (Table 6.5).

DIAGNOSIS OF FUNGAL INFECTIONS

These principles of diagnosis of fungal diseases are essentially the same as for bacterial and viral infections. Fungal diseases can be diagnosed by:
- examination of specimens by microscopy
- culture and identification of the pathogen
- serological investigations (both for antigen and antibody)
- molecular diagnostic methods.

Candidal infections

Smears, swabs and oral rinse samples are the common specimens received in the laboratory for the diagnosis of oral candidal infections. For this, the lesion is sampled with a dry swab and a smear is taken immediately thereafter (a smear is taken by scraping the lesion with the edge of a flat plastic

Table 6.5 Some applications of molecular amplification methods for rapid diagnosis of infections

Clinical example	Sample for direct examination	Organisms	Comment
Hepatitis C	Serum (frozen)	Hepatitis C virus	Detection of hepatitis C virus RNA by commercial PCR method
HIV-1 and HIV-2 infection	EDTA blood	HIV-1 and HIV-2	Diagnosis of HIV infection in infants or adults when serological tests are difficult to interpret
Tuberculosis	Sputum Other respiratory samples	*Mycobacterium tuberculosis*	Recommended for sputum smear-positive cases; standard commercial PCR methods — particularly useful for immunocompromised patients or when atypical clinical features of TB
Leprosy	Tissue biopsy	*Mycobacterium leprae*	PCR method available in reference centre to detect this 'non-cultivable' organism

EDTA, ethylenediaminetetraacetic acid; HIV, human immunodeficiency virus; PCR, polymerase chain reaction; RNA, ribonucleic acid; TB, tuberculosis.

instrument and transferring the sample to a glass microscope slide). In patients with possible *Candida*-associated denture stomatitis, a smear of the fitting surface of the denture as well as a swab should be taken.

In the laboratory, the smear is stained with the Gram stain or periodic acid–Schiff (PAS) reagent and examined microscopically to visualize the hyphae or blastospores of *Candida*. Their presence in **large numbers** suggests infection. The swabs are cultured on Sabouraud medium and incubated for 48–72 hours, when *Candida albicans* appears as cream-coloured large convex colonies. Other species of *Candida* co-infecting with *C. albicans* (e.g. *C. glabrata, C. krusei*) can be identified if the specimen is cultured in commercially available media, such as CHROMagar or Pagano–Levin agar, in which different species produce colonies with varying colours and hues (Fig. 6.13).

Yeasts so derived are speciated by **sugar fermentation and assimilation** tests and the **germ tube** test. The latter is a useful quick test to differentiate *C. albicans* and *C. dubliniensis* from the other *Candida* species such as *C. glabrata* and *C. krusei*.

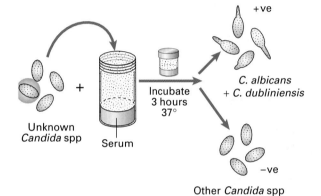

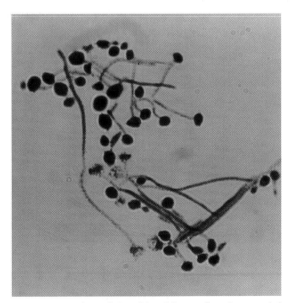

Fig. 6.14 Germ tube test: *Candida albicans* and *C. dubliniensis* produce short cylindrical extensions called 'germ tubes' when incubated in serum (3 h, 37°C); other *Candida* species are germ-tube negative, and need to be identified by sugar fermentation and assimilation reactions.

Fig. 6.15 Germ tubes of *Candida albicans* after Gram staining.

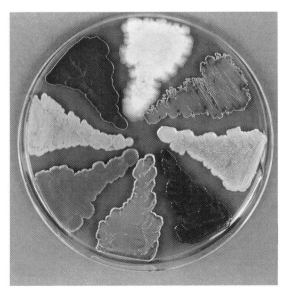

Fig. 6.13 Growth of different *Candida* species on Pagano–Levin agar exhibiting varying colony colours and hues.

Germ tube test

A small inoculum of the isolated yeast is incubated in serum at 37°C for about 3 hours and a few drops of the suspension are then examined microscopically. Virtually all strains of *C. albicans* and *C. dubliniensis* produce short, cylindrical extensions termed 'germ tubes', as opposed to the other *Candida* species, which do not exhibit this characteristic (Figs 6.14 and 6.15).

Histopathology

Incisional and excisional biopsies are useful in the diagnosis of persistent oral white lesions thought to be related to candidal infection. As a significant proportion of *chronic* candidal leucoplakic lesions are premalignant, a biopsy in addition to a swab is essential if the lesion does not resolve after antifungal therapy (see Ch. 35).

Other laboratory investigations

On occasions chronic candidal infections are associated with nutritional and haematological abnormalities and appropriate laboratory investigations (e.g. iron, vitamin levels) should also be carried out.

KEY FACTS

- *The main stages in the microbiological diagnosis of an infection are collection and transportation of appropriate specimens, clinical request and provision of clinical information to the microbiologist, laboratory analysis of the specimen, and interpretation of these results*
- Always **collect appropriate specimens** and transport them to the laboratory in a fresh state
- **During collection**, care must be taken to **avoid contamination** of the specimen with normal flora
- *Methods used in the laboratory diagnosis of infection can be broadly categorized into **non-cultural** (i.e. genomics), **cultural** and **immunological** techniques*
- *Some **appropriate specimens** for microbiological examination of important oral infections are aspirate of pus for purulent infections; deep gingival smear for acute ulcerative gingivitis; oral rinse for quantifying oral candida and coliform carriage; paper point samples of periodontal pockets, for molecular (PCR) diagnosis of periodontopathic bacterial infections*
- **Bacterial** species can be divided into **subtypes** using **serotyping, biotyping, phagetyping, bacteriocin typing**, etc.

- The action of an antimicrobial agent against an organism can be measured either **qualitatively** (disc diffusion tests) or **quantitatively** (minimum inhibitory concentration or minimum bactericidal concentration tests)
- The **minimum inhibitory concentration** (MIC) is the minimum concentration of the drug that will inhibit the visible growth of an organism (in a liquid culture)
- The **minimum bactericidal concentration** (MBC) is defined as the minimum concentration of drug that kills 99.9% of the test microorganisms in the original inoculum
- *The application of nucleic acid probes and PCR techniques are increasingly popular as rapid diagnostic methods of microbial infections*
- The major laboratory procedures for **identification of viruses** are (a) **direct microscopy** for **cytopathic effects** or for the presence of **viral antigens**, especially using **gene probes**; (b) **isolation** and **identification** of viruses grown in tissue culture; and (c) detection of virus specific **antibodies** in the patient's serum
- *Candida albicans* and *C. dubliniensis* can be differentiated from other *Candida* species as they are **germ-tube positive**

FURTHER READING

Collee, JG, Fraser, AG, Marmion, BP, and Simmons, A (1996). *Practical medical microbiology* (14th edn). Churchill Livingstone, Edinburgh.

De la Maza, LM, Pezzlo, MT, and Baron, EJ (1997). *Color atlas of diagnostic microbiology*. Mosby Year Book, St Louis.

Mims, C, Playfair, J, Roitt, I, Wakelin, D, and Williams, R (1998). Diagnostic principles of clinical manifestations. In *Medical microbiology* (2nd edn), sect. 13. Mosby, London.

Samaranayake, LP (1987). The wastage of microbial samples in clinical practice. *Dental Update* 14, 53–61.

Scully, C, and Samaranayake, LP (1992). *Clinical virology in oral medicine and dentistry*, Ch. 4. Cambridge University Press, Cambridge.

7 Antimicrobial chemotherapy

Antimicrobial compounds include antibacterial, antiviral, antifungal and antiprotozoal agents. All of these, apart from the last group, are prescribed in dentistry.

All antimicrobials demonstrate **selective toxicity**, i.e. the drug can be administered to humans with reasonable safety while having a marked lethal or toxic effect on specific microbes. The corollary of this is that all antimicrobials have adverse effects on humans and should therefore be used rationally and only when required.

Antimicrobial therapy aims to treat infection with a drug to which the causative organism is sensitive. Antimicrobials can be administered on a 'best guess' basis, with a sound knowledge of the:
- infectious disease
- most probable pathogen
- usual antibiotic sensitivity pattern of the pathogen.

This is called **empirical antibiotic therapy** and contrasts with **rational antibiotic therapy** in which antibiotics are administered after the sensitivity of the pathogen has been established by culture and in vitro testing in the laboratory. In general, empirical therapy is undertaken in a majority of situations encountered in dentistry.

BACTERIOSTATIC AND BACTERICIDAL ANTIMICROBIAL AGENTS

Antimicrobial agents are classically divisible into two major groups: **bactericidal agents**, which kill bacteria; and **bacteriostatic agents**, which inhibit multiplication without actually killing the pathogen. However, the distinction is rather hazy and is dependent on factors such as the **concentration of the drug** (e.g. erythromycin is bacteriostatic at low concentrations and bactericidal at high concentrations), the **pathogen** in question, and the **severity** of infection. Further, host defence mechanisms play a major role in eradication of pathogens from the body and it is not essential to use bactericidal drugs to treat most infections. A bacteriostatic drug which arrests the multiplication of pathogens and so tips the balance in favour of the host defence mechanisms is satisfactory in many situations.

Mode of action of antimicrobials

Antimicrobial agents inhibit the growth of or kill microorganisms by a variety of mechanisms. In general, however, one or more of the following target sites are involved:

- cell wall
- ribosomes
- cytoplasmic membrane
- nucleic acid replication sites.

A summary of the mode of action of commonly used antimicrobials is given in Table 7.1.

PRINCIPLES OF ANTIMICROBIAL THERAPY

Antimicrobial agents should be prescribed on a rational clinical and microbiological basis. In general, therapy should be considered for patients when one or more of the following conditions are present:
- fever and an acute infection
- spreading infection without localization
- chronic infection despite drainage or debridement
- infection in medically compromised patients
- cases of osteomyelitis, bacterial sialadenitis and some periodontal diseases, such as acute ulcerative gingivitis and localized aggressive periodontitis (previously localized juvenile periodontitis).

(*Note*: this is not an exhaustive list.)

Choice of drug

The choice of drug is strictly dependent upon the nature of the infecting organisms and their sensitivity patterns. However, in a clinical emergency such as septicaemia or Ludwig's angina, antimicrobial agents must be prescribed empirically until laboratory tests are completed. In general, another antimicrobial drug should be prescribed if the patient has had penicillin within the previous month because of the possible presence of penicillin-resistant bacterial populations previously exposed to the drug.

Spectrum of activity of antimicrobial agents

Antimicrobial agents can be categorized as **broad-spectrum** and **narrow-spectrum** antibiotics, depending on their activity against a range of Gram-positive and Gram-negative bacteria. For example, penicillin is a narrow-spectrum antibiotic with activity mainly against the Gram-positive bacteria, as is metronidazole, which acts almost entirely against strict anaerobes and some protozoa.

53

Table 7.1   Cellular target sites of antimicrobial drugs commonly used in dentistry

Target site	Drug	Bactericidal/static	Comments
Cell wall	Beta-lactams, e.g. penicillin, ampicillin, cephalosporin, cloxacillin	Cidal	Interfere with cross-linking of cell wall peptidoglycan molecules
	Bacitracin (topical)	Cidal	Inhibit peptidoglycan formation
Ribosomes	Erythromycin, fusidic acid (topical)	Static[a] or cidal[b]	Interfere with translocation, thus inhibiting protein synthesis
	Tetracycline	Static	Interferes with attachment of transfer RNA, thus inhibiting protein synthesis
Cytoplasmic membrane	Polyenes, e.g. nystatin, amphotericin	Static	Disrupts yeast cell membrane
Nucleic acid replication	Metronidazole	Cidal	Interferes with DNA replication
	Idoxuridine, aciclovir	Cidal	Interfere with DNA synthesis in DNA viruses

[a] Low concentrations.
[b] High concentrations.

Broad-spectrum antimicrobials (e.g. tetracyclines, ampicillins) are active against many Gram-positive and Gram-negative bacteria and they are often used for empirical or 'blind' treatment of infections when the likely causative pathogen is unknown. This unfortunately leads to 'abuse' of broad-spectrum agents, with the consequent emergence of resistance in organisms that were originally sensitive to the drug. The spectrum of activity of some broad-spectrum and narrow-spectrum antimicrobial agents is shown in Table 7.2.

Combination therapy

Whenever possible, a single antimicrobial agent should be used to reduce the:
- incidence of possible side-effects
- emergence of resistant bacteria
- drug costs.

However, there are certain clinical situations where a combination of drugs is valuable: for example, to achieve a high bactericidal level when treating patients with infective endocarditis; the use of gentamicin and metronidazole in the empirical treatment of a patient with serious abdominal sepsis; and combination therapy in the management of tuberculosis. **In dentistry, combination therapy should be avoided as far as possible.**

Antimicrobial prophylaxis

Antimicrobial prophylaxis is the use of a drug to prevent colonization or multiplication of microorganisms in a susceptible host. The value of prophylaxis depends upon a balance between:
- the benefit of reducing the infection risk and consequent secondary morbidity
- the possible toxic effects to the host, including alterations of the host commensal flora
- the cost effectiveness.

When used appropriately, prophylaxis can reduce morbidity and the cost of medical care. Irrational prophylaxis leads to a false sense of security, increased treatment cost and the possible emergence of resistant flora.

Table 7.2   Spectrum of activity of some commonly used antimicrobial agents

Drug	Spectrum
Phenoxymethylpenicillin (penicillin V)	1. Aerobic Gram-positives (e.g. streptococci, pneumococci, β-lactamase-negative staphylococci, lactobacilli, actinomyces) 2. Anaerobic Gram-positives (e.g. anaerobic streptococci) 3. Anaerobic Gram-negatives (e.g. most *Bacteroides*, fusobacteria, *Veillonella*)
Penicillinase-resistant penicillins (e.g. flucloxacillin)	All the above, including β-lactamase-producing staphylococci
Ampicillin	As for penicillin, also includes *Haemophilus* spp.
Cephalosporins	As for penicillin, also includes some coliforms
Erythromycin	Gram-positives mainly but some anaerobes not susceptible at levels obtained by oral administration
Tetracycline	Broad spectrum. Many Gram-positives and -negatives
Metronidazole	All strict anaerobes are sensitive, including some protozoa. Of questionable value for facultative anaerobes

Aims

The aims of antimicrobial prophylaxis are:

1. Eradication of the colonization of the host by virulent agents, e.g. chemoprophylaxis (with rifampicin) given to close contacts of patients with meningococcal meningitis (see Ch. 25).
2. Prevention of implantation and/or implanted organisms reaching a critical mass sufficient to produce infection, e.g. antimicrobial prophylaxis in infective endocarditis patients before surgical procedures.
3. Prevention of the emergence of latent infection, e.g. antifungal agents given either intermittently or continuously to prevent candidal infection in HIV-infected patients.

In dentistry, antibiotics are used as prophylactic agents before dental or surgical treatment of patients who:

- are at risk of infective endocarditis (see Ch. 24)
- have facial fractures or compound skull fractures, and cerebral rhinorrhoea
- are immunocompromised
- have recently received radiotherapy to the jaws (as they succumb to infection as a result of severe ischaemia of the bone caused by radiotherapy)
- have prosthetic hip replacements, ventriculoatrial shunts, insertion of implants or bone grafting.

However, the advantages and disadvantages of prophylactic antimicrobial therapy in the latter three groups should be carefully weighed as some consider this superfluous.

Prescribing an antimicrobial agent

The following should be considered before any antimicrobial agent is prescribed.

Is there an infective aetiology?

When there is no good clinical evidence of infection antimicrobial therapy is unnecessary, except in prophylaxis (discussed above).

Have relevant specimens been taken before treatment?

Appropriate specimens should be collected before drug therapy is begun as the population of pathogens may be reduced, and therefore less easily isolated, if specimens are collected after antimicrobial agents have been taken. Further, the earlier the specimens are taken, the more likely it is that the results will be useful for patient management.

When should the treatment be started?

In patients with life-threatening infections, e.g. Ludwig's angina, intravenous therapy should generally be instituted *immediately* after specimen collection. Antimicrobial therapy may be withheld in chronic infections until laboratory results are available (e.g. actinomycosis).

Which antimicrobial agent?

Consider the pharmacodynamic effects, including toxicity, when choosing a drug from a number of similar antimicrobial agents that are available to treat many infections (see below).

An adequate medical history, especially in relation to past allergies and toxic effects, should be taken before deciding on therapy.

PHARMACODYNAMICS OF ANTIMICROBIALS

Dosage

Antimicrobial agents should be given in therapeutic doses sufficient to produce a tissue concentration greater than that required to kill or inhibit the growth of the causative microorganism(s).

Duration of treatment

Ideally treatment should continue for long enough to eliminate all or nearly all of the pathogens, as the remainder will in most instances be destroyed by the host defences. Conventionally this cannot be precisely timed and standard regimens last for some 3–5 days, depending on the drug. However, a short-course, high-dose therapy of certain antibiotics such as amoxicillin (amoxycillin) is as effective as a conventional 5-day course. The other advantages of short courses of antimicrobial agents are good patient compliance and minimal disturbance to commensal flora, leading to an associated reduction in side effects such as diarrhoea.

Route of administration

In seriously ill patients drugs should be given by the parenteral route to overcome problems of absorption from the intestinal tract. All antimicrobial agents given by mouth must be acid-stable.

Distribution

The drug must reach adequate concentrations at the infective focus. Some antibiotics, such as clindamycin, that penetrate well into bone are preferred in chronic bone infections; in meningitis, a drug that penetrates the cerebrospinal fluid should be given.

Excretion

The pathway of excretion of an antimicrobial agent should be noted; e.g. drugs metabolized in the liver, such as erythromycin estolate, should not be given to patients with a history of liver disease because they may cause hepatotoxicity, leading to jaundice.

Toxicity

Most antimicrobials have side effects and the clinician should be aware of these (for examples, see the following section on individual antibiotic drugs).

Drug interactions

Drug interactions are becoming increasingly common owing to the extensive use of a variety of drugs. For instance, antibiotics such as penicillin and erythromycin can significantly

Table 7.3 Some drug interactions of antimicrobials commonly used in dentistry

Drug affected	Drug interacting	Effect
Penicillins	Probenecid, neomycin	May potentiate the effect of penicillin. Reduced absorption
Erythromycin	Theophylline	Increase theophylline levels, leading to potential toxicity
Cephalosporins	Gentamicin Frusemide (furosemide, Lasix)	Additive effect leading to nephrotoxicity Possible increase in nephrotoxicity
Tetracycline	Antacids, dairy products, oral iron, zinc sulphate	Reduced absorption
Metronidazole	Alcohol Disulfiram, phenobarbitone (phenobarbital), phenytoin	'Antabuse' effect Reduced effect

reduce the efficacy of some oral contraceptives, and antacids can interfere with the action of tetracyclines. All clinicians should therefore be aware of the drug interactions of any antimicrobial they prescribe. The major drug interactions of antimicrobials commonly used in dentistry are given in Table 7.3.

FAILURE OF ANTIMICROBIAL THERAPY

Consideration should be given to the following potential problems if an infection does not respond to drugs within 48 hours:

- inadequate drainage of pus or debridement
- inappropriateness of the antimicrobial agent, including bacterial resistance to the drug, dosage and drug interactions
- presence of local factors such as foreign bodies which may act as reservoirs of reinfection
- impaired host response, e.g. in patients who are immuno-compromised by drugs or HIV infection
- poor patient compliance
- possibility of an unusual infection or that the disease has no infective aetiology
- poor blood supply to tissues.

Antibiotic resistance in bacteria

Emergence of drug resistance in bacteria is a major problem in antibiotic therapy and depends on the organism and the antibiotic concerned. Whereas some bacteria rapidly acquire resistance (e.g. *Staphylococcus aureus*) others rarely do so (e.g. *Streptococcus pyogenes*). Resistance to some antibiotics is virtually unknown (e.g. metronidazole), but strains resistant to others (e.g. penicillin) readily emerge.

Antibiotic resistance develops when progeny of resistant bacteria emerge. As they will be at a selective advantage over their sensitive counterparts, and as long as the original antibiotic is prescribed, the resistant strains can multiply uninhibitedly (e.g. hospital staphylococci with almost universal resistance to penicillin). Such antibiotic resistance can be divided into:

- **primary (intrinsic) resistance**: where the organism is naturally resistant to the drug, i.e. its resistance is unrelated to contact with the drug (e.g. resistance of coliforms to penicillin)

- **acquired resistance**: either due to mutation within the same species or gene transfer between different species
- **cross-resistance**: when resistance to one drug confers resistance to another chemically related drug (e.g. bacteria resistant to one type of tetracycline may be resistant to all other types of tetracycline).

Mechanisms of antibiotic resistance

Inactivation of the drug. This is very common, e.g. production of β-lactamase by staphylococci. The enzyme, which is plasmid-coded, destroys the β-lactam ring responsible for the antibacterial activity of penicillins.

Altered uptake. The amount of drug that reaches the target is either reduced or completely inhibited (e.g. tetracycline resistance in *Pseudomonas aeruginosa*). This can be either due to altered permeability of the cell wall or to pumping of the drug out of the cell (efflux mechanism).

Modification of the active site of the drug (e.g. trimethoprim and sulphonamide resistance).

Most of the above are mediated by bacterial plasmids (Table 7.4).

Table 7.4 Plasmid-mediated antibiotic resistance

Antibiotic	Mechanism of resistance
Beta-lactams	Beta-lactamase breaks down the β-lactam ring to an inactive form
Aminoglycosides	Modifying enzymes cause acetylation, adenylation, phosphorylation
Chloramphenicol	Acetylation of the antibiotic to an inactive form
Erythromycin, clindamycin	Methylation of ribosomal RNA prevents antibiotic binding to ribosomes
Sulphonamides, tetracycline	Alteration of cell membrane decreases permeability to the antibiotic

ANTIMICROBIALS COMMONLY USED IN DENTISTRY

Although a large array of antimicrobial agents have been described and are available to medical practitioners, only a limited number of these are widely prescribed by dental practitioners. The following therefore is an outline of the major antimicrobials (antibacterials, antifungals and antivirals) used in dentistry.

ANTIBACTERIAL AGENTS

Penicillins

Penicillins are the most useful and widely used antimicrobial agents in dentistry. A wide array of penicillins have been synthesized by incorporation of various side-chains into the β-lactam ring (Table 7.5). The spectrum of activity and indications for the use of these penicillins vary widely. The more commonly used penicillins such as phenoxymethylpenicillin (penicillin V) are described below in some detail. Others such as the carboxypenicillins (carbenicillin and ticarcillin) and ureidopenicillins (azlocillin and piperacillin) which are active against Gram-negative organisms are rarely used in dentistry, except for amoxicillin (amoxycillin).

The commonly used penicillins are remarkably non-toxic but all share the problem of allergy. Minor reactions such as rashes are common, while severe reactions, especially anaphylaxis, although rare, can be fatal. Allergy to one penicillin is shared by all the penicillins and, in general, the drug should not be given to a patient who has had a reaction to any member of this group. Some 10% of patients sensitive to penicillin show cross-reactivity to cephalosporins.

Phenoxymethylpenicillin (penicillin V)

Administration. Oral, as it is acid-resistant.

Mode of action. Bactericidal; inhibits cell wall synthesis by inactivating the enzyme transpeptidase which is responsible for cross-linking the peptidoglycan cross-walls of bacteria; an intact β-lactam ring is crucial for its activity.

Spectrum of activity. Effective against a majority of α-haemolytic streptococci and penicillinase-negative staphy-

lococci. Aerobic Gram-positive organisms including *Actinomyces, Eubacterium, Bifidobacterium* and *Peptostreptococcus* spp. are sensitive, together with anaerobic Gram-negative organisms such as *Bacteroides, Prevotella, Porphyromonas, Fusobacterium* and *Veillonella* species. The majority of *Staphylococcus aureus* strains, particularly those from hospitals, are penicillinase producers and hence resistant to penicillin. (A small minority of α-haemolytic streptococci, and some *Actinobacillus actinomycetemcomitans* strains implicated in aggressive periodontitis, are resistant.)

Resistance. Very common owing to the β-lactamase produced by bacteria, which inactivates the drug by acting on the β-lactam ring.

Indications. As this drug can be administered orally it is commonly used by dental practitioners in the treatment of acute purulent infections, post-extraction infection, pericoronitis and salivary gland infections.

Pharmacodynamics. Phenoxymethylpenicillin is less active than parenteral benzylpenicillin (penicillin G) because of its erratic absorption from the gastrointestinal tract. Therefore in serious infections phenoxymethylpenicillin could be used for continuing treatment after one or more loading doses of benzylpenicillin, when clinical response has begun.

Toxicity. Virtually non-toxic; may cause severe reactions in patients who are allergic; anaphylaxis may occur very rarely. Other uncommon reactions include skin rashes and fever. Despite these drawbacks it is one of the cheapest and safest antibiotics.

Benzylpenicillin (penicillin G)

Administration. Intramuscular, intravenous.

Indications. Useful in moderate to severe infections (e.g. Ludwig's angina) as its parenteral administration results in rapid, high and consistent antibiotic levels in plasma.

Toxicity. Chances of allergy developing are increased by injection, and it is obligatory to ascertain the hypersensitivity status of the patient before the drug is administered. Benzylpenicillin may cause convulsions after high doses by intravenous injection or in renal failure.

Broad-spectrum penicillins susceptible to staphylococcal penicillinase

Ampicillin and amoxicillin. *Administration.* Oral (amoxicillin absorption is better than ampicillin), intramuscular, intravenous.

Spectrum of activity. Similar to penicillin but effective against a broader spectrum of organisms, including Gram-negative organisms such as *Haemophilus* and *Proteus* spp. Amoxicillin and ampicillin have similar antibacterial spectra.

Resistance. One drawback of amoxicillin is its susceptibility to β-lactamase, but if potassium clavulanate is incorporated with amoxicillin the combination (co-amoxiclav) is resistant to the activity of β-lactamase (Fig. 7.1).

Indications. Ampicillin is sometimes used in the empirical treatment of dentoalveolar infections when the antibiotic sensitivity patterns of the causative organisms are unknown. In dentistry, amoxicillin is the drug of choice for prophylaxis of infective endocarditis in patients undergoing surgical procedures and scaling (see Ch. 24). A short course of high-dose amoxicillin (oral) has been shown to be of value in the treatment of dentoalveolar infections.

Table 7.5	Types of penicillin
Group	**Type of penicillin**
Narrow-spectrum	Benzylpenicillin
	Phenoxymethylpenicillin
	Procaine penicillin
	Benzathine penicillin
Broad-spectrum	Ampicillin
	Amoxicillin
	Esters of ampicillin
Penicillinase-resistant	Methicillin
	Flucloxacillin
Antipseudomonal	Piperacillin
	Mezlocillin

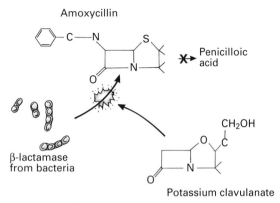

Fig. 7.1 Amoxycillin (amoxicillin) is broken down by β-lactamase of bacteria, to penicilloic acid. If potassium clavulanate (a product of *Streptomyces clavuligerus*) is incorporated with amoxycillin, it inhibits the β-lactamase activity. The combination drug is known as co-amoxiclav.

Toxicity. Associated with a higher incidence of drug rashes than penicillin, and hence should not be administered to patients with infectious mononucleosis (glandular fever) or lymphocytic leukaemia (because of the probability of a drug rash). Nausea and diarrhoea are frequent, particularly on prolonged administration; superinfection and colonization with ampicillin-resistant bacteria, such as coliforms and fungi, may also occur. The incidence of diarrhoea is less with amoxicillin.

Isoxazolyl penicillins: methicillin, cloxacillin and flucloxacillin

Administration. Oral, intramuscular, intravenous.

Spectrum of activity. Narrow-spectrum antistaphylococcal penicillins relatively resistant to β-lactamase produced by *Staphylococcus aureus*.

Indications. The main use of cloxacillin and flucloxacillin is in the treatment of confirmed infections due to β-lactamase-producing *S. aureus*.

Toxicity. These penicillins are safe and non-toxic even when used in high doses.

Sensitivity. When these antibiotics were introduced almost all strains of *S. aureus* were sensitive to these drugs. However, methicillin-resistant *S. aureus* (MRSA) strains are now emerging widely and hence these drugs should not be used indiscriminately.

Other penicillins

Other groups of penicillins, such as carboxypenicillins (e.g. ticarcillin), acylureidopenicillins (e.g. piperacillin) and amidinopenicillins (e.g. mecillinam), are not routinely prescribed in dentistry and hence are not described here.

Cephalosporins, cephamycins and other beta-lactams

This group of drugs now includes more than 30 different agents and newer agents are being manufactured each year. All cephalosporins are β-lactams similar to penicillin but are relatively stable to staphylococcal penicillinase; the degree of stability varies with different cephalosporins. The group includes cephalosporins (cefotaxime, cefuroxime, cephalexin and cephradine), cephamycins (cefoxitin), monobactams (aztreonam) and carbapenems (imipenem and meropenem).

Administration. Cephradine and cephalexin, which can be given by mouth, and cephaloridine belong to the first generation of cephalosporins and are used in dentistry. The vast majority of cephalosporins are given parenterally, hence they are virtually restricted to hospital use.

Spectrum of activity. Broad-spectrum; active against both Gram-positive and Gram-negative bacteria, although individual agents have differing activity against certain organisms.

Indications. Few absolute indications. In dentistry, cephalosporins should be resorted to as a second line of defence, depending on culture and antibiotic sensitivity test results.

Toxicity. Some 10% of penicillin-sensitive patients demonstrate cross-sensitivity; allergic reactions, including urticaria and rashes; possibly nephrotoxicity. Another disadvantage is that oral bacteria, including streptococci, may develop cross-resistance both to penicillins and cephalosporins. Hence, cephalosporins are not suitable alternatives for a patient who has recently had penicillin.

Erythromycin

The most popular member of the macrolide group of antibiotics.

Administration. Oral, intravenous.

Mode of action. Bacteriostatic.

Spectrum of activity. Similar, though not identical, to that of penicillin and is thus the first choice in dentistry for treating penicillin-allergic patients; in addition *Haemophilus influenzae* and *Bacteroides*, *Prevotella* and *Porphyromonas* spp. are sensitive; has an added advantage of being active against β-lactamase-producing bacteria. Not usually used as a first-line drug in oral and dental infections because obligate anaerobes are not particularly sensitive.

Toxicity. A few serious side effects, the main disadvantage being that high doses (given for prophylaxis of infective endocarditis) cause nausea; prolonged use (> 14 days) of erythromycin estolate may be hepatotoxic.

Clindamycin

Administration. Oral, intravenous or intramuscular.

Mode of action. Inhibits protein synthesis by binding to bacterial ribosomes.

Spectrum of activity. Similar to that of erythromycin (with which there is partial cross-resistance) and benzylpenicillin; in addition it is active against *Bacteroides* spp.

Indications. Mainly reserved, as a single dose, for prophylaxis of infective endocarditis in patients allergic to penicillin; particularly effective in penetrating poorly vascularized bone and connective tissue.

Toxicity. Mild diarrhoea is common. Although rare, the most serious side effect of clindamycin, which can sometimes be fatal, is pseudomembranous (antibiotic-associated) colitis, especially in the elderly and in combination with other drugs. The colitis is due to a toxin produced by *Clostridium difficile*, an anaerobe resistant to clindamycin. Allergy to these drugs is extremely rare and hypersensitivity to penicillin is not shared by them.

Tetracyclines

Formerly one of the most widely used antibiotic groups owing to their very broad spectrum of activity and infrequent side effects. Their usefulness has decreased as a result of increasing bacterial resistance. They remain, however, the treatment of choice for infections caused by intracellular organisms such as chlamydiae, rickettsiae and mycoplasmas, as they penetrate macrophages well. A range of tetracyclines is available, although tetracycline itself remains the most useful for dental purposes.

Administration. Mostly oral.

Mode of action. Bacteriostatic; interfere with protein synthesis by binding to bacterial ribosomes.

Spectrum of activity. Have a wide spectrum of activity against oral flora, including *Actinomyces, Bacteroides, Propionibacterium, Actinobacillus, Eubacterium* and *Peptococcus* spp.

Indications. In dentistry, tetracyclines are used with some success as adjunctive treatment in localized aggressive periodontitis (formerly localized juvenile periodontitis); they are effective against many organisms associated with these diseases (see Ch. 33). They are also useful as mouthwashes to alleviate secondary bacterial infection associated with extensive oral ulceration, especially in compromised patients.

Pharmacokinetics. Widely distributed in body tissues, and incorporated in bone and developing teeth (Fig. 7.2); particularly concentrated in gingival fluid. Absorption of oral tetracycline is decreased by antacids, calcium, iron and magnesium salts.

Toxicity. Because of the deposition of tetracycline within developing teeth, its use should be avoided in children up to 8 years of age and in pregnant or lactating women, otherwise unsightly tooth staining may occur. Diarrhoea and nausea may occur after oral administration, as a result of disturbance to bowel flora. However, when reduced dosages are used, even for prolonged periods (e.g. for acne), few side effects are apparent. Serious hepatotoxicity may occur with excessive intravenous dosage.

Metronidazole

The exquisite anaerobic activity of this drug, which was first introduced to treat protozoal infections, makes it exceedingly effective against strict anaerobes and some protozoa.

Administration. Oral, intravenous, rectal (suppositories).

Mode of action. Bactericidal; it is converted by anaerobic bacteria into a reduced, active metabolite which inhibits DNA synthesis.

Spectrum of activity. Active against almost all strict anaerobes, including *Bacteroides* spp., fusobacteria, eubacteria, peptostreptococci and clostridia.

Indications. The drug of choice in the treatment of acute necrotizing ulcerative gingivitis; also used, either alone or in combination with penicillin, in the management of dentoalveolar infections.

Pharmacokinetics. Well absorbed after oral (or rectal) administration; widely distributed and passes readily into most tissues, including abscesses, and crosses the blood–brain barrier into cerebrospinal fluid. The drug is metabolized in the liver.

Toxicity. Minor side effects of metronidazole include gastrointestinal upset, transient rashes and metallic taste in the mouth. Metronidazole interferes with alcohol metabolism and, if taken with alcohol, may cause severe nausea, flushing and palpitations (disulfiram-type effect). It potentiates the effect of anticoagulants and, if used for more than a week, peripheral neuropathy may develop, notably in patients with liver disease; allergenicity is very low.

Sulphonamides and trimethoprim

These drugs interfere with successive steps in the synthesis of folic acid (an essential ingredient for DNA and RNA synthesis). They are widely used in combination because of in vitro evidence of synergism.

Co-trimoxazole

A combination of sulphamethoxazole (sulfamethoxazole) and trimethoprim in a 5 : 1 ratio.

Administration. Oral, intramuscular, intravenous.

Mode of action. Bacteriostatic (see above).

Spectrum of activity. Broad; active against both Gram-positive and Gram-negative bacteria.

Indications. Use now mainly confined to infections in HIV-infected persons.

Pharmacokinetics. A major advantage of sulphonamides is their ability to penetrate into the cerebrospinal fluid; contraindicated in pregnancy or liver disease.

Fusidic acid

A narrow-spectrum antibiotic with main activity against Gram-positive bacteria, particularly *Staphylococcus aureus.* Angular cheilitis associated with *S. aureus* is a specific indication for the use of fusidic acid in the form of a topical cream. A small percentage of *S. aureus* strains show resistance to fusidic acid.

Other antimicrobial agents

The foregoing describes the major antimicrobials prescribed by dentists; the student is referred to recommended texts for details of other antibiotics, such as aminoglycosides and antituberculous drugs, and a comprehensive review of this subject.

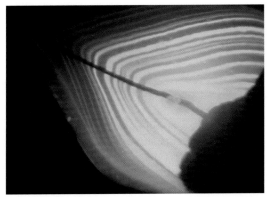

Fig. 7.2 Tetracycline stains in a deciduous tooth visualized by polarizing light microscopy. Each yellow band represents an episode of drug administration.

ANTIFUNGAL AGENTS

In contrast to the wide range of antibacterial agents, the number of effective antifungals is limited. This is because selective toxicity is much more difficult to achieve in eukaryotic fungal cells, which share similar features with human eukaryotic cells. Polyenes and the azoles are the most commonly used antifungals in dentistry. Nystatin and amphotericin are polyene derivatives; miconazole and fluconazole are two examples of a variety of azole antifungals currently available (Table 7.6).

Polyenes

Nystatin

Administration. Too toxic for systemic use; not absorbed from the alimentary canal and hence used to prevent or treat mucosal candidiasis; it is available in the form of pastilles, ready-mixed suspensions, ointments and powder.

Mode of action. Polyene binds to the cytoplasmic membrane of fungi, altering cell-wall permeability with resultant leakage of cell contents and death; in very low doses it is fungistatic.

Indications. Widely used in the treatment of oral candidiasis. Patient compliance is superior with the flavoured pastille formulation, as opposed to the bitter-tasting oral suspension or lozenge.

Spectrum of activity. Nystatin resistance in candidiasis is unknown.

Toxicity. Nausea, vomiting and diarrhoea are rare side effects; no adverse effects have been reported when the topical route is used.

Amphotericin

Amphotericin is the other polyene group antifungal. It is used essentially in the same way as nystatin; lozenges, ointment and oral suspensions are available. As with nystatin, its absorption from the gut is minimal on topical administration. Amphotericin is the drug of choice for the treatment of systemic candidiases and other exotic mycoses (e.g. histoplasmosis, coccidioidomycosis).

Azoles

Miconazole

Administration. An imidazole available as an oral gel or cream.

Mode of action. This drug, like other imidazoles, acts by interfering with the synthesis of chemicals needed to form the plasma membrane of fungi, resulting in leakage of cell contents and death.

Indications. Its dual action against yeast and staphylococci is useful in the treatment of angular cheilitis.

Spectrum of activity. Both fungicidal and bacteriostatic for some Gram-positive cocci, including *Staphylococcus aureus*. Resistance only rarely occurs.

Fluconazole

Fluconazole is a triazole drug that is highly popular because of its wide spectrum of activity on yeasts and other fungi. Specifically used to prevent *Candida* infection in HIV-infected individuals as intermittent or continuous therapy.

Administration. Oral; because of its long half-life it is administered once a day, so patient compliance is good.

Mode of action. See above.

Indications. As a second-line antifungal for recalcitrant oral *Candida* infections; drug of choice for prophylaxis of oral and systemic candidal infections in HIV-infected patients.

Pharmacokinetics. Weak protein binding, water-soluble, long half-life.

Toxicity. Minor: gastrointestinal irritation, allergic rash, elevation of liver enzymes (common to all azoles). Interacts with anticoagulants, terfenadine, cisapride and astemizole.

Itraconazole

Another azole with properties similar to fluconazole; useful for candidiasis in HIV infection.

ANTIVIRAL AGENTS

Few antiviral drugs with proven clinical efficacy are available, in contrast to the great range of successful antibacterial agents. The shortage of antivirals is mainly due to the difficulty of interfering with the viral activity within the cell without damaging the host. Most antiviral agents achieve maximum benefit if given early in the disease. Immunocompromised patients with viral infections generally benefit from active antiviral therapy, as these infections may spread locally and systemically.

Other problems associated with the therapy of virus infections are:

- The incubation period of most viral infections is short, and by the time the patient shows signs of illness, the virus has already done most of the damage. Furthermore,

Table 7.6 Common antifungal agents and their activity

Drug group	Example	Target	Mechanism
Polyenes	Nystatin Amphotericin	Cell membrane function	Bind to sterols in cell membrane causing leakage of cell constituents and cell death
Azoles	Miconazole Ketoconazole Fluconazole	Cell membrane synthesis	Inhibit ergosterol synthesis
DNA analogues	Flucytosine	Nucleic acid synthesis	Inhibit DNA synthesis and central protein synthesis

laboratory diagnosis of virus infections takes several days. However, advances in the rapid viral diagnostic methods using molecular techniques should help overcome this problem.

- Viruses that are latent in cells and not actively replicating (e.g. herpesviruses in the trigeminal ganglion) are immune to antivirals.

Aciclovir is the major antiviral drug prescribed in dentistry.

Aciclovir

Aciclovir is an efficient, highly selective antiviral agent useful in the treatment of primary as well as secondary herpetic stomatitis and herpes labialis.

Administration. Topical (cream), oral (tablets, suspensions), intravenous.

Mode of action. Aciclovir blocks viral DNA production at a concentration of some thousand times less than that required to inhibit host cell DNA production (Fig. 7.3).

Indications. Topical aciclovir (5% cream) can be prescribed for recurrent herpetic ulcers; primary herpetic gingivostomatitis can be treated with either aciclovir cream or tablets. Treatment must be started in the prodromal phase (when there is a local tingling or burning sensation). Application at later stages of infection will reduce the length, discomfort and the viral shedding period correspondingly. Aciclovir tablets or

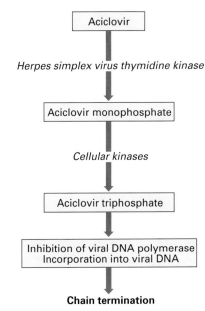

Fig. 7.3 Mode of action of aciclovir in herpesvirus-infected cells.

oral suspension may be given for severe herpetic stomatitis or herpes zoster.

An alternative agent for herpetic ulcerations is penciclovir cream.

KEY FACTS

- All **antimicrobials** demonstrate **selective toxicity** and should be used only **rationally** and **when necessary**
- Antibiotic therapy can be either **empirical**, when the antibiotic is prescribed on a 'best guess' basis, or **rational**, when the prescription is dictated by the known antibiotic sensitivity of the offending pathogen
- Antimicrobials are **classified** by their **target sites** and their **chemical family**
- There are four possible **target areas** of antimicrobials: **the cell wall, ribosomes** (protein synthesis), **cytoplasmic membrane** and the **nucleic acid replication sites**
- **Whenever possible, use a single antimicrobial** drug (and not multiple agents) to reduce the incidence of possible

side effects, emergence of resistant bacteria and the drug costs

- **Antibiotic resistance** in bacteria can be either **primary** (intrinsic) or **acquired**; acquired resistance arises either due to mutation or gene transfer
- Major **mechanisms of antibiotic resistance** include the production **of drug-destroying enzymes, altering the drug uptake** and **target site modification**
- Selective toxicity is much more difficult to achieve with antifungal agents because the eukaryotic fungal cells share similar features with human eukaryotic cells
- The shortage of antiviral agents is mainly due to the difficulty of interfering with the viral activity within the cell without damaging the host

---

FURTHER READING

Ellepola, ANB, and Samaranayake, LP (2000). Oral candidal infections and antimycotics. *Critical Reviews in Oral Biology and Medicine* 11, 172–198.

Levy, SB (1992). *The antibiotic paradox. How miracle drugs are destroying the miracle.* Plenum, New York.

Mims, C, Playfair, J, Roitt, I, Wakelin, D, and Williams, R (1998). Antimicrobial agents and chemotherapy. In *Medical microbiology* (2nd edn), Ch. 30. Mosby, London.

O'Grady, F, Lambert, HP, Finch, RG, and Greenwood, D (1997). *Antibiotics and chemotherapy: their use in therapy* (7th edn). Churchill Livingstone, Edinburgh.

Samaranayake, LP, and Johnson, N (1999). Guidelines for the use of antimicrobial agents to minimise the development of resistance. *International Dental Journal* 49, 189–195.

Basic immunology

Immunology is a vast and complex subject. What is presented here is a highly
abbreviated account of basic immune mechanisms and how they operate when
microbes assault the body systems. Students are strongly recommended to consult
the books and articles listed at the end of each chapter in order to broaden their
understanding of these topics.

- The immune system
- The immune response
- Immunity and infection

8 The immune system

Immunology is the branch of biology concerned with the body's defence reactions. The word 'immunology' is derived from the Latin *immunis* meaning 'free of burden'. In essence, the immune system exists to maintain the integrity of the body by excluding or removing the myriad potentially burdensome or threatening microorganisms which could invade from the environment. Internally derived threats, mutant cells with malignant potential, may also be attacked by the immune system.

There are two kinds of immunological defence:
- **natural** or **innate immunity**, comprising mainly pre-existing antigen non-specific defences
- **adaptive immunity**, during which the immune system responds in an antigen-specific manner to efficiently neutralize the threat, and retains a memory of the threat so that any future encounter with the same threat will result in an accelerated and heightened protective response.

During its development, the immune system must be educated specifically to avoid reacting against all normal components of the body (**tolerance**). Immunology can be considered 'the science of self–non-self discrimination'.

The vital importance of the immune system is evident in the life-threatening infections suffered by patients with immune defects (**immunodeficiency**). In other situations there may be too much immunity. A byproduct of a successful immune response may be damage to normal 'bystander' cells, but this is normally limited by stringent immune regulatory mechanisms. Deficiencies of immunoregulation may be the root causes of **hypersensitivity** diseases such as **autoimmunity** and **allergy**.

These concepts are summarized in Figure 8.1.

THE INNATE IMMUNE SYSTEM

Mechanical and chemical barriers

Intact skin is usually impenetrable to microorganisms. Membranous linings of the body tracts are protected by mucus, acid secretions and enzymes such as lysozyme, which breaks down bacterial cell-wall proteoglycan.

Phagocytosis

If the mechanical defences are breached, phagocytic cells able to engulf particles form the next barrier. These include polymorphonuclear leucocytes (**polymorphs**) and **macro-phages**. The former are short-lived circulating cells which can invade the tissues, while the latter are the mature, tissue-resident stage of circulating **monocytes**.

Macrophages are found in areas of blood filtration where they are most likely to encounter foreign particles, e.g. liver sinusoids, kidney mesangium, alveoli, lymph nodes and spleen. Phagocytes attach to microorganisms by non-specific cell membrane 'threat' receptors, after which pseudopodia extend around the particle and internalize it into a phagosome. Lysosomal vesicles containing proteolytic enzymes fuse with the phagosome and oxygen and nitrogen radicals are generated, which kill the microbe.

Natural killer cells

Natural killer (NK) cells are non-phagocytic lymphocytes that have a special role in the killing of virus-infected and malignant cells (Fig. 8.2). These cells have two kinds of receptors with opposing action: antigen receptors able to recognize specific molecules on target cells, through which **activation** signals are transmitted, and receptors that recognize self major histocompatibility complex type I antigens (MHC-I, see below) through which **inactivation** signals are transmitted. Activation of NK cells can only occur when there is no inactivation signal, so virus-infected and tumour cells with downregulated MHC-I antigens are susceptible to NK cytotoxicity, but normal MHC-I-positive cells are protected. The killing mechanism is activated by **cytokines** released by virus-infected cells, tissue cells, lymphocytes and NK cells themselves. The NK cells are also important in the adaptive immune response, being the effector cells for killing antibody-coated microorganisms (**antibody-dependent cell-mediated cytotoxicity, ADCC**).

Acute-phase proteins

The concentration of several proteins in body fluids increases rapidly during tissue injury or infection:
- **C-reactive protein** can bind to bacteria and promote their removal by phagocytosis
- α_1-**antitrypsin** neutralizes proteases released by bacteria or damaged tissue.

Inflammation

Injured or infected tissues become inflamed in order to direct components of the immune system to where they are needed. 65

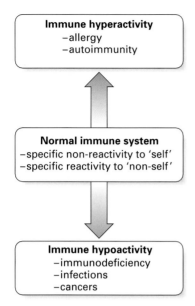

Fig. 8.1 Normal and aberrant immunity.

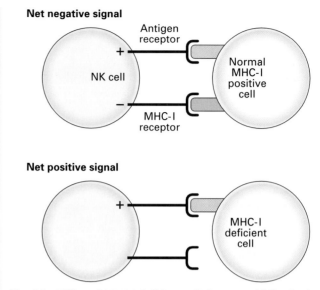

Fig. 8.2 Killing of MHC-I deficient cells by natural killer (NK) cells. MHC, major histocompatibility complex.

The blood supply to the tissues is increased, capillaries become more permeable to soluble mediators and leucocytes, and the latter migrate towards the site of infection as a result of the production of **chemotactic factors**.

COMPLEMENT

The complement system is very much involved in the inflammatory response and is one of the key effector mechanisms of the immune system. It consists of at least 30 components — enzymes, regulators and membrane receptors — which interact in an ordered and tightly regulated manner to bring about phagocytosis or lysis of target cells.

Complement components are normally present in body fluids as inactive precursors. The **alternative pathway** of complement activation can be stimulated directly by microorganisms and is important in the early stages of the infection before the production of antibody. It is part of the innate immune system. The **classical pathway** requires antibody, which may take weeks to develop. Both pathways can lead to the lytic or **membrane attack pathway**. During the course of complement activation, numerous split products of complement components, with important biological effects, are produced.

Alternative activation

Complement factor C3 is the central component of both the classical and alternative pathways (Fig. 8.3). Products of C3 activation, C3b and inactivated C3b (iC3b) bind to microorganisms and are recognized by complement receptors (CR)

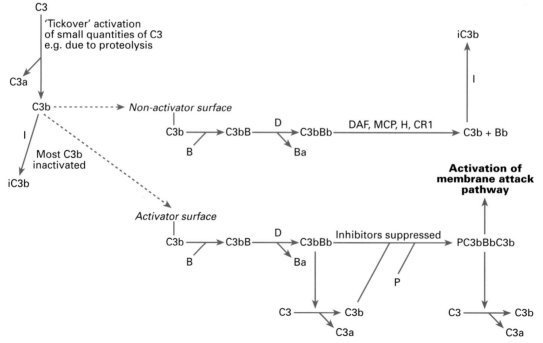

Fig. 8.3 Alternative pathway of complement activation. B, factor B; CR, complement receptor; D, factor D; DAF, decay accelerating factor; H, β₁H-globulin; I, C3 inactivator; MCP, membrane co-factor protein; P, properdin.

on phagocytes. Complement receptor 1 binds C3b, while CR3 and CR4 bind iC3b; CR2 is found on B cells and is involved in B-cell activation. Small amounts of C3b are produced, even in the absence of infection, when a small fragment, C3a, is released from the native C3 molecule. Almost all of it is immediately inactivated by factor I. If any C3b molecules bind to a normal host cell surface they can then bind the next component in the sequence, factor B. Factor D (the only complement factor present in body fluids as an active enzyme) splits off a small fragment, Ba, leaving an active C3 convertase, C3bBb, on the cell surface. However, the normal host cell is able actively to dissociate and inactivate C3bBb. This is achieved by the concerted action of regulatory proteins decay acceleration factor (DAF), membrane co-factor protein (MCP), β_1H globulin (factor H), CR1 and factor I.

Activator surfaces are those that inhibit the regulatory proteins, allowing C3bBb to remain intact. For example, bacterial endotoxins and lipopolysaccharides inhibit factor H. The enzyme C3bBb converts C3 into C3a and C3b. The latter is incorporated, along with properdin (factor P), to form PC3bBbC3b. This is a stable enzyme whose substrates are C3 and C5. It amplifies C3b production and activates the membrane attack pathway.

Classical activation

Classical pathway complement activation (Fig. 8.4) is initiated mainly by complexes of antigen with antibody. Antibodies of the IgG1, IgG2, IgG3 and IgM classes, but not IgG4, IgA, IgD or IgE, can activate the classical pathway.

The first component of the classical pathway, C1, is actually a complex of C1q (whose structures can be likened to a bunch of six tulips), two molecules of C1r and two molecules of C1s. This complex can bind very weakly to monomeric IgG, but when IgG complexes with antigen in such a way that adjacent IgG molecules are close together, C1q binds firmly

between the two molecules. The C1 complex can bind strongly to a single molecule of pentameric IgM, but only after the conformation of the latter has been altered by binding to antigen.

The binding of C1q(rs)$_2$ to antibody alters the conformation of the complex so that a normally hidden esterase enzymic site on C1s is revealed. The activated C1 complex is regulated by C1 inhibitor, which can bind C1r and C1s and strip them away from C1q.

Activated C1 reacts with fluid phase C4 and C2, splitting off small peptides C4a and C2a. The resulting C4b2b is deposited on a surface and performs a similar job to C3bBb of the alternative pathway: it can convert C3 into C3a and C3b, and the latter can either opsonize particles for phagocytosis or bind to C4b2b. Cell-bound C4b2b3b is more stable than C4b2b, being somewhat protected from the regulatory proteins DAF and C4-binding protein. Like PC3bBbC3b, it activates the membrane attack pathway.

Membrane attack

The peptides Bb and C2b, bound into their respective alternative (PC3bBbC3b) and classical (C4b2b3b) pathway enzymic complexes, initiate membrane attack (Fig. 8.5) by splitting a small peptide, C5a, from C5 to form C5b. This molecule binds C6 and C7. The trimolecular C5b67 has a transient binding site for cell membranes, but if it fails to bind rapidly to a target cell it is neutralized by S-protein. Cell-bound C5b67 acts as a template for the binding of one molecule of C8 and up to 18 molecules of C9. The C8 molecule is assembled in such a way as to begin to penetrate the cell membrane; polymerization of C9 within the complex completes the perturbation of the lipid membrane bilayer. Normal cells in the body are largely protected from bystander lysis by homologous restriction factor (HRF), which intercepts C8 and C9 before they can be properly assembled into the membrane attack complex (MAC). The MAC, with a molecular weight of $1-2 \times 10^6$, forms

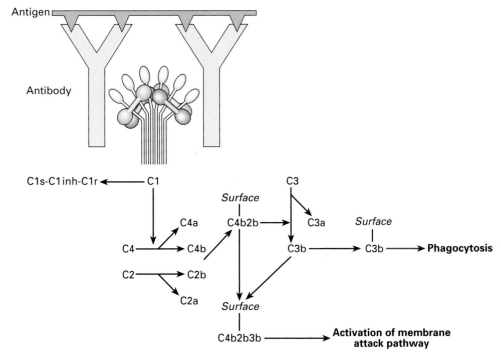

Fig. 8.4 Classical pathway of complement activation.

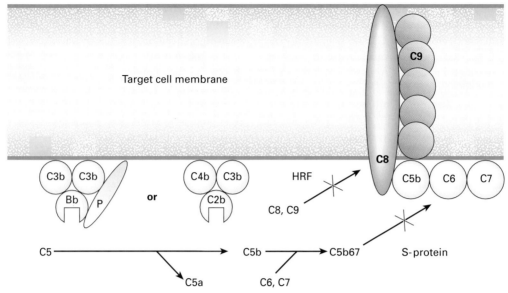

Fig. 8.5 Membrane attack pathway. HRF, homologous restriction factor; P, properdin.

transmembrane channels which permit osmotic influx so that the target cell swells up and bursts.

Biological effects of complement activation

Probably the most important function of the complement system is to **opsonize** antigen-antibody (immune) complexes, microorganisms and cell debris for phagocytosis (Fig. 8.6). This is achieved by deposition of C3b and iC3b on the particle. Phagocytes bind to the particle via CR1, CR3 and CR4. Also, CR1 is found on erythrocytes, which can bind immune complexes coated with C3b and transport them to the spleen or liver for digestion by macrophages.

The peptides C3a, C4a and C5a are **anaphylatoxins** which cause mast cell degranulation and smooth muscle contraction. They increase vascular permeability, which permits cells and fluids to enter the tissues from the circulation. They are regulated by anaphylatoxin inactivator, which splits off the C-terminal arginine so that binding to cellular receptors can no longer occur.

Further important properties of C5a are:
- inducing **adherence** of blood phagocytes to vessel endothelium, following which they are able to migrate into the tissues
- **upregulating** CR1, CR3 and CR4
- attracting phagocytes (**chemotaxis**) towards the site of complement activation.

Certain microorganisms, notably Gram-negative bacteria, can be lysed directly by the membrane attack complex. Gram-positive bacteria, however, are protected by their thick peptidoglycan cell walls.

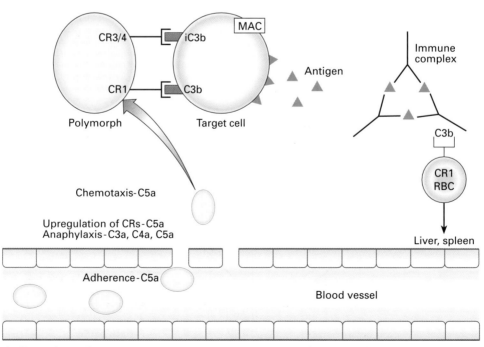

Fig. 8.6 Biological effects of complement. CR, complement receptor; MAC, membrane attack complex; RBC, red blood cell.

CELLS OF THE IMMUNE SYSTEM

All the cells of the immune system (Fig. 8.7) are derived from self-regenerating **haematopoietic stem cells** present in bone marrow and fetal liver. These differentiate along either the **myeloid** or the **lymphoid** pathway. Myeloid precursor cells give rise to mast cells, erythrocytes, platelets, dendritic cells, polymorphs (eosinophils, basophils, neutrophils) and mononuclear phagocytes (monocytes in the blood, macrophages in the tissues). Lymphoid precursor differentiation gives rise to T (thymus-dependent) lymphocytes, B (bone marrow-derived) lymphocytes and natural killer lymphocytes.

Dendritic cells and monocyte/macrophages play key roles in the immune system as **antigen-presenting cells** (APC). The B lymphocytes are responsible for secreting immunoglobulin antibodies and can also function as highly efficient APCs for T lymphocytes. The latter are divided into two major subsets: **T helper cells**, which usually bear the 'cluster of differentiation' marker CD4, and **T cytotoxic cells**, which usually carry CD8. The T helper cells are required for activating the effector function of B cells, other T cells, NK cells and macrophages. They do this by transmitting signals via cell-to-cell contact interactions and/or via soluble hormone-like factors called **lymphokines**. The T cytotoxic cells kill target cells such as virus-infected host cells. Another functional property of some T lymphocytes is to downregulate immune responses. These **T suppressor cells** are usually CD8-positive.

The lymphoid organs

The **primary** sites of lymphocyte production are the **bone marrow** and **thymus**. Immature lymphocytes produced from stem cells in the bone marrow may continue their development within the bone marrow (B lymphocytes, NK cells) or migrate to the thymus and develop into T lymphocytes. 'Education' within the primary lymphoid organs ensures that emerging lymphocytes can discriminate self from non-self. They migrate through the blood and lymphatic systems to the **secondary lymphoid organs** — spleen, lymph nodes and mucosa-associated lymphoid tissue (MALT) of the alimentary, respiratory and urinogenital tracts. Here lymphocytes encounter foreign antigens and become activated effector cells of the immune response.

The spleen acts as a filter for blood and is the major site for clearance of opsonized particles. It is an important site for production of antibodies against intravenous antigens. The lymph nodes form a network of strategically placed filters which drain fluids from the tissues and concentrate foreign antigen on to APCs and subsequently to lymphocytes. Spleen and lymph nodes are encapsulated organs, whereas MALT is non-encapsulated dispersed aggregates of lymphoid cells positioned to protect the main passages by which microorganisms gain entry into the body. Gut-associated lymphoid tissue (GALT) includes Peyer's patches of the lower ileum, accumulations of lymphoid tissue in the lamina propria of the intestinal wall, and the tonsils.

Mature lymphoid cells continually circulate between the blood, lymph, lymphoid organs and tissues until they encounter an antigen which will cause them to become activated (see Ch. 9).

Antigen recognition

The T and B lymphocytes are responsible for **specificity** in the immune response. They have cell surface receptors whose purpose is to recognize foreign antigens. Each receptor usually binds only to a single antigen, though there may be a degree of **cross-reactivity** with other antigens of very similar structure. Since all antigen receptors on a given lymphocyte are identical, each B or T cell can usually recognize only one antigen. A single cell, on encountering its specific antigen, must proliferate to form a clone of identical cells able to deal with the offending antigen (**clonal selection**).

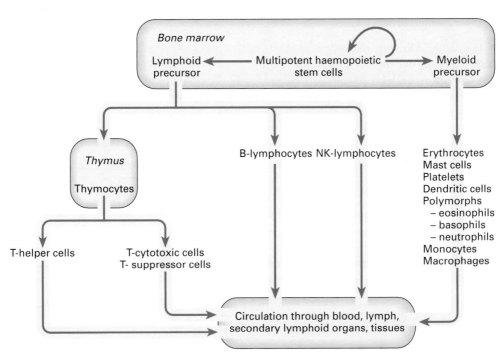

Fig. 8.7 Cells and organs of the immune system. NK, natural killer.

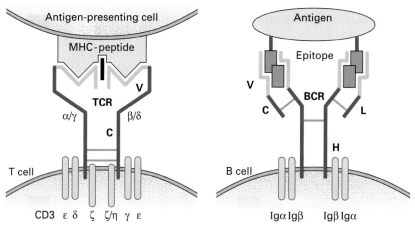

Fig. 8.8 Antigen recognition by T and B cells. V, variable; C, constant; H, heavy chain; L, light chain; TCR, T-cell receptor; BCR, B-cell receptor; MHC, major histocompatibility complex.

The T-cell antigen receptor (TCR) recognizes linear peptides bound to MHC molecules on the surface of APCs. The B-cell receptor (BCR) binds directly to often non-linear antigenic determinants (**epitopes**) and does not require MHC presentation (Fig. 8.8).

Major histocompatibility complex

In humans, products of the highly polymorphic MHC genetic loci on chromosome 6 are known as histocompatibility locus antigens (HLAs). These antigens are responsible for tissue transplant rejection when recipient and donor are not matched for HLA phenotype. This, however, is not the *raison d'être* of MHC molecules. Their function is to bind APC-processed short antigenic peptides and to present them on the APC surface to T cells.

There are two classes of HLA molecules:

- HLA-A, -B and -C (class I) are found on all nucleated cells in the body
- HLA-DQ, -DR and -DP (class II) molecules are usually found only on monocyte/macrophages, B cells, dendritic cells (i.e. APCs), some epithelial cells and activated T cells.

One HLA-A, -B, -C, -DQ, -DR and -DP antigen is inherited from each parent, so each individual expresses up to six class I and six class II antigens. Each HLA molecule can bind a large number of different antigenic peptides. However, the complement of HLA antigens possessed by an individual will determine the range of antigenic peptides that can be presented by APCs.

Class I HLA antigens consist of a single polymorphic α chain which is closely associated with a molecule of non-MHC-encoded β_2-microglobulin. Class II antigens consist of two distinct polypeptide chains, α and β, which are non-covalently joined. Both classes of molecules bind peptides during their intracellular assembly and the HLA-peptide complex is transported to the APC surface. Class I molecules present peptides to $CD8^+$ T lymphocytes, while $CD4^+$ T cells are restricted to MHC class II.

The T-cell receptor and generation of T-cell diversity

The T-cell receptor is a two-chain structure comprising polypeptides derived from TCR α and TCR β genes. Less frequently a subset of T cells will use TCR γ and TCR δ instead (Fig. 8.9). Each chain consists of a **variable** (V) region and a **constant** (C) region. The two adjacent V regions make contact with antigenic peptides and the presenting MHC. The α and δ genes are on chromosome 14q11, TCR β on chromosome 7q32–34 and TCR γ on chromosome 7p14–15.

The genetic template for the α chain is created by joining one of many Vα genes with one of the more than 40 J (joining) α genes and a single C gene. The β-chain template is similarly created by joining one of the large number of Vβs, one of two D (diversity) βs, one of 2 Jβs and one of the two Cβ genes. The number of different αβ V regions that can be created is high, and the repertoire is further increased by the random addition of small numbers of template-independent nucleotides (**n-region additions**) at junctions between gene

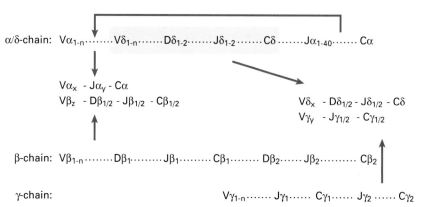

Fig. 8.9 Generation of T-cell diversity. V, variable; C, constant; D, diversity; J, joining.

segments, which is catalysed by **terminal deoxynucleotidyl transferase (TdT)**.

The TCR γδ receptor is also produced by selecting from Vγ, Jγ, Cγ, Vδ, Dδ, Jδ and Cδ segments. The theoretical Vγδ repertoire is smaller than the Vαβ repertoire, indicating that γδ T cells recognize a more limited variety of peptides.

The TCR αβ and γδ chains have short cytoplasmic tails and cannot transmit signals to the T-cell nucleus following binding of antigen. This function is achieved by CD3, comprising γ, δ, ε, ζ and η, or γ, δ, ε, ζ and ζ chains (see Fig. 8.8). The ζ chain can become phosphorylated by a tyrosine kinase attached to the attendant CD4 and CD8 molecules (p56^{lck}), and this sets off complex biochemical pathways which lead to nuclear triggering.

The B-cell receptor, generation of B-cell diversity and isotype selection

The B-cell receptor is a cell membrane-bound form of immunoglobulin antibody and recognizes the same antigenic specificity as the antibody that will eventually be secreted by the B cell. It is a four-chain structure comprising two identical heavy (H) chains which anchor the receptor in the plasma membrane, and two identical light (L) chains. The whole molecule projects out from the B-cell surface in the shape of a Y.

Like TCR chains, each H and L chain consists of V and C regions (Fig. 8.10). The antigen-binding site is created by juxtaposition of V regions from one H and one L chain, and there are two such sites per BCR. Their tertiary structure creates a pocket which accommodates an epitope with the mirror-image configuration.

The V_L region genetic template is created by selecting from V and J genes, while the V_H chain is derived from V, D and J genes. Additional diversity is created by n-region additions. Furthermore, point mutations can be introduced into V genes, which tend to increase the strength of binding of an antibody or BCR to its antigen (**affinity maturation**).

The L chains can be one of two types, kappa (κ) or lambda (λ), depending on which C_L gene is used. The κ light chain gene is on chromosome 2p11 and the λ light chain gene on chromosome 22q11. There are nine C_H genes on chromosome 14q32 arranged in the order 5′-μ-δ-γ₃-γ₁-α₁-γ₂-γ₄-ε-α₂-3′. The class, or *isotype*, of immunoglobulin depends on which C_H gene is used: μ gives IgM, δ IgD, γ₃ IgG₃, α₁ IgA₁, ε IgE. Immature B cells use only μ and express IgM, while mature but unstimulated B cells express IgM and IgD. Following stimulation by antigen, B cells can delete 5′ genes, for example

μ, δ, γ₃, and express the next most 5′ C_H gene, in this case γ₁ (IgG₁). Switching to particular C_H genes is largely under the control of regulatory T cells.

Like the TCR, BCRs have associated molecules (see Fig. 8.8). Two polypeptide chains, Igα and Igβ, are associated with each of the IgH chains and assist in the transmission of signals to the nucleus following binding of antigen by V-BCR.

Deletion of anti-self reactivities

Random usage of all the possible TCR and BCR V gene combinations would result in a large fraction of the repertoire being directed against self. This fraction of the repertoire must be purged in order to prevent immune damage to the body. This is achieved largely during late embryonic and early neonatal development. Following seeding of the primary lymphoid organs by lymphoid precursors, differentiation along defined developmental pathways occurs, accompanied by rapid cell proliferation and also massive cell loss due to depletion of anti-self reactivities.

Thymic differentiation

The most immature thymocytes are TCR⁻CD3⁻CD4⁻CD8⁻ (Fig. 8.11). These first differentiate into TCR⁻CD3⁻CD4⁺CD8⁺ and then rearrange TCR αβ or TCR γδ genes and express CD3; TCR⁺CD3⁺CD4⁺CD8⁺ are then selected for MHC reactivity. Thymocytes with TCRs that bind **weakly** to MHC antigens on thymic cortical epithelial or stromal cells are allowed to survive (**positive selection**); those with no MHC reactivity die 'of neglect'. Thymocytes with **strong** reactivity against self MHC + self peptides (there will have been little exposure to foreign peptides in utero) expressed on medullary dendritic cells and macrophages are signalled to undergo **programmed cell death** by apoptosis (**negative selection**).

If the weak reactivity with MHC that results in positive selection is against MHC class I, the T cell, when fully mature, will respond only to peptides presented on class I. It will stop expressing CD4 but continue to express CD8, which itself has the ability to bind to a monomorphic site on MHC-I and functions as an important coreceptor to strengthen adhesion between the T cell and the APC. The mature T cell will be TCR⁺CD3⁺CD4⁻CD8⁺ and function as a T cytotoxic or T suppressor cell. Alternatively, selection on MHC-II will produce class II restricted TCR⁺CD3⁺CD4⁺CD8⁻ T helper cells. CD4 strengthens the adhesion between the T cell and the APC by binding to MHC-II.

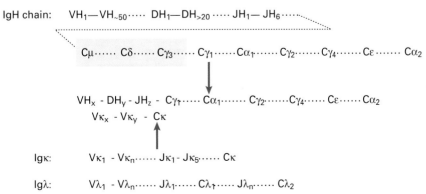

Fig. 8.10 Generation of B-cell diversity. V, variable; C, constant; D, diversity; J, joining.

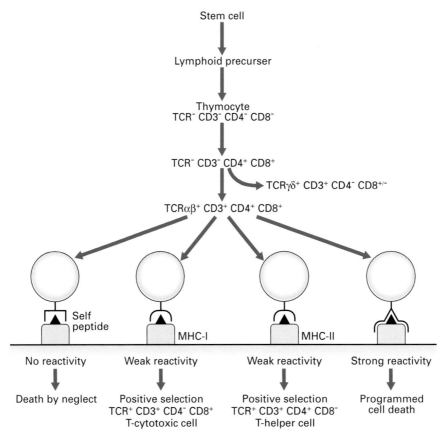

Fig. 8.11 Thymic differentiation. TCR, T-cell receptor; CD, cluster of differentiation; MHC, major histocompatibility complex.

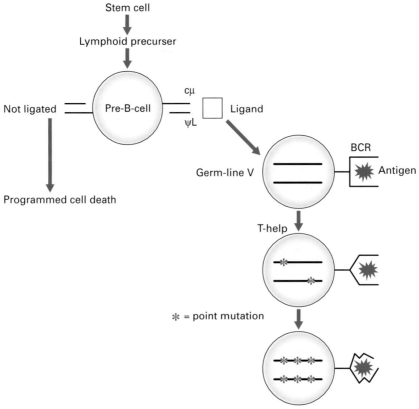

Fig. 8.12 The process of B-cell differentiation. *, point mutation; V, variable; BCR, B-cell receptor.

Fewer than 10% of thymocytes survive the selection process. Those that do have the ability to bind weakly to MHC on APCs and the potential to bind **strongly** to MHC + non-self peptides.

Differentiation of B cells

The need to delete anti-self BCRs is probably less than the need to delete anti-self TCRs, since B cells require T-cell help to produce high-affinity antibodies, and deletion of anti-self T helper cells should be sufficient to prevent activation of anti-self B cells. Furthermore, it is desirable to have low-affinity autoantibodies able to opsonize tissue breakdown products for clearance by phagocytes, which would ensure removal of previously sequestered tissue antigens before they could activate T cells.

Pre-B cells in fetal liver or bone marrow are not yet able to rearrange V(D)J genes, but can produce the C region of IgM H chain ($C\mu$). This is found in abundance in the pre-B cell cytoplasm and is also expressed on the cell surface in conjunction with 'surrogate' light chains (ΨL). If this primitive BCR ($C\mu$-ΨL) is not ligated, the pre-B cell will undergo programmed cell death, but if it is ligated it survives and rearranges Ig genes. Once H and L chains are produced, a complete BCR, consisting of IgM plus Igα and Igβ, will be expressed on the surface.

At this stage the V genes of the BCR are in **germ-line configuration**, i.e. they have not incorporated any point mutations. Products of germ-line V genes generally have low affinity for antigen and can bind weakly to several different antigens (polyreactivity). Weak binding of antigen plus receipt of signals from T helper cells induces low-affinity B cells to proliferate. The V gene point mutations introduced at cell division alter the strength of binding to antigen, with retention of B cells with higher-affinity BCRs (**affinity maturation**) (Fig. 8.12).

Peripheral tolerance

Thymic deletion of T cells bearing self-reactive TCRs is undoubtedly the most important mechanism for ensuring non-reactivity to self. Nevertheless, not all self antigens are represented in the thymus, so extrathymic tolerance induction is also needed.

Autoreactive T cells are most likely to encounter extrathymic self peptides on epithelial cells rather than professional APCs. The activation signal through the TCR will therefore not be followed by co-stimulatory signals required for full activation. Such an interaction may result either in apoptosis of the T cell or it may become **anergic**, i.e. it survives but in a non-reactive state, often with downregulated expression of TCR, CD3 and CD4/CD8.

The **T suppressor cells** are probably required to regulate anti-self reactions when there is failure of thymic or peripheral tolerance induction. Their mechanism of action is poorly understood, but it is likely that they operate mainly by inhibiting T helper cells.

KEY FACTS

- The immune system exists to protect the body against threats from outside (pathogens) and inside (cancer)
- Various natural or **innate** defence mechanisms initiate protection, but **specific** or **adaptive responses**, with **memory**, are required to fully neutralize most threats
- Deficient immunological function results in increased susceptibility to infection
- The immune system must learn not to react against 'self' components, otherwise **autoimmune disease** results
- Components of the innate immune system include **phagocytes, natural killer cells**, the **alternative complement pathway** and **inflammation**
- The adaptive immune response requires **antigen-presenting cells** (macrophages, dendritic cells, B cells) to process antigen into peptides displayed on MHC molecules on the cell surface
- The T lymphocytes are of two types: **T helper cells**, which are CD4-positive and recognize peptides presented by MHC-II molecules, and **T suppressor/cytotoxic** cells, which are CD8-positive and recognize MHC-I-peptide complexes
- Both B cells and T cells recognize antigen through specific receptors. These receptors have variable regions which are derived by selection and recombination of germ-line genes
- Those T cells whose antigen receptors react strongly to self molecules in the thymus are deleted, while those that recognize self molecules outside the thymus are usually made non-reactive

---

FURTHER READING

Janeway, CA Jr, Travers, P, Hunt, S, and Walport, M (1999). Manipulating the immune response to fight infection. In *Immunobiology* (4th edn). Current Biology Ltd, Churchill Livingstone, Gorland Publishing Inc., London.

Roitt, IM (1997). *Roitt's Essential immunology* (9th edn). Blackwell, Oxford.

Roitt, I, Brostoff, J, and Male, D (1997). *Immunology* (5th edn). Mosby, London.

Staines, N, Brostoff, J, and James, K (1994). *Introducing immunology* (2nd edn). Mosby, London.

The immune response

Chapter 8 described the development of B and T cell repertoires. At birth the immature immune system consists of B cells selected for low-affinity polyreactive antibody production, while the T cell repertoire consists of T-cell antigen receptors (TCRs) potentially able to recognize foreign but usually not self peptides presented by major histocompatibility complex (MHC) molecules on antigen-presenting cells (APCs). The latter must also provide co-stimulatory signals for full T-cell activation.

During the vulnerable few months following birth, while immune system maturation is continuing, the infant receives protection against pathogens from the mother's 'experienced' immune system. Maternal immunoglobulin G (IgG) antibodies cross the placenta and provide **passive immunity**. The IgA antibodies in mother's milk protect the infant's digestive system. By the age of 9 months, all maternal IgG antibodies will have been catabolized and suckling may have been terminated. The infant must now be able to mobilize its own adaptive immune response mechanisms to fight off potential pathogens.

ANTIBODIES

Antibodies, or immunoglobulins (Ig), are the secreted products of B lymphocytes which have become activated following binding of antigen to their B-cell receptors (BCR). The specificity for antigen of the secreted antibody is the same as that of the BCR, so they will bind to the same antigen that induced their production. The formation of the antigen–antibody complex may result in:

- neutralization of the antigen (e.g. soluble toxins, viruses)
- removal of the complex by phagocytic cells, which bind via **Fc receptors** (FcRs) to the Ig constant region
- killing of antigen-bearing cells by the membrane attack complex of complement or by natural killer (NK) cells, monocyte/macrophages or granulocytes which bind antibody-coated cells via FcRs.

The basic Y-shaped, four-chain structure of the antibody molecule is shown in Figure 9.1. Antigen-binding specificity is provided by the combined variable (V) regions of heavy (H) and light (L) chains. Since the basic Ig unit has two such pairings, the molecule can bind two identical epitopes, i.e. is bivalent. The Ig heavy chain constant region, particularly domains 2 and 3 which make up the Fc region, largely determine the biological activity of the molecule.

There are five distinct classes of Ig (IgG, IgA, IgM, IgD, IgE), four subclasses of IgG (IgG1, IgG2, IgG3, IgG4) and two subclasses of IgA (IgA1, IgA2). These are derived from usage of different heavy chain genes, as described in Chapter 8. The different structures and properties of Ig molecules are summarized in Figure 9.2.

CYTOKINES

Cytokines are hormone-like glycoproteins involved in communication between cells, particularly those of the immune system. Lymphocyte-derived cytokines are known as **lymphokines**, those produced by monocyte/macrophages as **monokines**. They are required for the initiation and regulation of all stages of the immune response, from stem cell differentiation to effector cell activation. Their action is mediated by binding to specific receptors on target cells; often the receptor may be released from the target cell in soluble form so that it may intercept the cytokine and act as an inhibitor. There are also other forms of cytokine inhibitors responsible for keeping these molecules under tight regulation. Each cytokine has several different activities (**pleiotropy**), and the same activity may be produced by several different cytokines (**redundancy**). The response of a cell to an individual cytokine depends on the context in which it receives the signal, e.g. its state of differentiation and activation and the presence of other cytokines in the microenvironment.

Chemokines are a family of low molecular weight, structurally related cytokines that promote adhesion of cells to endothelium, chemotaxis and activation of leucocytes. They are involved in leucocyte trafficking, providing specific signals for lymphocyte entry into lymphoid and other tissue.

Table 9.1 outlines the main sources and activities of cytokines. It is not exhaustive, and new cytokines and activities are undoubtedly awaiting discovery. The exciting field of cytokine research has led to the isolation of genes for cytokines and their receptors and inhibitors and the ability to manufacture these molecules by recombinant DNA technology. There is optimism that therapeutic use of these reagents will, in the near future, benefit patients with infections, autoimmunity, allergy and other immunologically mediated diseases.

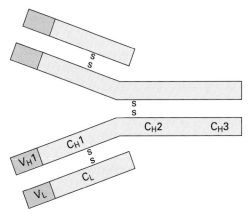

Fig. 9.1 Structure of the immunoglobulin molecule. C, constant region; H, heavy chain; L, light chain; C_H1, C_H2, C_H3 are globular domains with different biological properties; V, variable region.

ANTIGEN PROCESSING AND PRESENTATION

The T lymphocytes use their TCRs to recognize short antigenic peptides bound to MHC class I or class II molecules. This requires that protein antigens be processed and directed to the site of MHC assembly within an MHC-expressing cell. While virtually any cell type can process peptides on to MHC-I molecules, 'professional' APCs (monocyte-macrophages, dendritic cells, B lymphocytes) are usually the only cell types to present MHC-II + peptide (Fig. 9.3).

Antigen-presenting cells express a variety of adhesion molecules which bind to counterstructures on T cells during engagement of the TCR. This maintains the necessary intercellular contact for transfer of activation signal 1. Adhesion molecules include intercellular adhesion molecules ICAM-1 (CD54) and ICAM-2 (CD102) and leucocyte function-associated antigen LFA-3 (CD58) on APCs and LFA-1 (CD11a/CD18), which binds ICAM-1 or -2, and LFA-2 (CD2), which binds LFA-3, on T cells.

Professional APCs also express the B7.1 (CD80) and B7.2 (CD86) co-stimulator molecules which both interact with CD28 and cytotoxic T-lymphocyte-associated antigen (CTLA-4) on T cells. While CD28 transmits activation signal 2 to the responding T cell, CTLA-4 appears to be involved in termination of activation. Interaction between CD40 on APC and CD40 ligand (CD40L, CD154) on responding T cells is

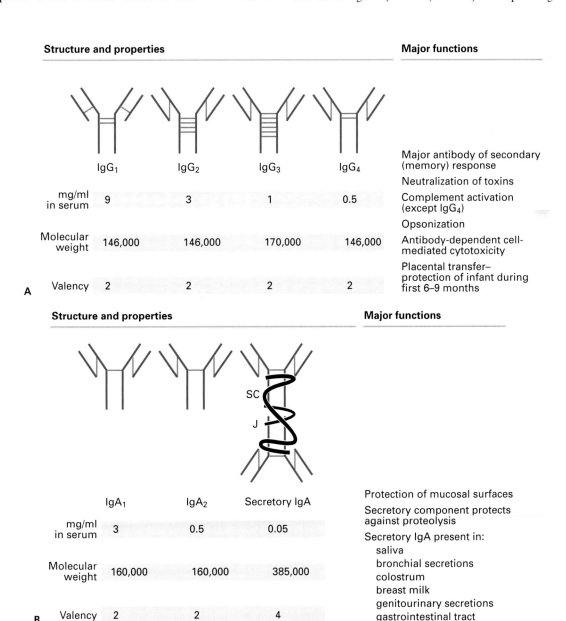

Structure and properties | **Major functions**

	IgG$_1$	IgG$_2$	IgG$_3$	IgG$_4$
mg/ml in serum	9	3	1	0.5
Molecular weight	146,000	146,000	170,000	146,000
Valency	2	2	2	2

Major functions:
- Major antibody of secondary (memory) response
- Neutralization of toxins
- Complement activation (except IgG$_4$)
- Opsonization
- Antibody-dependent cell-mediated cytotoxicity
- Placental transfer–protection of infant during first 6–9 months

A

Structure and properties | **Major functions**

	IgA$_1$	IgA$_2$	Secretory IgA
mg/ml in serum	3	0.5	0.05
Molecular weight	160,000	160,000	385,000
Valency	2	2	4

Major functions:
- Protection of mucosal surfaces
- Secretory component protects against proteolysis
- Secretory IgA present in:
  - saliva
  - bronchial secretions
  - colostrum
  - breast milk
  - genitourinary secretions
  - gastrointestinal tract

B

Fig. 9.2 Structure, properties and functions of different classes of immunoglobulins. SC, secretory component; J, joining chain.

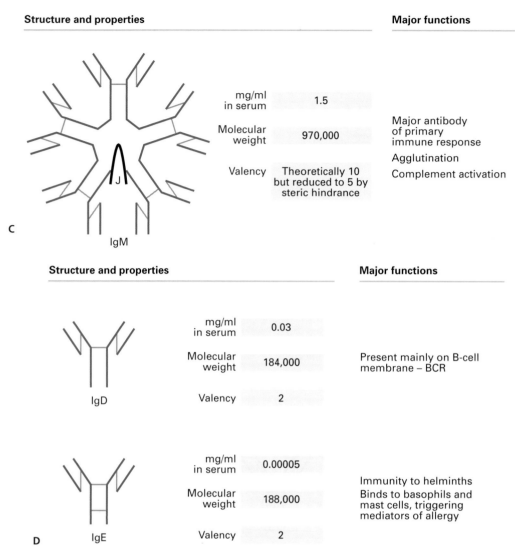

Structure and properties

Major functions

mg/ml in serum	1.5	
Molecular weight	970,000	Major antibody of primary immune response
Valency	Theoretically 10 but reduced to 5 by steric hindrance	Agglutination Complement activation

C   IgM

Structure and properties

Major functions

mg/ml in serum	0.03	
Molecular weight	184,000	Present mainly on B-cell membrane – BCR
Valency	2	

IgD

mg/ml in serum	0.00005	Immunity to helminths
Molecular weight	188,000	Binds to basophils and mast cells, triggering mediators of allergy
Valency	2	

D   IgE

Fig. 9.2 (*Continued*). Structure, properties and functions of IgM (C), and IgD and IgE (D).

another important signal 2 for activation. Cells other than professional APCs, despite expression of MHC-I + peptide, cannot usually stimulate T cells because they lack B7 and CD40.

The MHC + peptide, adhesion molecules and co-stimulator molecules on APCs interact with clusters of TCRs and ligands on T cells, forming an organized interface termed the **immunological synapse**. It is the overall strength of this multipoint interaction that determines the strength of the activation signal received by the T cell. Strong signals lead to full activation while weak signals may induce partial or no activation.

There are two separate pathways of antigen processing for endogenous and exogenous antigens. Endogenous antigens are usually processed on to MHC-I and presented to CD8+ cytotoxic T cells; exogenous antigens are processed on to MHC-II and presented to CD4+ T helper cells.

Processing of endogenous antigens

Cellular cytoplasmic proteins, including cell surface molecules which are recycled to the cytoplasm, undergo proteolysis to small peptides in the **proteosome** and the peptides are then taken to the endoplasmic reticulum, which is the site of production of MHC-I molecules, by the **transporter associated with antigen processing** (TAP). The assembly of the complete class I molecule, α chain + β_2-microglobulin, requires the introduction of an 8–11 amino acid peptide into the peptide-binding groove. 'Empty' MHC molecules are highly unstable. Once assembled, MHC-I + peptide is transported to the cell surface.

The vast majority of cell surface MHC-I molecules contain endogenously processed self peptides, but peptides arising from proteolysis of intracellular pathogens (e.g. viruses) and recycled cell-surface tumour antigens can also come to occupy the peptide-binding groove. Those T cells bearing TCRs reactive with MHC + self peptide are deleted during thymic differentiation, so normally only foreign peptides are targets for the T-cell immune system.

Endogenous antigen presentation leads to expression of a target structure recognizable only by CD8+ T cells, since recognition of MHC-I and CD8 expression are co-selected in the thymus (see Ch. 8). The CD8 molecule binds to MHC-I and helps to generate an intracellular signal of TCR engage-

Table 9.1 Main producers and major actions of cytokines

Cytokine	Main producers	Major actions
IL-1	Macrophages	Mediator of inflammation; augments immune response
IL-2	T cells	T-cell activation and proliferation
IL-3	T cells	Haematopoiesis (early progenitors)
IL-4	T cells	T-cell, B-cell, mast cell proliferation; IgE production
IL-5	T cells	B-cell proliferation; IgA production; eosinophil, basophil differentiation
IL-6	Macrophages, T cells	Mediator of inflammation; B-cell differentiation
IL-7	Bone marrow cells, thymic stroma	Haematopoiesis (lymphocytes)
IL-8	Macrophages	Neutrophil chemotaxis
IL-9	T cells	T-cell proliferation
IL-10	Macrophages, T cells	Inhibitor of cytokine production
IL-11	Bone marrow stromal cells	Haematopoiesis (early progenitors)
IL-12	Macrophages	T-cell differentiation
IL-13	T cells	Similar to IL-4
IL-14	T cells	Proliferation of activated B cells
IL-15	Stromal cells	Similar to IL-2
IL-16	T cells	T-cell chemotaxis
IL-17	T cells	Mediator of inflammation and haematopoiesis
IL-18	Macrophages	Similar to IL-12
IFNα IFNβ IFNγ	Leukocytes Fibroblasts T cells, NK cells	Activation of macrophages, NK cells; upregulation of MHC expression; protection of cells against virus infection
LT	T cells	Mediator of inflammation; killing of tumour cells
TGFβ	Macrophages, lymphocytes, endothelial cells, platelets	Wound healing; IgA production; suppression of cytokine production
TNFα	Macrophages, T cells	Mediator of inflammation; killing of tumour cells
gCSF	Macrophages	Haematopoiesis (granulocytes)
mCSF	Monocytes	Haematopoiesis (monocyte/macrophages)
gmCSF	T cells	Haematopoiesis (granulocytes, monocyte/macrophages)

IL, interleukin; IFN, interferon; LT, lymphotoxin; TGF, transforming growth factor; TNF, tumour necrosis factor; CSF, colony stimulating factor; g, granulocyte; m, monocyte/macrophage.

ment. Endogenous processing of intracellular pathogen thus leads to activation of cytotoxic effector cells able to destroy the infected cell.

Processing of exogenous antigen

Phagocytic or endocytic uptake of exogenous antigens such as extracellular pathogens results in proteolysis within the endosomal compartment. Here peptides encounter MHC-II molecules consisting of α and β chains held together by the **invariant chain**. Peptides of 15–18 amino acids can replace the invariant chain. MHC-II + peptide is transported to the cell surface to be 'seen' by the TCR of a CD4$^+$ T helper cell. Engagement of the TCR induces signal 1 for T-cell activation, interaction of adhesion molecules and of CD4 with MHC-II

helps to transfer this signal to the nucleus, and B7–CD28 and/or CD40–CD40L interaction generates signal 2. The activated T helper cell responds to further signals from cytokines released by the APC, notably interleukin (IL) 1, which in turn stimulates expression of IL-2 receptors, release of IL-2 and cell proliferation. A clone of activated T helper cells is produced, each member of which can recognize the original MHC-II + peptide and is able to secrete various lymphokines for activation of other immune effector mechanisms.

T HELPER SUBSETS

The nature of the immune effector response is largely determined by the range of lymphokines secreted by activated T

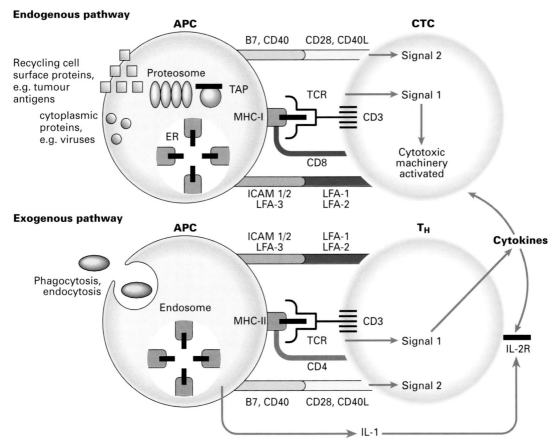

Fig. 9.3 Antigen processing and presentation to cytotoxic T cells (CTC) and T helper cells (T_H). APC, antigen-presenting cell; ER, endoplasmic reticulum; ICAM, intercellular adhesion molecule; IL, interleukin; LFA, leucocyte function-associated antigen; TAP, transporter associated with antigen processing; TCR, T-cell receptor; MHC, major histocompatibility complex; R, receptor.

helper cells. Upon initial stimulation, an activated T helper cell will secrete a wide range of lymphokines (T_H0 phenotype), but, depending on the type of APC and the environment in which T helper activation is taking place, the lymphokine secretion profile will usually polarize towards production of either IL-2, interferon γ (IFNγ) and lymphotoxin (LT) (T_H1) or IL-4, IL-5 and IL-10 (T_H2). While T_H1 lymphokines stimulate mainly macrophage and dendritic cell activation, T_H2 lymphokines stimulate B-cell activation and antibody production (Fig. 9.4).

If the APC is a macrophage or dendritic cell it will normally be stimulated to produce IL-12 during T helper cell activation. Neighbouring NK cells and possibly other cell types respond to IL-12 by producing IFNγ, which stimulates the T_H1 and suppresses the T_H2 secretion profile. If the APC is a non-IL-12 producing cell, such as a B cell, or if T_H0 activation takes place in an environment containing IL-4-secreting cells (possibly NK-T cells, a poorly understood population of lymphocytes bearing both NK- and T-cell markers), IL-4 will be the dominant early lymphokine. Interleukin 4 stimulates production of T_H2- and suppresses T_H1-type lymphokines.

ACTIVATION OF MACROPHAGES

Macrophages receive activation signal 1 when they bind pathogens to threat receptors (Fig. 9.5). When they present MHC-II + peptide and provide activation signals 1 and 2 for T helper cells, they also receive a second signal for their own activation. Macrophage-derived IL-12 induces T helper cells

of the T_H1 phenotype. Interferon γ released by T_H1 induces macrophages to express receptors for TNFα. These can bind membrane-bound TNFα expressed by T_H1, inducing the activated state. Activated macrophages secrete autocrine TNFα for maintaining this state, along with the inflammatory cytokines IL-1 and IL-6.

Following activation, macrophages express increased levels of Fc and complement receptors and thereby have higher phagocytic capability. They also increase expression of MHC

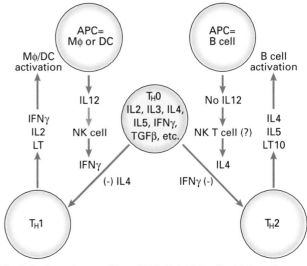

Fig. 9.4 Secretion profiles of T_H0, T_H1, T_H2 cells. APC, antigen-presenting cell; DC, dendritic cell; IFN, interferon; IL, interleukin; NK, natural killer; LT, lymphotoxin; Mφ, macrophage; NKT, natural killer T-cell; TGF, transforming growth factor.

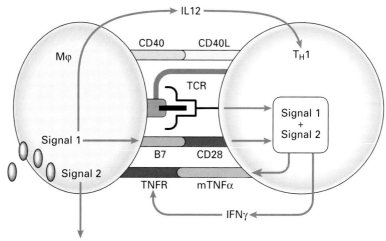

Fig. 9.5 Activation of macrophages. CR, complement receptor; FcR, Fc receptor; IFN, interferon; IL, interleukin; Mφ, macrophage; R, receptor; TNF, tumor necrosis factor.

and adhesion molecules, increasing the efficiency of antigen presentation. Their ability to kill pathogens increases as a result of raised levels of intracellular and secreted enzymes. Most importantly, powerful microbicidal mechanisms involving generation of reactive oxygen intermediaries ($^{\cdot}OH$, $O^{\cdot}$, O_2^{-}, H_2O_2) and nitric oxide (NO) are induced.

B-CELL ACTIVATION

B cells are highly efficient antigen-presenting cells. They receive signal 1 for activation by binding antigen, often concentrated on the surface of follicular dendritic cells within lymph node germinal centres, to the BCR, and then proceed to internalize antigen and process peptides on to MHC-II molecules for presentation to T helper cells (Fig. 9.6). They are then induced to express co-stimulatory B7 and can therefore provide signal 2 for T helper cell activation through CD28. Activated T helper cells are induced to express CD40L for binding to B cell CD40. Interaction between these two molecules induces B-cell activation, Ig production and isotype switching.

Interleukin 12 is not usually the dominant cytokine at the site of B–T$_H$ interaction, so T helper cells induced by B–APC will generally be of the T$_H$2 type, secreting IL-4, IL-5 and IL-10. These lymphokines further promote B-cell proliferation, activation and isotype switching.

TARGET CELL KILLING

Cytotoxic T cells carrying CD8, activated via the endogenous antigen presentation pathway, are able to recognize and kill target cells, such as virus-infected cells, expressing MHC-I + foreign peptide (Fig. 9.7). Both CD8 and various adhesion proteins are important in enhancing and maintaining target cell–effector cell contact.

When a cytotoxic T cell makes contact with its specific target, cytoplasmic granules polarize to the contact point and are released into the narrow gap between the cells. Cytotoxic granules contain perforin and granzymes. **Perforin** is related to complement C9, with which it shares the ability to polymerize on the target cell surface, forming transmembrane channels. **Granzymes** are granular proteases which gain

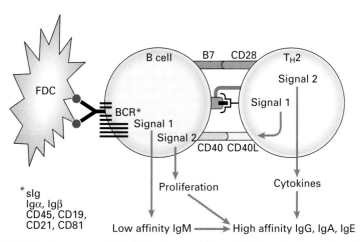

Fig. 9.6 Activation of B cells. BCR, B-cell receptor; FDC, follicular dendritic cell; L, ligand; sIg, surface immunoglobin.

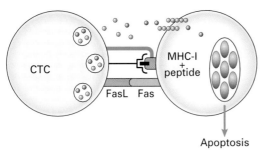

Fig. 9.7 Target cell killing. CTC, cytotoxic T cell; L, ligand; MHC, major histocompatibility complex.

entry into the target cell through perforin pores. Granzymes activate the target cell's suicide programme (**apoptosis**), which leads to nuclear fragmentation and packaging of products of nuclear distintegration into apoptotic bodies, which are efficiently removed by phagocytosis.

Target cell apoptosis can also be induced by binding of Fas ligand (FasL), induced during activation of cytotoxic effector T cells, with the death receptor Fas (CD95) on target cells.

Natural killer cells and γδ T cells also employ perforin and granzymes to kill target cells. The γδ TCR can apparently receive signal 1 for activation without participation of classical MHC-I or -II molecules, and γδ T cells are either CD8⁻ or express CD8αα rather than the usual CD8αβ. The γδ T cells are important in defence against infection, and experimental animals depleted of γδ T cells eliminate microbes inefficiently.

Natural killer cells are apparently responsible for killing target cells that express lower than normal levels of MHC-I molecules, such as some malignant or virus-infected cells (see Fig. 8.2). Cells deficient in MHC-I cannot be attacked by cytotoxic T cells; however, production of IFN-γ by activated NK cells will promote expression of MHC-I on target cells and permit the more efficient T cell cytotoxicity to proceed.

REGULATION OF THE IMMUNE RESPONSE

The specific immune response involving activation and clonal expansion of B cells and T cells brings into play a variety of non-specific effector mechanisms involving complement, cytokines, granulocytes, macrophages, mast cells, etc. These have the potential to damage normal host tissues, so it is crucial that the specific immune response be swiftly curtailed once the initiating foreign invader has been effectively neutralized.

Anti-idiotypic antibody

The variable regions, or **idiotypes** (ids), of antibodies, BCRs and TCRs represent novel molecules not previously experienced by the immune system. Tolerance will not have been induced against them and, if present in sufficient quantity, as occurs during a clonally expanded immune response, they will be immunogenic and induce **anti-idiotypic antibodies** (anti-ids).

Secreted antibody may be recognized by B cells bearing BCRs with anti-id reactivity. This usually takes place on the surface of follicular dendritic cells and transmits activation signal 1 to the anti-id B cell. Further activation signals are received following processing of the id and presentation of its peptides to a specific T_H2 cell. The fully activated anti-idiotypic B cell undergoes clonal expansion and secretes anti-id (Fig. 9.8). This will form immune complexes with circulating id which will be removed by phagocytes.

Anti-id will also bind to id (BCR) on the surface of B cells. This will lead to cross-linking of BCRs and FcRs, which generates an inactivation signal (Fig. 9.8).

The TCR on clonally expanded activated T cells can also lead to the generation of anti-id, which could induce tolerogenic signals when it binds to cell-bound TCR, perhaps by inducing activation signal 1 in the absence of signal 2.

T suppressor cells

Activation of immune effector mechanisms involving B cells, cytotoxic T cells, macrophages or NK cells all require participation of T helper cells and their secreted lymphokines. Termination of a successful immune response could therefore be effectively achieved by silencing the driving T helper cells.

The phenomenon of T helper inactivation by **T suppressor cells** (Fig. 9.9) has been difficult to prove, and although most immunologists now accept the existence of this specialized T-cell subset, its mode of action is still unclear. As T helper cells recycle their TCRs and process TCR id peptides on to MHC-I, CD8⁺ T cells with appropriate anti-id TCRs might bind to and inactivate the T helper cell by a cytotoxic mechanism or by transmitting 'off' signals through membrane interactions.

An important mechanism of immune suppression is induction of a different cytokine profile from the one driving the

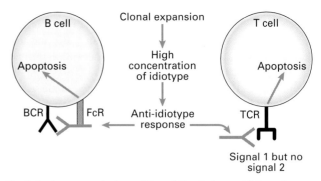

Fig. 9.8 Downregulation of B and T cells by anti-idiotypic antibody. BCR, B-cell receptor; FcR, Fc receptor; TCR, T-cell receptor.

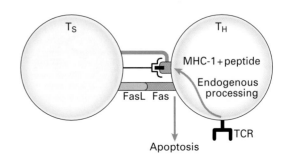

Fig. 9.9 A possible mechanism of T suppression. MHC, major histocompatibility complex; L, ligand; TCR, T-cell receptor.

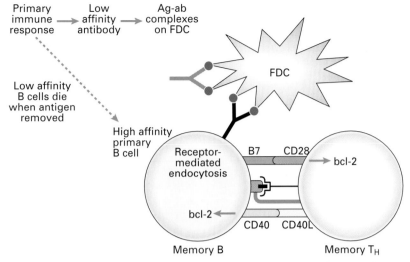

Fig. 9.10 Induction of memory cells. Ag–ab, antigen–antibody; FDC, follicular dendritic cell; L, ligand.

ongoing reaction, e.g. suppression of cell-mediated immunity by type 2 cytokines or suppression of humoral immunity by type 1 cytokines (**immune deviation**). A population of **T regulatory cells** that secrete mainly TGFβ and/or IL-10 also suppresses cytokine-dependent immune reactions.

IMMUNOLOGICAL MEMORY

The initial encounter with foreign antigen leads to an immune response which evolves slowly over days or weeks and eventually neutralizes and eliminates the invader. Although effector mechanisms are switched off once they are no longer required, the original antigenic experience is not forgotten. Long-lived T and B memory cells are selected for survival and mount an accelerated and enhanced response on encountering the antigen for a second time (Fig. 9.10).

Memory B cells

The primary B cell response leads to production of mainly low-affinity IgM antibodies, but some responding B cells undergo heavy chain class switching and V region somatic mutation to produce higher-affinity IgG, IgA or IgE antibodies. Memory B cells are selected from this latter population because their BCRs can interact with antigen–antibody complexes formed during the primary response. These remain for long periods on the surface of follicular dendritic cells within germinal centres of secondary lymphoid tissue. High-affinity BCRs compete successfully with the lower-affinity antibody within the complex and bind antigen.

Signalling between B cell CD40 and CD40L on activated T cells also appears to be required for memory B-cell survival.

This interaction induces activation of the *bcl*-2 oncogene, an inhibitor of programmed cell death.

When memory B cells re-encounter their specific antigen, they rapidly produce high-affinity IgG, IgA or IgE. This requires fewer T helper cells and lower levels of lymphokines than the primary response.

Memory T cells

Memory T cells cannot be distinguished from naive T cells on the basis of isotype switch or affinity maturation because TCRs do not undergo these processes. Memory and naive T cells, at least those of the CD4$^+$ T helper subset, can at present best be distinguished by expression of different isoforms of the common leucocyte antigen CD45, CD45RO on the former and CD45RA on the latter. The two isoforms of CD45 are also segregated on subsets of CD8$^+$ cells.

While CD4$^+$CD45RO$^+$ memory T cells provide help for B-cell activation, CD4$^+$CD45RA$^+$ naive cells preferentially induce T suppressor cells. This may be related to the different lymphokine secretion profiles of the two subsets, with naive T cells producing mainly IL-2 and memory T cells producing multiple lymphokines.

Memory T cells express higher levels of various adhesion and co-stimulatory molecules than naive T cells and are much more efficient at interacting with other cell types.

As with memory B cells, long-term survival of memory T cells is triggered by re-exposure to antigen. Antigen is retained in the body for prolonged periods mainly in the form of immune complexes on the surface of follicular dendritic cells and is available only to the high-affinity BCRs of memory B cells. Therefore selection of memory T cells probably requires recognition, processing and presentation of MHC-II + peptide by memory B cells.

KEY FACTS

- Antibodies, the secreted products of B lymphocytes, neutralize antigens, induce killing of target cells by complement and natural killer cells and opsonize particles for phagocytosis

- **Cytokines** and **chemokines** mediate intercellular communication within the immune system, being required for initiation and regulation of all stages of the immune response. Type 1 cytokines induce mainly macrophage activation, type 2 cytokines induce mainly antibody secretion

- T cells and B cells require two signals for activation, the first through the TCR/BCR, the second through B7–CD28 or CD40–CD40L interaction. Receipt of only the first signal usually results in anergy or cell death

- Macrophages are activated when they process exogenous antigen onto MHC-II and present peptides to T helper cells. The latter become activated and secrete type 1 cytokines, including interferon-γ, a powerful macrophage activator. Activated macrophages secrete inflammatory cytokines and are highly efficient at phagocytosis, antigen presentation and microbial killing

- B cells are activated when they present antigen to T helper cells and receive both a first signal through the BCR and a second signal from CD40L binding to CD40. Type 2 cytokines, including IL-4, stimulate clonal proliferation, antibody secretion, affinity maturation and isotype switching of antibody

- Cytotoxic T cells become activated when they encounter endogenous antigen processed onto MHC-I and are stimulated by signal 1, signal 2 and type 1 cytokines. They kill by secreting perforin and granzymes towards the target cell or by inducing apoptosis of Fas-expressing cells

- Termination of the immune response is essential to prevent widespread damage to healthy tissues. **Anti-idiotypic antibodies** bind to BCRs and TCRs and switch off activated cells; T suppressor cells switch off T helper cells. Type 1 cytokine production can be suppressed by induction of type 2 cytokines, and vice versa

- At the end of an immune response, responding high-affinity B cells and T cells survive in a resting state for long periods and respond rapidly and efficiently on re-encountering the same antigen (**immunological memory**)

FURTHER READING

Janeway, CA Jr, Travers, P, Hunt, S, and Walport, M (1999). *Immunobiology* (4th edn). Current Biology Ltd, Churchill Livingstone, Gorland Publishing Inc., London.

Mims, C, Playfair, J, Roitt, I, Wakelin, D, and Williams, R (1998). Vaccination. In *Medical microbiology* (2nd edn), Ch 15 Mosby Year Book, St Louis.

Roitt, IM (1997). *Roitt's Essential immunology* (9th edn). Blackwell, Oxford.

Roitt, I, Brostoff, J, and Male, D (1997). *Immunology* (5th edn). Mosby, London.

Staines, N, Brostoff, J, and James, K (1994). *Introducing immunology* (2nd edn). Mosby, London.

10 Immunity and infection

Bacterial, viral, parasitic and fungal infections are major causes of morbidity and mortality worldwide, especially in poorer societies with less access to medicines and vaccines, greater exposure to infectious agents and poorer nutrition. Infectious and parasitic diseases were responsible for 29.6% of the world's disease burden in 1999, according to the World Health Organization (Table 10.1).

All of the immunological mechanisms described in the previous two chapters are called upon to limit and eliminate infectious agents. However, pathogens have developed a remarkable variety of strategies to evade the host's immune defences, and the immune response itself may damage host tissues.

IMMUNITY TO BACTERIA

Summary of defence mechanisms

- The bacterial cell-wall proteoglycan can be attacked by lysozyme.
- Bacteria release peptides which are chemotactic for polymorphs.
- Polymorphs and macrophages use receptors for bacterial sugars to bind and slowly phagocytose them.
- Bacteria induce macrophages to release inflammatory cytokines such as interleukins 1 and 6 and tumour necrosis factor α (TNFα).
- Bacterial lipopolysaccharides and endotoxins activate the alternative complement pathway, generating opsonizing C3b and iC3b on the bacterial surface. The membrane attack complex (MAC) can lyse Gram-negative but not Gram-positive bacteria.
- Bacterial polysaccharides (e.g. pneumococcal) with multiple repeated epitopes may activate B cells independently of T helper cells because of their ability to cross-link B-cell receptors (BCRs). The resultant mainly IgM antibodies efficiently agglutinate bacteria and activate the classical complement pathway.
- Exogenous processing of phagocytosed bacteria by macrophages results in presentation of peptide epitopes in the context of MHC-II to T_H1 cells. These induce macrophage activation for efficient bacterial killing.
- Processing of bacterial antigens by B cells induces T_H2 responses and high-affinity antibody production: IgG antibodies neutralize soluble bacterial products such as toxins; IgA antibodies protect mucosal surfaces from bacterial attachment. Immune complexes activate the classical complement pathway. Phagocytic uptake of bacteria coated with C3b/iC3b and antibody is rapid and efficient.

Bacterial evasion strategies

Many bacteria have developed ways of interfering with phagocytosis. Encapsulated bacteria do not display sugar molecules for recognition by receptors on phagocytes. They are only phagocytosed when coated with antibodies, so can proliferate in non-immune individuals in the first few days after infection. Even when taken up by phagocytes, many encapsulated bacteria resist digestion (e.g. *Haemophilus influenzae*, *Streptococcus pneumoniae*, *Klebsiella pneumoniae*, *Pseudomonas aeruginosa*) or can even kill phagocytes (e.g. streptococci, staphylococci, *Bacillus anthracis*). *Mycobacterium*, *Listeria* and *Brucella* spp. are able to survive within the cytoplasm of non-activated macrophages and can only be killed by a cell-mediated immune response driven by T_H1 macrophage-activating lymphokines.

Damage caused by immune responses to bacteria

Group A β-haemolytic streptococci cause sore throat and scarlet fever which resolve on induction of specific antibody. Certain components of some strains of streptococci contain epitopes which are cross-reactive with epitopes present on heart tissue. Antibodies that eliminate the infecting bacteria can bind to heart tissue and cause complement-mediated lysis and antibody-dependent cellular cytotoxicity (rheumatic heart disease). Furthermore, circulating immune complexes can deposit in synovia and glomeruli, causing complement-mediated joint pain and glomerulonephritis, respectively. Induction of cross-reacting anti-heart antibody by group A streptococci is illustrated in Figure 10.1.

Other examples of postbacterial immune complex diseases include subacute bacterial endocarditis, infected ventriculo-arterial shunts, secondary syphilis, and gonococcal and meningococcal septicaemia.

Persistent infection of macrophages, e.g. with *Mycobacterium tuberculosis* or *M. leprae*, provokes a chronic, local, cell-mediated immune reaction due to continuous release of antigen. Lymphokine production causes large numbers of macrophages to accumulate, many of which give rise to epithelioid cells or fuse to form giant cells (syncytia). Incorporation of fibroblasts also occurs and the persisting pathogen becomes walled off inside a fibrotic, necrotic **granuloma**. 83

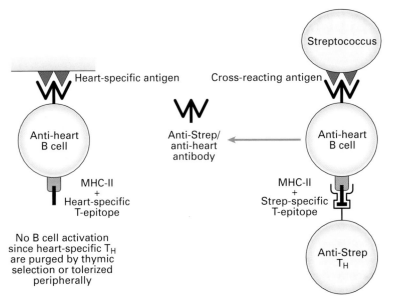

Fig. 10.1 Induction of anti-heart antibodies by group A streptococci.

Non-functional granulomas may replace extensive areas of normal tissue, e.g. in the lungs of tuberculosis patients.

IMMUNITY TO VIRUSES

Viruses cannot proliferate outside a host cell. The infectious virion must attach to a suitable cell via a specific membrane receptor and enter the cell cytoplasm. Viral replication may or may not destroy the host cell. Viral genes may become incorporated within the host cell genome and remain in a state of **latency** for long periods. In some cases, integrated viral genes activate cellular oncogenes and induce malignant transformation.

Summary of defence mechanisms

- Viral proliferation induces infected cells to produce interferons α and β which protect neighbouring cells from pro-

ductive infection. Interferons induce enzymes that inhibit messenger RNA translation into proteins and degrade both viral and host cell messenger RNA, effectively preventing the host cell from supporting replication of the virus or replicating itself.

- Some viruses, notably Epstein–Barr virus, bind C1 and activate the classical complement pathway, resulting in MAC-induced lysis.
- Macrophages readily take up viruses non-specifically and kill them. Some viruses, however, are able to survive and multiply in macrophages. Viruses do not usually induce macrophages to release inflammatory cytokines.
- Processing of viral antigens by B cells and presentation to T_H2 cells induces high-affinity antibody production. Antibodies are effective against free rather than cell-associated viruses. Antibodies specific for epitopes responsible for binding to cellular receptors prevent attachment and penetration. These are mainly IgG antibodies in extracellular fluids, IgM antibodies in the blood and IgA antibodies at mucosal surfaces. Antibody-coated viruses may be destroyed by the classical complement activation pathway or may be taken up by phagocytes bearing Fc or complement receptors.
- Intracellular viral antigens are processed by the endogenous pathway and viral peptides presented on MHC-I molecules can be recognized by $CD8^+$ T cytotoxic cells. These effector cells efficiently destroy virus-infected cells and provide long-term protection against subsequent infection with the same virus.
- Free virions taken up by macrophages and processed by the exogenous pathway stimulate specific T_H1 cells to release interferon (IFN) γ, which, like IFNα and IFNβ, protects neighbouring cells from productive infection.
- Virally infected cells may downregulate MHC molecules and become susceptible to killing by natural killer (NK) cells. Antibody-coated virus-infected cells, whose cytotoxic T-cell epitopes may be masked by antibody, can be killed by NK cells which bind via Fc receptors. Interferon γ activates the killing mechanism of NK cells, but paradoxically induces re-expression of MHC antigens on the target cells and suppression of NK cytotoxicity. However, such target cells would then be susceptible to T-cell cytotoxicity.

Table 10.1 Leading causes of infectious diseases worldwide

Infectious disease	Cause	Annual deaths
Acute respiratory infections (mostly pneumonia)	Bacterial or viral	4 300 000
Diarrhoeal diseases	Bacterial or viral	3 200 000
Tuberculosis	Bacterial	3 000 000
Hepatitis B	Viral	1 000 000 to 2 000 000
Malaria	Protozoan	1 000 000
AIDS	Viral	1 000 000
Measles	Viral	900 000
Neonatal tetanus	Bacterial	600 000
Pertussis (whooping cough)	Bacterial	360 000

From *The World Health Report* (1999) Geneva: WHO.

Viral evasion strategies

Certain viruses can modify the structure of components that are targets for the immune response (**antigenic variation**). Point mutations in the genes encoding viral antigens cause minor structural changes (**antigenic drift**), while exchange of large segments of genetic material with other viruses changes the whole structure of the antigen (**antigenic shift**). Antigenic drift of influenza A virus haemagglutinin occurs before each winter's minor influenza epidemic, while major epidemics, such as those of 1918, 1957, 1968 and 1977, were the result of antigenic shift of haemagglutinin and/or neuraminidase.

Viruses that can integrate their genes within the host cell genome, such as human herpesviruses, provoke only low-level immunity which fails to clear the latently infected cells. Periodic cycles of activation and replication occur when the equilibrium between the virus and the host defence is upset by other infections, metabolic disturbances, immunosuppressive treatment, or extreme physical or psychological stress.

Viruses that infect cells of the immune system may inhibit their function, e.g. Epstein–Barr virus (B cells); measles, human T lymphotropic virus type I, human immunodeficiency virus (HIV) (T cells); dengue, lassa, Marburg–Ebola, HIV (macrophages).

Some herpesviruses and poxviruses can secrete proteins that mimic and interfere with key immune regulators such as cytokines and cytokine receptors.

Damage caused by immune responses to viruses

Epstein–Barr virus is a potent T-cell-independent polyclonal activator of B cells. It induces B cells, including those with anti-self BCRs which are normally inactive due to purging of the corresponding anti-self T helper cells, to secrete antibodies. Several viruses, notably hepatitis B virus, can cause chronic autoimmune disease due to release of previously sequestered (i.e. non-tolerogenic) self antigens following tissue damage. Complexes of antivirus antibodies with antigen can activate complement in the blood vessels, joints and glomeruli, causing vasculitis, arthritis and glomerulonephritis. Cytotoxic T cells may destroy essential host cells displaying viral antigens, e.g. coxsackievirus (myocarditis), mumps virus (meningoencephalitis) and viruses causing damage to the myelin nerve sheath (postviral polyneuritis).

HIV and AIDS

By the beginning of the year 2001, approximately 36 million people worldwide had become infected with human immunodeficiency virus (HIV) and approximately 22 million had died of the acquired immune deficiency syndrome (AIDS) (see also Ch. 30). The virus causes depletion of CD4$^+$ T helper lymphocytes over many years. Patients eventually succumb to opportunistic infections (*Pneumocystis carinii*, *Mycobacterium tuberculosis*, atypical mycobacteria, *Histoplasma*, *Coccidioides*, *Cryptococcus*, *Cryptosporidium* and *Toxoplasma* spp., herpes simplex, cytomegalovirus, etc.) and may develop Kaposi's sarcoma, B-cell lymphomas and other malignancies. Infection of the brain by HIV can cause dementia and encephalitis.

The major route of transmission of HIV is by sexual intercourse: male to female, female to male and male to male. It can also be transmitted from mother to fetus across the placenta, during delivery or by breast-feeding. Direct injection into the bloodstream, e.g. by multiple use of needles and syringes for injection of drugs, also transmits HIV.

The life cycle of HIV is shown in Figure 10.2. The virus gains entry into target cells by binding its surface gp120 molecule (glycoprotein of 120 kDa) to CD4 on T helper cells and a subset of macrophages. The latter can also take up opsonized HIV via Fc or complement receptors. A coreceptor is also required for infection of target cells: CXCR4, also known as fusin or LESTR, is the receptor for the chemokine SDF-1 and is the coreceptor for infection of T cells by HIV; CCR5, the receptor for chemokines RANTES, MIP-1α and MIP-1β, is the coreceptor for infection of macrophages. Viral gp41 causes fusion with the cell membrane and injection into the target cell of two strands of viral genetic information, which is RNA. One strand is destroyed by viral ribonuclease H and viral reverse transcriptase converts the surviving strand into a DNA copy. This forms the template for synthesis of the complementary second strand by cellular DNA polymerase. The double-stranded DNA is then integrated into host cell DNA by viral integrase.

Integrated proviral DNA remains dormant until the latently infected cell receives immune activation stimuli. The cytokines interleukin 6 (IL-6) and TNFα can bind to a transactivation response region (TAR) within the 5' long terminal repeat (LTR), initiating expression of viral genes. These include structural genes (*gag*, *pol*, *env*, which give rise to core proteins, viral enzymes and envelope gp41 and gp120, respectively) and a variety of regulatory genes which promote transcription (*tat*, *rev*, *vpr*), production of full-length genomic RNA (*rev*), budding of virions from the cell surface (*vpu*, *nef*) and infectivity of cell-free virus (*vif*). Genomic RNA and viral enzymes are packaged inside the core proteins, while the envelope glycoproteins are transported to the cell membrane. New complete virions are formed by budding from the infected cell surface.

The virus is usually transmitted from person to person within macrophages (infected macrophages are more numerous than infected T helper cells in genital secretions) or as cell-free virus. Infected macrophages contain HIV virions within cytoplasmic vacuoles; probably IL-6 and TNFα produced in response to phagocytic uptake induce constant slow production of virions from integrated proviral DNA. When infected macrophages enter the new host they are destroyed, releasing HIV. Dendritic cells transport HIV to draining lymph nodes where they infect CD4$^+$ cells.

Proliferation of HIV within lymph nodes occurs throughout the long period of clinical latency, even though the patient remains well and is not deficient in T helper cells. Eventually the lymph node architecture becomes damaged and generalized release of HIV causes rapid destruction of T helper cells.

Budding of HIV from an infected T helper cell destroys the integrity of the cell membrane. In addition to this direct form of killing of infected cells, HIV can apparently destroy or inactivate uninfected T helper cells by various indirect mechanisms, most of which remain theoretically possible rather than of proven clinical relevance. These possible pathogenic mechanisms are shown in Figures 10.3 to 10.7.

Some AIDS patients show evidence of superantigen-mediated loss of T cells bearing particular Vβ TCRs. **Superantigens** activate large numbers of T helper cells by binding

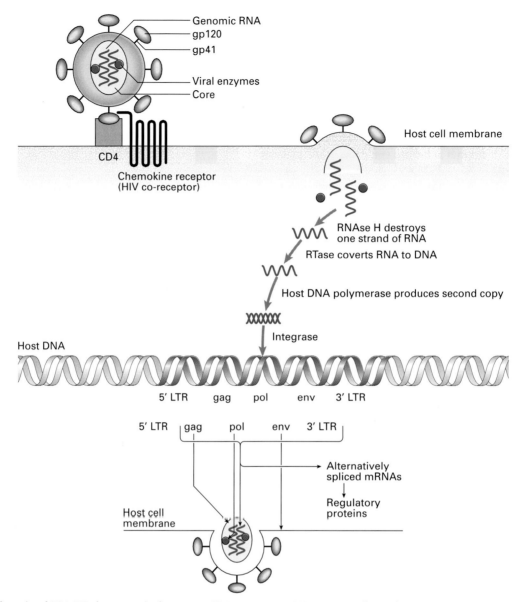

Fig. 10.2 Life cycle of HIV. LTR, long terminal repeat; mRNA, messenger RNA; RNAse, ribonuclease; RTase, reverse transcriptase.

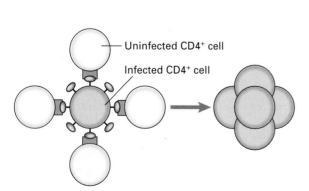

Fig. 10.3 Giant cell formation induced by HIV. Glycoprotein gp120 present on the surface of HIV-infected cells binds to CD4 on uninfected cells; gp41 induces fusion of adjacent cells and production of non-functional, infected giant cells (syncytia). Thus HIV can pass from cell to cell without being exposed to the host's immune response.

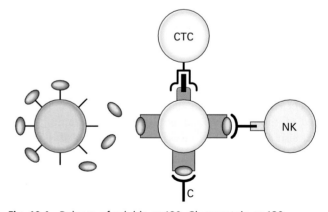

Fig. 10.4 Release of soluble gp120. Glycoprotein gp120 released from HIV-infected cells can bind to CD4 of uninfected cells which can then be destroyed by antibody-dependent complement or natural killer (NK) cell cytotoxicity after binding of anti-gp120 antibody. Processing of gp120 onto MHC-I forms a target structure for cytotoxic T cells (CTC).

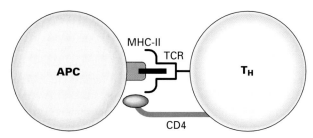

Fig. 10.5 Inhibition of T helper cell (T$_H$) activation: gp120 inhibits CD4–MHC-II and TCR–MHC-II-peptide interaction. APC, antigen-presenting cell; TCR, T-cell receptor.

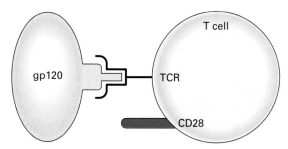

Fig. 10.6 Inactivation of T cell: gp120 has sequence homology with MHC-II and can bind to T-cell receptors (TCRs). Transmission of signal 1 without signal 2 (B7–CD28) inactivates the cell or induces apoptosis.

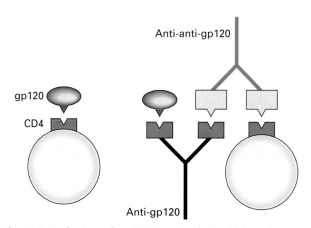

Fig. 10.7 Induction of anti-CD4 antibody. Anti-idiotypic antibody against anti-gp120 cross-reacts with CD4. Antibody-coated CD4-positive cells are destroyed by antibody-dependent complement or cellular cytotoxicity.

to MHC-II and TCR in a non-peptide-specific way, in contrast to the small number of cells activated by specific peptide. Following high-level T-cell activation, which is a hallmark of HIV infection, superantigen-activated T cells undergo apoptosis. However, HIV has not conclusively been shown to possess superantigens and this form of T helper cell destruction also remains unproved. Binding of HIV to chemokine receptors may also signal T-cell activation, viral proliferation and eventually apoptotic cell death.

Throughout the period of clinical latency there is massive infection, destruction and replacement of CD4$^+$ T cells, with billions of new cells being infected and killed every day. Ultimately the processes leading to replacement of T helper cells become exhausted, the cell number drops and immune function deteriorates. The virus may reduce replenishment of T cells from haematopoietic stem cells following infection of the bone marrow. Furthermore, destroyed CD4$^+$ cells can be replaced by CD4$^+$ or CD8$^+$ T cells with equal likelihood, so the representation of the latter gradually increases compared with the former and immune suppressor activity will come to dominate over helper activity. Virus-infected macrophages are deficient in IL-12 production and therefore cannot induce T$_H$1 responses. Instead, the dominant T$_H$2 response leads to hypergammaglobulinaemia and production of autoantibodies and B-cell lymphomas.

Newly available, highly active drug combinations interfere with virus proliferation and T-cell destruction and delay disease progression.

IMMUNITY TO PARASITES

Summary of defence mechanisms

- Protozoan parasites such as *Plasmodium* (malaria), *Leishmania* (leishmaniasis) and *Trypanosoma* (Chagas' disease, sleeping sickness) induce macrophages to release inflammatory IL-1, IL-6 and TNFα.
- Protozoa that survive within macrophages (e.g. *Trypanosoma cruzi*, *Leishmania*) can be killed following macrophage activation by T$_H$1 cells.
- IgG and IgM antibodies are effective against parasites that circulate freely in blood (e.g. *T. brucei*, plasmodium sporozoite and merozoite stages) and against parasite-infected cells that display parasite antigens on the surface. Complement activation leads to target cell lysis and opsonization for phagocytosis.
- IgE antibodies are of major importance against helminths such as *Schistosoma*, *Trichinella*, *Strongyloides* and *Wucheria*. T$_H$2 cells produce IL-4 and IL-5 in response to helminth antigens presented by B cells. Interleukin 4 stimulates switching to IgE production, while IL-5 induces eosinophilia. Immunoglobulin E binds to mast cell or basophil Fc$_\varepsilon$ receptors and cross-linking of IgE by parasite antigens leads to release of eosinophil chemotactic factor. Eosinophils attracted to the parasite release eosinophil cationic protein and major basic protein which damage the tegument of the parasite.

Parasite evasion strategies

Trypanosoma brucei possesses variant surface glycoproteins (VSG). There are several genes for different VSGs, only one of which is expressed at any given time. After antibodies have been produced against one VSG it is shed from the surface and a new VSG gene is expressed (**antigenic variation**). Leishmania cap off their surface antigens when exposed to antibody (**antigenic modulation**). Schistosomes synthesize host-like antigens such as α$_2$-macroglobulin to mask their own foreignness and also adsorb host molecules, such as red blood cell antigens, MHC antigens, complement factors and immunoglobulins, on to their surface (**antigenic disguise**).

Parasites have various immune suppressor capabilities: *Trypanosoma brucei* induces T suppressor cell activation. *Plasmodium* and *Leishmania* release soluble antigens which intercept antiparasite antibodies and saturate phagocytes. *Trypanosoma cruzi* produces molecules that inhibit or accelerate the decay of C3 convertases. *Leishmania* downregulates MHC-II expression on parasitized macrophages, reducing their ability to present antigenic peptides to CD4+ T cells. *Toxoplasma* prevents fusion of phagocytic vacuoles with lysosomes. *Leishmania* inhibits the respiratory burst of macrophages. Schistosomes release peptidases that cleave bound immunoglobulin, and other factors that inhibit T-cell proliferation, release of IFNγ and eosinophil activation.

Damage caused by immune responses to parasites

Helminths induce not only parasite-specific IgE but also polyclonal IgE, which can give rise to manifestations of allergy such as urticaria and angioedema. Sudden release of large amounts of parasite antigen can trigger fatal anaphylactic shock.

Parasite antigens that cross-react with host antigens (e.g. *T. cruzi* antigens cross-reactive with cardiac antigens) and parasites coated with host antigens can induce autoimmune attack against host tissues (cf. Fig. 10.1).

Circulating immune complexes containing parasite antigens cause some of the tissue damage seen in malaria, trypanosomiasis and schistosomiasis. Portal fibrosis and pulmonary hypertension in schistosomiasis are due to T-cell-mediated granulomatous responses to schistosome eggs.

IMMUNITY TO FUNGI

Fungal infections may be **superficial** (e.g. ringworm caused by *Trichophyton rubrum*, oral thrush and vulvovaginitis caused by *Candida albicans*), **subcutaneous** (e.g. abscesses and ulceration caused by *Sporothrix schenkii*) or **systemic** (e.g. histo-plasmosis, coccidioidomycosis, systemic candidiasis, cryptococcosis, aspergillosis).

In healthy individuals, and even in immunodeficient patients with defects in antibody production, fungal infections generally remain localized and resolve rapidly. In contrast, patients with T-cell or neutrophil defects may suffer chronic infections, indicating that these are the important effector cells in immunity to fungi.

Production of antifungal antibodies may result in IgE-mediated allergic disease, e.g. allergic bronchopulmonary aspergillosis, or IgG-mediated immune complex disease, e.g. when aspergillus grows to form an aspergilloma in pre-existing lung cavities. *Histoplasma*, *Coccidioides* and *Cryptococcus* can induce granuloma formation in the lungs.

VACCINATION

Natural infection often produces lifelong protection, with development of memory T and B cells able to respond rapidly on subsequent challenges with the same agent. Many infections cause severe clinical symptoms and even death, which could be prevented by inducing memory cells *before* exposure to pathogens occurs (Fig. 10.8).

Passive immunization

Passive transfer of maternal antibodies during pregnancy and breast-feeding provides limited protection for the newborn baby, but following catabolism of these antibodies protection is lost. Vaccination to induce memory B cells is not successful during the neonatal period because maternal antibodies neutralize vaccine antigens, although induction of memory T cells can be achieved at this time.

Short-term protection can also be achieved later in life by passive transfer of immune globulin. Immunoglobulin G antibodies decay with a half-life of about 3 weeks, so regular infusions must be given over prolonged periods to individuals at risk. Patients with humoral immune deficiencies should receive doses of 200–400 mg intravenous immunoglobulin per kilogram bodyweight every 4 weeks. Short-term passive

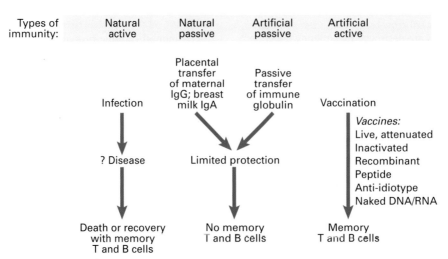

Fig. 10.8 Natural and artificial immunization.

immunization using hyperimmune globulin or monoclonal antibodies can be useful as post-exposure prophylaxis, e.g. following exposure to rabies virus.

Active immunization

Memory T and B cells can be induced most successfully using **live vaccines** containing microorganisms that have been attenuated to reduce their virulence. A single dose is usually sufficient to induce both systemic and mucosal immunity. Immunocompromised patients must not be given live vaccines because of the danger of disseminated infection.

Inactivated vaccines consist of killed whole organisms, products of organisms, or subunits of organisms. Since there is no replication of the organism to provide immune stimulation over several days, inactivated vaccines must be given in multiple doses in the presence of an **adjuvant**. The most widely used adjuvant for human vaccines is alum, which forms a precipitate with protein antigens from which the antigens are slowly released to the immune system.

Toxoids consist of bacterial exotoxins rendered harmless by treatment with formaldehyde. Antigenicity can be increased by combination with suspensions of other bacteria containing endotoxins, for example diphtheria–tetanus–pertussis triple vaccine (see also Ch. 36).

Vaccines currently available for active immunization are shown in Table 10.2, and recommended vaccination schedules in Table 10.3.

New approaches to vaccine development

Proven, effective vaccines are still not available against many of today's leading killers, notably malaria, parasitic diseases and HIV. Even the vaccines in regular use cannot be considered 100% effective. Most of them induce antibody effectively but are less able to stimulate cell-mediated immunity. It has

Table 10.2 Currently available active immunizing agents

Vaccine	Formulation
Anthrax	Inactivated *Bacillus anthracis*
BCG (tuberculosis)[a]	Live attenuated *Mycobacterium bovis*
Cholera	Inactivated *Vibrio cholerae*
Diphtheria[a]	Toxoid
Haemophilus influenzae	Capsular polysaccharide conjugated to protein
Hepatitis B virus[a]	Recombinant viral protein
Influenza[a]	Inactivated virus
Measles[a]	Live attenuated virus
Meningococcus	Capsular polysaccharide
Mumps[a]	Live attenuated virus
Pertussis	Killed whole *Bordetella pertussis*
Plague	Inactivated *Yersinia pestis*
Pneumococcus	Capsular polysaccharide of *Streptococcus pneumoniae*
Polio[a]	Inactivated or live attenuated virus
Rabies	Inactivated virus
Rubella[a]	Live attenuated virus
Tetanus[a]	Toxoid
Typhoid	Inactivated or live attenuated *Salmonella typhi*
Yellow fever	Live attenuated virus

[a] Vaccines available for dental care workers.
BCG, bacille Calmette–Guérin.

Table 10.3 Recommended immunization schedules

Age	BCG	Polio	HBV	Haem	DTP	DT	Tet	MMR	Rub	Pneu	Flu
Birth	√		√								
1 mo			√								
2–4 mo		√		√	√						
3–5 mo		√	√	√	√						
4–6 mo		√		√	√						
12 mo								√			
18 mo				√	√						
5–6 yr						√		√			
10–14 yr	√[a]					√			√		
15–18 yr		√					√[+]				
50 yr										√	
65 yr											√

[a] If negative by Mantoux skin test. [+] Repeat every 10 years.
Key: BCG, bacille Calmette–Guérin; Polio, poliomyelitis; HBV, hepatitis B virus; Haem, *Haemophilus influenzae*; DTP, diphtheria–tetanus–pertussis; DT, diphtheria–tetanus; Tet, tetanus; MMR, measles–mumps–rubella; Rub, rubella; Pneu, pneumococcus; Flu, influenza. Note: These immunization schedules are relatively standard, though minor geographic variations in policy may occur due to disease prevalence.

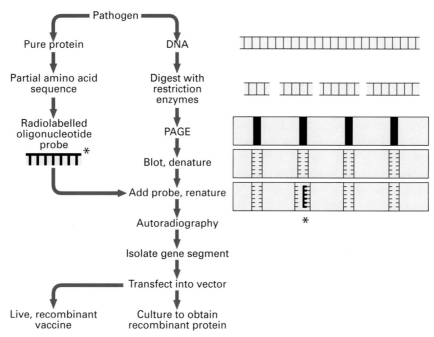

Fig. 10.9   Recombinant vaccines. PAGE, polyacrylamide gel electrophoresis.

even been suggested that current vaccines given early in life polarize cytokine production towards type 2 rather than type 1 responses and that the increasing prevalence of asthma and allergies could be partly a consequence of immunization with IL-4-inducing vaccines. However, new approaches to vaccine development promise greater control of infectious diseases in the not-too-distant future.

One way of improving the efficacy of inactivated vaccines would be to develop more effective **adjuvants**. Freund's complete adjuvant, which contains oil, detergent and mycobacteria, stimulates powerful B-cell and T-cell responses in experimental animals, but is too toxic for human use. The active principle of mycobacteria, muramyl dipeptide, strongly enhances macrophage activity, is non-toxic, and may become useful in human vaccines. Immunostimulating complexes (ISCOMs), prepared from saponin, cholesterol and phosphatidylcholine, provide a vehicle for presenting proteins to the immune system and induce T- and B-cell memory.

Inactivated vaccines made from whole microorganisms may contain proteins that stimulate both protective and non-protective — or even suppressive — immune responses. Subunit vaccines containing only protection-inducing proteins should be much more effective than cruder preparations.

Modern subunit vaccines are now being produced by **recombinant DNA technology** (Fig. 10.9). Candidate protein antigens must first be identified and purified so that a partial amino acid sequence can be determined. An oligonucleotide probe consisting of the corresponding nucleotide sequence is then constructed and labelled with radioisotope.

Next, DNA is extracted from the pathogen, digested with restriction enzymes and the DNA fragments separated by polyacrylamide gel electrophoresis (PAGE). After blotting on to nitrocellulose the DNA is denatured by heating. The probe is added and binds to its complementary sequence when the temperature is lowered, thereby identifying the relevant gene segment. Autoradiography reveals its position on the blot and the original polyacrylamide gel can be sliced to obtain the gene. This is then transfected into the DNA of suitable host cells (bacterial, yeast, insect or human). When the host cells are cultured, recombinant as well as host proteins are synthesized.

This technology is particularly useful for producing antigenic proteins from viruses that are difficult to culture, and a highly effective recombinant hepatitis B vaccine is already in routine use.

Synthetic peptide vaccines containing only relevant epitopes of the antigenic protein have also been produced and shown to be effective in animal models. In theory it should be possible to construct vaccines containing both B-cell and T-cell epitopes on a carrier molecule such as poly-L-lysine. For pathogens that undergo antigenic variation, notably HIV, it might be possible to construct peptide vaccines containing sufficiently large arrays of peptides to protect against most variants of the pathogen.

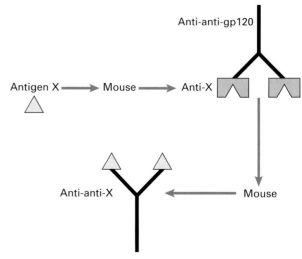

Fig. 10.10   Anti-idiotype vaccines.

Live recombinant vaccines also hold considerable promise. Gene segments coding for pathogen proteins can be inserted into attenuated vectors such as vaccinia, BCG or adenovirus. Immunizing pathogen proteins are released during the time the vector replicates in the host. Live, replication-incompetent microorganisms can be engineered for use as vaccines by removing some of the genes involved in replication, though later reversion to full pathogenicity would be difficult to rule out.

Anti-idiotypic antibodies can be used as vaccines instead of pathogen proteins. The protein antigen (X) is used to raise monoclonal antibodies in mice; V regions of anti-X are then used to immunize a second mouse. The resultant monoclonal anti-anti-X has similar antigenic properties to X itself (Fig. 10.10). By isolating the V genes from the hybridoma producing anti-anti-X, anti-idiotypic vaccines can be produced using recombinant DNA technology.

Recent progress in production of **genetic vaccines** using RNA or DNA coding for specific pathogen proteins has been encouraging. When injected intramuscularly, the genetic information remains unintegrated in muscle cells but gives long-term expression of properly folded and glycosylated immunogenic protein and strong cell-mediated, as well as humoral, immunity. In mice, DNA vaccines have been shown to induce protective cell-mediated immunity against leishmaniasis, tuberculosis and malaria. A trial of a DNA vaccine against malaria in humans showed induction of malaria-specific cytotoxic T cells. An oral DNA vaccine containing the gene for peanut allergen protected mice against rapidly fatal peanut-induced anaphylaxis, indicating that DNA vaccines could protect against IL-4-induced allergic disease by inducing IFNγ.

KEY FACTS

- Infectious diseases are responsible for 30% of the world's disease burden
- AIDS, caused by HIV, is responsible for 5% of the world's disease burden
- All of the immunological mechanisms described in the previous two chapters are involved in defence against pathogens
- Microorganisms have developed various strategies to avoid host defences
- The immune response against pathogens may secondarily cause damage to host tissues
- Natural infection may produce lifelong protection against reinfection with the same pathogen, with induction of memory T and B lymphocytes

- Some, but by no means all, infectious diseases can be prevented by vaccination in childhood with live attenuated or inactivated pathogens or their products
- Currently available vaccines are better at inducing type 2 rather than type 1 cytokines, and hence induce humoral immunity but often little cell-mediated immunity
- New approaches are required to produce stronger vaccines against today's leading killer infections. Genetic vaccines appear to offer promise in this regard, inducing powerful cell-mediated as well as humoral immune responses in animal and human studies

FURTHER READING

Janeway, CA Jr, Travers, P, Hunt, S, and Walport, M (1999). *Immunobiology* (4th edn). Current Biology Ltd, Churchill Livingstone, Gorland Publishing Inc., London.

Mims, C, Playfair, J, Roitt, I, Wakelin, D, and Williams, R (1998). Vaccination. In *Medical microbiology* (2nd edn), Ch. 15. Mosby Year Book, St Louis.

Powell, MF, and Newman, HJ (eds) (1995). *Vaccine design*. Plenum, New York.

Roitt, IM (1997). *Roitt's Essential immunology* (9th edn). Blackwell, Oxford.

Roitt, I, Brostoff, J, and Male, D (1997). Vaccination. In *Immunology* (5th edn), Ch. 19. Mosby, London.

Salisbury, DM, and Begg, NT (1996). *Immunisation against infectious disease*. HMSO, London.

Microbes of relevance to dentistry

This section outlines the characteristic features of important microbes that are particularly relevant to dentistry. The information given here relates intimately to the diseases described in the rest of the book: the chapters in this section should therefore be reviewed in conjunction with those on systemic and oral diseases in Parts 4 and 5.

- Streptococci, staphylococci and micrococci
- Lactobacilli, corynebacteria and propionibacteria
- Actinomycetes, clostridia and *Bacillus* species
- Neisseriae, *Veillonella*, parvobacteria and *Capnocytophaga*
- Enterobacteria
- Vibrios, campylobacters and *Wolinella*
- *Bacteroides*, *Porphyromonas* and *Prevotella*
- Fusobacteria, *Leptotrichia* and spirochaetes
- Mycobacteria and legionellae
- Chlamydiae, rickettsiae and mycoplasmas
- Viruses of relevance to dentistry
- Fungi of relevance to dentistry

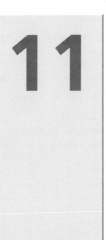

11 Streptococci, staphylococci and micrococci

Streptococci comprise a diverse group of Gram-positive cocci which continuously undergo taxonomic revision. They are distributed widely in humans and animals, mostly forming part of their normal flora. A few species cause significant human morbidity. The **oral streptococci**, which include the cariogenic *mutans* group, are important members of the genus. Another common group of cocci, the **staphylococci**, live on the skin but are infrequently isolated from the oral cavity and are significant agents of many pyogenic (pus-producing) human infections.

STREPTOCOCCI

General properties

Characteristics

Catalase-negative, Gram-positive spherical or oval cocci in pairs and chains; 0.7–0.9 μm in diameter. Chain formation is best seen in liquid cultures or pus.

Culture

These cocci grow well on blood agar, although enrichment of media with glucose and serum may be necessary. Typical haemolytic reactions are produced on blood agar (Fig. 11.1):
- **α-haemolysis**: narrow zone of partial haemolysis and green (viridans) discoloration around the colony, e.g. viridans streptococci
- **β-haemolysis**: wide, clear, translucent zone of complete haemolysis around the colony, e.g. *Streptococcus pyogenes*
- **no haemolysis** (γ-haemolysis), e.g. non-haemolytic streptococci.

Serology

The carbohydrate antigens found on the cell walls of the organisms are related to their virulence. Hence serogrouping, termed Lancefield grouping, is useful in identification of the more virulent β-haemolytic species. Currently 20 Lancefield groups are recognized (A–H and K–V) but not all are equally important as human pathogens. The following are worthy of note:
- **group A** includes the important human pathogen *Streptococcus pyogenes*

- **group B** contains one species, *S. agalactiae*, an inhabitant of the female genital tract; it causes infection in neonates
- **group C** mainly causes diseases in animals
- **group D** includes the enterococci (*S. faecalis*, etc.) and ranks next to group A in causing human disease.

Streptococcus pyogenes (group A)

Habitat and transmission

The normal habitat of this species is the human upper respiratory tract and skin; it may survive in dust for some time. Spread is by airborne droplets and by contact.

Characteristics

Found as a commensal in the nasopharynx of a minority of healthy adults, but more commonly (about 10%) in children. Grows well on blood agar, with a characteristic halo of β-haemolysis. Some strains produce mucoid colonies as a result of having a hyaluronic acid capsule. This may contribute to virulence by offering resistance to phagocytosis.

Exotoxins and enzymes. Produces a large number of biologically active substances, such as:
- **streptokinase**: a proteolytic enzyme which lyses fibrin
- **hyaluronidase**: attacks the material that binds the connective tissue, thereby causing increasing permeability (hence called the 'spreading factor')
- **DNAases** (streptodornases): destroy cellular DNA
- **haemolysins** (streptolysins, leucocidins): phage-mediated and are responsible for the characteristic erythematous rash in scarlet fever.

(*Note*: not all these products are produced by every strain; the combined action of enzymes and toxins contribute to the pathogenicity.)

Culture and identification

Culture on blood agar yields characteristic β-haemolytic colonies (lysis of blood due to streptolysins O and S). A Gram-stained smear may show characteristic cocci in chains (Fig. 11.2); these are more developed in liquid than in solid media. The isolate can be presumptively identified as *Streptococcus pyogenes* if it is sensitive to bacitracin.

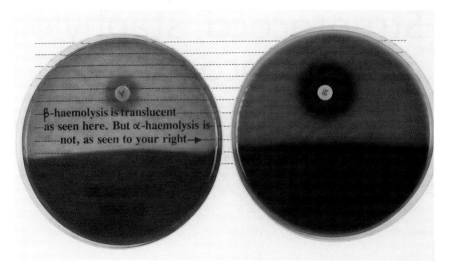

Fig. 11.1 Alpha- and beta-haemolysis: β-haemolytic colonies (e.g. *Streptococcus pyogenes*) produce complete translucence of blood agar, whereas α-haemolytic colonies (e.g. *Streptococcus pneumoniae*) do not. Note also the sensitivity of *S. pneumoniae* to a disc impregnated with optochin.

If rheumatic fever is suspected, then testing the patient's antistreptolysin O (ASO) antibody titre will demonstrate previous exposure to *S. pyogenes*.

Pathogenicity

Streptococcus pyogenes causes a number of infections; the most notable are:
- tonsillitis and pharyngitis
- peritonsillar abscess (now rare)
- scarlet fever
- mastoiditis and sinusitis
- otitis media (middle-ear infection)

- wound infections leading to cellulitis and lymphangitis
- impetigo (a skin infection).

Complications. After an episode of infection some patients develop complications, such as rheumatic fever, glomerulonephritis and erythema nodosum, which may have long-lasting effects. Note that:
- in cellulitis, hyaluronidase ('spreading factor') mediates the subcutaneous spread of infection
- erythrogenic toxin causes the rash of scarlet fever
- post-streptococcal infection, manifesting as rheumatic fever, is caused by immunological cross-reaction between

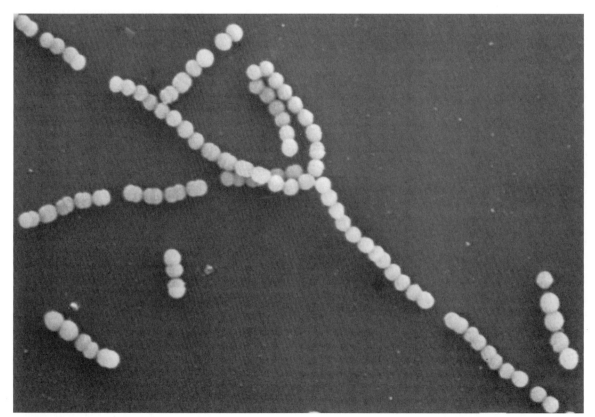

Fig. 11.2 Scanning electron micrograph of a chain of streptococci.

bacterial antigen and human heart tissue, and acute glomerulonephritis is caused by immune complexes bound to glomeruli (see Ch. 23).

Treatment and prevention

Penicillin is the drug of choice; erythromycin is suitable for patients hypersensitive to penicillin. No vaccine is available.

Streptococcus agalactiae (group B)

This species is increasingly recognized as a human pathogen, especially as a cause of neonatal meningitis and sepsis.

Habitat and transmission

Found in the human vagina; sometimes anorectal carriage occurs. Babies acquire infection from the colonized mother during delivery or during nursing.

Characteristics

Gram-positive cocci in chains.

Culture and identification

Gram-stained smear and culture yielding β-haemolytic colonies on blood agar; colonies on blood agar are generally larger than *S. pyogenes*. Lancefield group is determined by antiserum against cell-wall polysaccharide.

Pathogenicity

No toxins or virulence factors have been identified. This species causes neonatal meningitis and septicaemia; it is also associated with septic abortion and gynaecological sepsis.

Treatment and prevention

Penicillin is the drug of choice; erythromycin is suitable for patients hypersensitive to penicillin. Prophylactic antibiotics may be given to neonates if the mother is culture-positive.

Oral streptococci

Oral streptococci, which live principally in the oropharynx, are a mixed group of organisms with variable characteristics.

Table 11.1 Some recognized species of oral streptococci

Group	Species
mutans group	S. mutans, serotypes c, e, f S. sobrinus, serotypes d, g S. cricetus, serotype a S. rattus, serotype b and others
salivarius group	S. salivarius S. vestibularis
anginosus group	S. constellatus S. intermedius S. anginosus
mitis group	S. sanguis S. gordonii S. parasanguis S. oralis and others

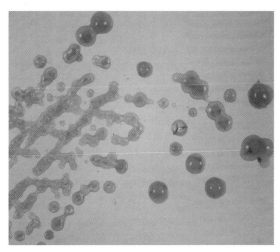

Fig. 11.3 Gelatinous colonies of *mutans* streptococci mainly comprising extracellular polysaccharides.

Together with the application of new typing techniques, particularly those based on molecular biology, this means that the nomenclature of oral streptococci is in a constant state of flux. They typically show α-haemolysis on blood agar, but this is not a constant feature as some strains are non-haemolytic and others β-haemolytic. Oral streptococci can be divided into four main 'species groups' as follows:

- *mutans* group
- *salivarius* group
- *anginosus* group
- *mitis* group.

Each of these groups comprises a number of species (Table 11.1).

Habitat and transmission

Streptococci make up a large proportion of the resident oral flora. It is known that roughly one-quarter of the total cultivable flora from supragingival and gingival plaque and half of the isolates from the tongue and saliva are streptococci. They are vertically transmitted from mother to child. Infective endocarditis caused by these organisms (loosely termed viridans streptococci) is generally a result of their entry into the bloodstream during intraoral surgical procedures (e.g. tooth extraction), and sometimes even during tooth brushing.

Culture and identification

Gram-positive cocci in chains; α-haemolytic; catalase-negative. Growth not inhibited by bile or optochin (ethylhydrocupreine hydrochloride), in contrast to pneumococci. Commercially available kits are highly useful in laboratory identification of these organisms.

Pathogenicity

The *mutans* group of streptococci are the major agents of dental caries (but in the absence of predisposing factors, such as sucrose, they cannot cause caries). They have a characteristic ability to produce voluminous amounts of sticky, extracellular polysaccharides in the presence of dietary carbohydrates (Fig. 11.3); these help tenacious binding of the organisms to enamel and to each other.

They are also important agents of infective endocarditis and some 60% of cases are due to this organism. Usually bacteria released during dental procedures settle on damaged heart valves, causing infective endocarditis (see Ch. 24).

Treatment and prevention

In patients at risk of infective endocarditis (e.g. those with damaged or prosthetic heart valves), prophylactic antibiotic cover should always be given before dental procedures (see Ch. 24).

See Chapter 32 for caries.

Streptococcus mutans

Streptococcus mutans gained notoriety in the 1960s when it was demonstrated that caries could be experimentally induced and transmitted in animals by oral inoculation with the organism. The name 'mutans' results from its frequent transition from coccal phase to coccobacillary phase. Currently seven distinct species of human and animal *mutans* streptococci and eight serotypes (*a–h*) are recognized, based on the antigenic specificity of cell-wall carbohydrates. The term *Streptococcus mutans* is limited to human isolates belonging to three serotypes (*c, e* and *f*).

Other oral streptococci

A group of oral organisms previously classified as **nutritionally variant streptococci** (*S. adjacens, S. defectivus*) and isolated under appropriate environmental conditions have been assigned to a new genus called *Abiotrophia*. Their role in oral disease is not well characterized.

Streptococcus pneumoniae (pneumococcus)

This organism causes a number of common diseases, such as pneumonia and meningitis in adults and otitis media and sinusitis in children.

Habitat and transmission

A normal commensal in the human upper respiratory tract; up to 4% of the population carry this bacteria in small numbers. Transmission is via respiratory droplets.

Characteristics

Gram-positive 'lancet-shaped' cocci in pairs (diplococci) or short chains; cells are often capsulate; α-haemolytic on blood agar; catalase-negative; facultative anaerobe (i.e. grows under both aerobic and anaerobic conditions).

Culture and identification

Forms α-haemolytic colonies. After incubation for 2 days the colonies appear typically as 'draughtsmen' because of their central indentation (a result of spontaneous autolysis of older bacteria in the centre of the colony). The species is differentiated from other α-haemolytic streptococci by its sensitivity to optochin and solubility in bile (Fig. 11.1). Observation for the capsular swelling with type-specific antiserum (quellung reaction) confirms the identity and is the standard reference method. The latex agglutination test (see Fig. 6.7) for capsular antigen in spinal fluid can be diagnostic.

Pathogenicity

Although no exotoxins are known, this organism induces an inflammatory response. The substantive polysaccharide capsule retards phagocytosis. Vaccination with antipolysaccharide vaccine helps provide type-specific immunity. Viral respiratory infection predisposes to pneumococcal pneumonia by damaging the mucociliary lining of the upper respiratory tract (the mucociliary escalator). Other common diseases caused by pneumococci include lobar pneumonia, acute exacerbation of chronic bronchitis, otitis media, sinusitis, conjunctivitis, meningitis and, in splenectomized patients, septicaemia.

Treatment and prevention

Penicillin or erythromycin is very effective. However, resistance to penicillin is rapidly emerging as a global concern.

Gram-positive anaerobic cocci

Gram-positive anaerobic cocci (GPAC), currently belonging to the genus *Peptostreptococcus*, can often be isolated from dental plaque and the female genital tract. They are also found in carious dentine, subgingival plaque, dentoalveolar abscesses and in advanced periodontal disease, usually in mixed culture. Their pathogenic role is still unclear. The representative species belong to *P. anaerobius, P. magnus* and *P. micros*. There are moves afoot to revise the nomenclature of these organisms, hence the description GPAC is used here.

STAPHYLOCOCCI

Staphylococci too are Gram-positive cocci, but unlike the chains of streptococci, they are arranged in characteristic grape-like clusters. The *Staphylococcus* genus contains more than 15 different species, of which the following are of medical importance: *S. aureus, S. epidermidis* and *S. saprophyticus*.

Staphylococci cause a variety of both common and uncommon infections, such as abscesses of many organs, endocarditis, gastroenteritis (food poisoning) and toxic shock syndrome. They are infrequently isolated from the oral cavity. Higher proportions of *S. aureus* are found in the saliva of healthy subjects older than 70 years.

Staphylococcus aureus

Habitat and transmission

The habitat is the human skin, especially the anterior nares and the perineum. Domesticated animals also carry staphylococci. Higher carriage rates are seen in hospital patients and staff. These bacteria are disseminated through air and dust and are always present in the hospital environment. The usual transmission route is via the hands.

Characteristics

Gram-positive cocci in clusters (cluster formation is due to their ability to divide in many planes); non-sporing, non-motile; some strains are capsulate.

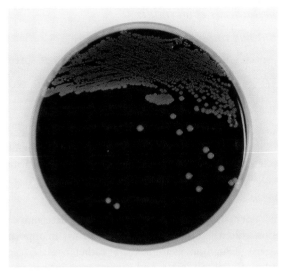

Fig. 11.4 Golden-yellow colonies of *Staphylococcus aureus*.

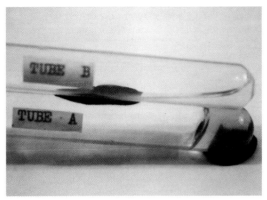

Fig. 11.5 A positive tube coagulase test (tube A).

Culture and identification

Grows aerobically as yellow or gold colonies on blood agar (Fig. 11.4); catalase-positive (this differentiates them from the catalase-negative streptococci).

Other tests used to differentiate the more virulent *S. aureus* from the less pathogenic *S. epidermidis* include the following.

Coagulase test. *Staphylococcus aureus* coagulates dilute human serum or rabbit plasma (i.e. it is coagulase-positive), whereas *S. epidermidis* does not (coagulase-negative). This test could be done either in a test tube (the tube test), which requires overnight incubation (Fig. 11.5), or on a slide (the slide test), which is a rapid test.

Protein A — latex agglutination test. Protein A, synthesized by almost all strains of *S. aureus*, has a special affinity to the Fc fragment of immunoglobulin G (IgG). Hence when latex particles coated with IgG (and fibrinogen) are mixed with an emulsified suspension of *S. aureus* on a glass slide, visible agglutination of the latex particles occurs; no such reaction is seen with *S. epidermidis* (Fig. 11.6).

Other tests. These include the phosphatase test, DNAase test and mannitol fermentation test (most strains of *S. aureus* form acid from mannitol, while few *S. epidermidis* do so).

Typing of Staphylococcus aureus

Typing is important to determine the source of an outbreak of infection. This is commonly done by the pattern of susceptibility to a set of more than 20 bacteriophages — **phage typing**. The bacteria can also be serotyped using surface antigenic characteristics; this is not commonly used.

Pathogenicity

A variety of enzymes and toxins are produced by *Staphylococcus aureus*, although no one strain produces the whole range listed in Table 11.2. The two most important are coagulase and enterotoxin. Coagulase is the best correlate of pathogenicity. Some of the diseases caused by *S. aureus* are:

● superficial infections: common agent of boils, carbuncles, pustules, abscesses, conjunctivitis and wound infections; rarely causes oral infections; may cause angular cheilitis (together with the yeast *Candida*) at the angles of the mouth
● food poisoning (vomiting and diarrhoea) caused by enterotoxins
● toxic shock syndrome, also caused by an enterotoxin

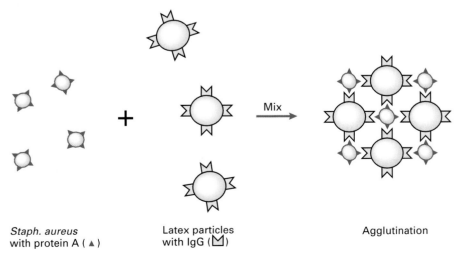

Staph. aureus
with protein A (▲)

Latex particles
with IgG (Ⓜ)

Agglutination

Fig. 11.6 Identification of *Staphylococcus aureus*. Protein A of *S. aureus* has a special affinity for IgG; when latex particles coated with IgG are mixed with a suspension of the organism, visible agglutination of latex particles occurs.

Table 11.2 Toxins and enzymes produced by *Staphylococcus aureus*

Toxin/enzyme	Activity
Toxins	
Cytotoxins (α, β, γ, δ)	Cell lysis
Leucocidin	Kills leucocytes
Epidermolytic toxin	Exfoliation and splitting of epidermis
Toxic shock syndrome toxin	Shock, rash, desquamation
Enterotoxin (A–E)	Induces vomiting and diarrhoea
Enzymes	
Coagulase	Clots plasma
Catalase	Affects bactericidal activity of polymorphs
Hyaluronidase	Connective tissue breakdown
DNAase (nuclease)	DNA hydrolysis
Lipase	Breaks lipids of cell membranes
Penicillinase	Breaks down β-lactam drugs
Protein A	Antiphagocytic

- deep infections; osteomyelitis, endocarditis, septicaemia, pneumonia.

Predisposing factors for infection are minor and major breaks in the skin, foreign bodies such as sutures, low neutrophil levels, and injecting drug abuse.

Treatment and prevention

The vast majority (> 80%) of strains are resistant to β-lactam drugs, and some to a number of antibiotics. The latter phenomenon (**multiresistance**) is common, particularly in strains isolated from hospitals; these cause hospital (**nosocomial**) infection. Penicillin resistance is due to the production of β-lactamase encoded by plasmids. The enzyme destroys the efficacy of antibiotics with a β-lactam ring (i.e. the penicillin group drugs).

Antibiotics active against *Staphylococcus aureus* include penicillin for sensitive isolates, flucloxacillin (stable against β-lactamase), erythromycin, fusidic acid (useful for skin infections), cephalosporins and vancomycin.

Cleanliness, hand-washing and aseptic management of lesions reduce the spread of staphylococci.

Staphylococcus epidermidis

Habitat and transmission

This species is found on the skin surface, and is spread by contact.

Culture and identification

Grows as white colonies on blood agar, hence the earlier name *S. albus*; catalase-positive; coagulase-negative; biochemically characterized by commercially available kits (e.g. APIStaph).

Pathogenicity

Being a normal commensal of the skin, this bacterium causes infection only when an opportunity arises (it is an opportunist pathogen). Common examples are catheter-related sepsis, infection of artificial joints, and urinary tract infections.

Treatment

Staphylococcus epidermidis exhibits resistance to a number of drugs (multiresistance), including penicillin and methicillin. It is sensitive to vancomycin.

Staphylococcus saprophyticus

This organism causes urinary tract infections in women, an infection especially associated with intercourse. It has the ability to colonize the periurethral skin and the mucosa. The organism can be differentiated from *S. epidermidis* (both grow as white colonies on blood agar) by the mannitol fermentation reaction and other biochemical tests.

MICROCOCCI

Micrococci are catalase-positive organisms similar to staphylococci. They are coagulase-negative and usually grow as white colonies on blood agar, although some species are brightly pigmented — pink, orange or yellow.

Stomatococcus mucilagenosus, formerly classified in the genus *Micrococcus*, is found in abundance on the lingual surface. This species has the ability to produce an extracellular slime which correlates with its predilection for the lingual surface. Its role in disease, if any, is unknown.

KEY FACTS

- **Streptococci are Gram-positive** and appear as **spherical** or oval cocci in **chains and pairs**
- Streptococci can be **classifed** according to (i) the **degree of haemolysis** on blood agar (α, mild; β, complete; γ, no haemolysis) and (ii) the cell-wall carbohydrate antigens into **Lancefield groups** (20)
- *Lancefield group A contains the important human pathogen Streptococcus pyogenes; the latter infection leads to rheumatic fever and rheumatic carditis which makes the endocardium susceptible to future episodes of infection*
- **Oral streptococci** are a **mixed group** of organisms and typically show α-**haemolysis** on blood agar

- *Oral streptococci can be divided into four main 'species groups' and of these the mutans group bacteria are the major agents of dental caries*
- **Staphylococci** resemble streptococci in appearance but are arranged in **grape-like clusters** and are all **catalase-positive** (all streptococci are catalase-negative)
- **Staphylococcus aureus** *is a common pathogen causing localized skin infections and serious systemic infections; it produces numerous toxins and enzymes as virulence factors*

FURTHER READING

Beighton, D, Hardie, J, and Whiley, RA (1991). A scheme for the identification of viridans streptococci. *Journal of Medical Microbiology* 35, 367–372.

Greenwood, D, Slack, R, and Peutherer, J (eds) (1997). *Medical microbiology* (15th edn), Chs 15–17. Churchill Livingstone, Edinburgh.

Jone, D, Board, RG, and Sussman, M (1990). *Staphylococci*. Society for Applied Microbiology Symposium Series, no. 19. Blackwell Scientific, Oxford.

Murdoch, DA (1993). Gram-positive anaerobic cocci. *Clinical Microbiology Reviews* 11, 81–120.

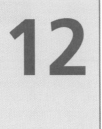

12 Lactobacilli, corynebacteria and propionibacteria

LACTOBACILLI

Lactobacilli are saprophytes in vegetable and animal material (e.g. milk). Some species are common animal and human commensals inhabiting the oral cavity and other parts of the body. They have the ability to tolerate acidic environments and hence are believed to be associated with the carious process.

The taxonomy of lactobacilli is complex. They are characterized into two main groups: **homofermenters**, which produce mainly lactic acid (65%) from glucose fermentation (e.g. *Lactobacillus casei*), and **heterofermenters**, which produce lactic acid as well as acetate, ethanol and carbon dioxide (e.g. *L. fermentum*). *Lactobacillus casei* and *L. rhamnosus*, *L. acidophilus* and the newly described species, *L. oris*, are common in the oral cavity. It should be noted that the taxonomy of lactobacilli is under constant revision.

Habitat and transmission

Lactobacilli are found in the oral cavity, gastrointestinal tract and female genital tract. In the oral cavity they constitute less than 1% of the total flora. Transmission routes are unknown.

Characteristics

These organisms ferment carbohydrates to form acids (i.e. they are **acidogenic**) and can survive well in acidic milieu (they are **aciduric**); they may be homofermentative or heterofermentative. The question as to whether they are present in carious lesions because they prefer the acidic environment, or whether they generate an acidic milieu and destroy the tooth enamel, has been debated for years (the classic 'chicken and egg' argument).

Culture and identification

Lactobacilli grow under microaerophilic conditions in the presence of carbon dioxide and at acidic pH (6.0). Media enriched with glucose or blood promote growth. A special selective medium, tomato juice agar (pH 5.0), promotes the growth of lactobacilli while suppressing other bacteria. Identification is by biochemical reactions.

Pathogenicity

Lactobacilli are frequently isolated from deep carious lesions where the pH tends to be acidic. Indeed, early workers believed that lactobacilli were the main cariogenic agent (a theory that has been disproved), so much so that the number of lactobacilli in saliva (the **lactobacillus count**) was taken as an indication of an individual's caries activity. Although this test is not very reliable, it is useful for monitoring the dietary profile of a patient because the level of lactobacilli correlates well with the intake of dietary carbohydrate.

CORYNEBACTERIA

The genus *Corynebacterium* contains many species which are widely distributed in nature. These Gram-positive bacilli demonstrate pleomorphism (i.e. coccobacillary appearance) and are non-sporing, non-capsulate and non-motile. In common with *Mycobacterium* and *Nocardia* spp., they have a cell-wall structure containing mycolic acid. A number of species are important human pathogens and commensals. The sometimes fatal upper respiratory tract infection of childhood diphtheria, is caused by *Corynebacterium diphtheriae*. It is important to distinguish this, and other pathogens within the genus, from commensal corynebacteria.

Corynebacterium diphtheriae

Habitat and transmission

Human throat and nose, occasionally skin; patients carry toxigenic organisms up to 3 months after infection. Transmission is via respiratory droplets.

Characteristics

Pleomorphic, Gram-positive, club-shaped (tapered at one end) bacilli, 2–5 μm in length, arranged in palisades. They divide by 'snapping fission' and hence are arranged at angles to each other, resembling Chinese characters. The rods have a beaded appearance, with the beads comprising an intracellular store of polymerized phosphate. The granules stain **metachromatically** with special stains such as Neisser methylene blue stain (i.e. the cells are stained with blue and the granules in red).

Culture and identification

A non-fastidious, facultative anaerobe which grows well at 37°C. Grows on blood agar but selective media are helpful for isolation from clinical specimens. In blood tellurite agar, commonly used for this purpose, corynebacteria produce distinctive grey-black colonies after 48 hours' incubation at 35°C. Preliminary identification is helped by the shape and size of the colonies on tellurite agar. Specific identification is by biochemical reactions and demonstration of toxin production.

The test for toxin production is important as some corynebacteria are non-toxigenic (and hence non-virulent) and are normal skin or throat commensals. Methods such as phage typing and bacteriocin typing are used for detection of the source of infection in epidemiological studies of outbreaks of diphtheria.

Toxin production

The exotoxin responsible for virulence can be demonstrated either by a gel precipitation test or guinea-pig inoculation (not popular). The gel precipitation test uses the **Elek plate**. In this test a filter paper soaked in diphtheria antitoxin is incorporated into serum agar before it has set; the test strain of *C. diphtheriae* under investigation is then streaked on to the agar at right angles to the filter-paper strip and incubated at 37°C. After 24 hours white lines of precipitation will be visible as a result of the combination of the antitoxin and the antigen (i.e. the toxin) if the strain is a toxigenic isolate (Fig. 12.1).

Diphtheria toxin. This exotoxin — produced by strains carrying bacteriophages with the *tox* gene — inhibits protein biosynthesis in all eukaryotic cells. The toxin has two components: subunit A, which has the ADP ribosylating activity, and subunit B, which binds the toxin to cell surface receptors. Essentially the toxin blocks protein synthesis of host cells by inactivating an elongation factor.

Macroscopically, its action on the respiratory mucosa results in the production of a grey, adherent pseudomembrane comprising bacteria, fibrin and epithelial and phagocytic cells. This may obstruct the airway and the patient may die of asphyxiation. When the toxin permeates into the bloodstream it acts systemically, affecting motor nerves of the myocardium and the nervous system.

The toxin can be converted to a **toxoid** (i.e. made non-toxic but still antigenic) by treatment with formaldehyde; the toxoid can then be used for prophylactic immunization — the first component of the DTP (diphtheria–tetanus–pertussis) vaccine.

Antitoxin, produced by injecting the toxin into horses, neutralizes the toxin (see below).

Pathogenicity

Corynebacterium diphtheriae is the agent of diphtheria; it usually affects the mucosa of the upper respiratory tract, and sometimes the skin. Cutaneous infections are especially seen in the tropics and are usually mixed infections with *Staphylococcus aureus* and/or *Streptococcus pyogenes*. Serious systemic manifestations are the result of the absorption of the exotoxin.

Treatment and prevention

In the acute phase, supportive therapy to maintain the airway is critical. Antitoxin is given to neutralize the toxin and penicillin to kill the organisms. Antibiotics have little effect once the toxin has spread, but will eliminate the toxigenic focus of bacteria. In epidemic outbreaks carriers are given either penicillin or erythromycin.

Immunization is highly effective in preventing diphtheria. A special test (**the Schick test**) is used to demonstrate immunity. Here, the circulating level of antibody after immunization (or clinical/subclinical infection) is assessed by inoculating a standardized dose of the toxin.

Other corynebacteria

Corynebacterium ulcerans is responsible for diphtheria-like throat lesions, but it does not cause toxaemia.

Corynebacterium (formerly *Bacterionema*) *matruchotti* is the only true coryneform organism in the oral cavity. It resembles a whip ('whip-handle cell'), with a short, fat body and a long filament at one end.

Diphtheroids

Bacilli that morphologically resemble diphtheria bacilli are called diphtheroids (e.g. *Corynebacterium hofmannii*, *C. xerosis*). They are normal inhabitants of the skin and conjunctiva and are occasional opportunistic pathogens in compromised patients (e.g. endocarditis in prosthetic valves).

PROPIONIBACTERIA

Propionibacteria are obligate anaerobic, Gram-positive rods, sometimes called 'diphtheroids' for the reasons given above. *Propionibacterium acnes* is part of the normal skin flora and may also be isolated from dental plaque. The pathogenesis of facial acne is closely related to the lipases produced by *P. acnes*, hence the name.

A new member of this genus is *P. propionica* (formerly *Arachnia propionica*), morphologically similar to *Actinomyces israelii* (except for the production of propionic acid from glucose by the former).

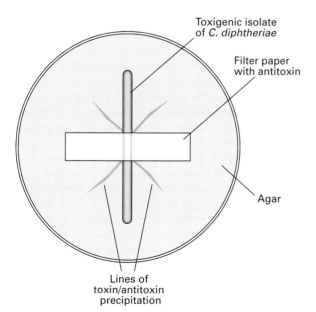

Fig. 12.1 Elek test for toxin-producing *Corynebacterium diphtheriae*. A filter paper impregnated with diphtheria antitoxin is incorporated into agar and the unknown (test) and the known (control) toxin-producing *C. diphtheriae* are streaked at right angles; after 24 hours' incubation white lines of precipitation are produced due to the combination of the antigen (toxin) and the antibody.

KEY FACTS

- Lactobacilli are **acidogenic** and **aciduric**
- Lactobacilli are common constituents of oral flora and are regular isolates from **dentinal caries lesions**
- *The numbers of lactobacilli in saliva correlate positively with caries activity*
- *Toxigenic strains of* Corynebacterium diphtheriae *are responsible for diphtheria, the sometimes fatal upper respiratory tract infection of childhood*

- *The diphtheria toxin is toxoidable, and is a component of the triple (DTP) vaccine*
- *Propionibacterium acnes* (loosely termed **'diphtheroids'**) is a significant component of the normal skin flora

FURTHER READING

Christie, AN (1987). *Infectious diseases* (4th edn), vol. 2, pp. 1183–1209. Churchill Livingstone, Edinburgh.

Greenwood, D, Slack, R, and Peutherer, J (eds) (1997). *Medical microbiology* (15th edn), Ch. 18. Churchill Livingstone, Edinburgh.

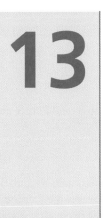

13 Actinomycetes, clostridia and *Bacillus* species

Actinomycetes, which were formally thought to be fungi, are true bacteria with long, branching filaments analogous to fungal hyphae. The two important genera of this group are *Actinomyces* and *Nocardia*. The chemical structure of the cell wall of these organisms is similar to that of corynebacteria and mycobacteria, and some are acid-fast. *Actinomyces* spp. are microaerophilic or anaerobic; *Nocardia* spp. are aerobic organisms.

Actinomyces spp.

Although most *Actinomyces* are soil organisms, the potentially pathogenic species are commensals of the mouth in humans and animals. They are a major component of dental plaque, particularly at approximal sites of teeth, and are known to increase in numbers in gingivitis. An association between root surface caries of teeth and *Actinomyces* has been described. Other sites colonized are the female genital tract and the tonsillar crypts.

A number of *Actinomyces* species are isolated from the oral cavity. These include *A. israelii*, *A. gerencseriae*, *A. odontolyticus*, *A. naeslundii* (genospecies 1 and 2), *A. myeri* and *A. georgiae*. A close relationship between *A. odontolyticus* and earliest stages of enamel demineralization, and the progression of small caries lesions have been reported. The most important human pathogen is *A. israelii*.

Actinomyces israelii

Habitat and transmission

This organism is a commensal of the mouth and possibly of the female genital tract. It is a major agent of human actinomycosis.

Characteristics

Gram-positive filamentous branching rods. Non-motile, non-sporing and non-acid-fast. Clumps of the organisms can be seen as yellowish 'sulphur granules' in pus discharging from sinus tracts; or the granules can be squeezed out of the lesions. (Strains belonging to *A. israelii* serotype II are now in a separate species, *A. gerencseriae*, a common but minor component of healthy gingival flora.)

Culture and identification

Grows slowly under anaerobic conditions, on blood or serum glucose agar at 37°C. After about a week it appears as small, creamy-white, adherent colonies on blood agar. The colonies resemble breadcrumbs or the surface of 'molar' teeth (Fig. 13.1). Because of the exacting growth requirements and the relatively slow growth, isolating this organism from clinical specimens is difficult, particularly because the other, faster-growing bacteria in pus specimens tend to obscure the slow-growing actinomycetes. 'Sulphur granules' in lesions are a clue to their presence. When possible, these granules should be crushed, Gram-stained and observed for Gram-positive, branching filaments, and also cultured in preference to pus.

Pathogenicity

Most (70–80%) actinomycotic infections are chronic, granulomatous, endogenous infections of the orofacial region (Fig. 13.2). Typically the lesions present as a chronic abscess, commonly at the angle of the lower jaw, with multiple external sinuses. There is usually a history of trauma such as a tooth extraction or a blow to the jaw. Actinomycetes are also isolated from infections associated with intrauterine devices, but their pathogenic role is unclear.

While the majority of the lesions (60–65%) are in the cervicofacial region, some 10–20% are abdominal (usually ileocaecal) and others are in the lung (thoracic). Although most infections are **monomicrobial** in nature (i.e. with *Actinomyces* alone causing the disease), a significant proportion of infections could be **polymicrobial**, with other bacteria such as *Actinobacillus actinomycetemcomitans*, *Haemophilus* spp. and anaerobes acting as co-infecting agents.

Treatment and prevention

Sensitive to penicillin, but prolonged courses up to 6 weeks are necessary for chronic infections. Oral penicillins such as amoxicillin (amoxycillin) are now popular. Recalcitrant lesions respond well to tetracycline because of its good bone penetration. Surgical intervention may be necessary in chronic jaw lesions.

Prevention of these infections is difficult because of their endogenous nature.

Nocardia

Nocardia species are soil saprophytes and cause nocardiosis in humans, especially in immunocompromised patients. These

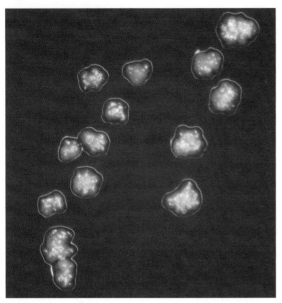

Fig. 13.1 Molar tooth-shaped colonies of *Actinomyces israelii*, on blood agar.

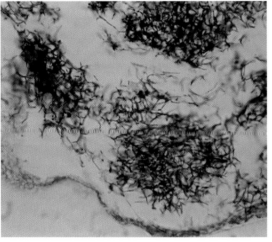

Fig. 13.2 A histopathological section from an actinomycetic lesion of the mandible showing a branching filamentous mass of *Actinomyces* spp. infiltrating the bony cortex.

organisms are aerobic, Gram-positive rods, which form thin, branching filaments. *Nocardia asteroides* causes the most common form of human nocardiosis, which is essentially a pulmonary infection that progresses to form abscesses and sinus tracts.

CLOSTRIDIA

Clostridia comprise many species of Gram-positive, anaerobic spore-forming bacilli (but spores are not found in infected tissues); a few are aerotolerant. They are an important group of pathogens widely distributed in soil and in the gut of humans and animals. There are four medically important species (*Clostridium tetani*, *C. botulinum*, *C. perfringens* and *C. difficile*) which cause significant morbidity and mortality, especially in developing countries. The major diseases caused by these organisms are listed in Table 13.1.

Clostridium spp.

Habitat

Soil, water, decaying animal and plant matter, and human and animal intestines.

Characteristics

Gram-positive rods; but older cultures may stain irregularly. All species form characteristic endospores which create a bulge in the bacterial body, for instance the drumstick-shaped *Clostridium tetani* (this shape is useful in laboratory identification of the organisms). Some species are motile with peritrichous flagella (e.g. *C. tetani*), while others (e.g. *C. perfringens*) have a capsule.

Culture and identification

Grow anaerobically on blood agar or Robertson's cooked meat medium (liquid culture). Although *Clostridium tetani* and *C. novyi* are strict anaerobes, *C. histolyticum* and *C. perfringens* can grow in the presence of limited amounts of oxygen (aerotolerant). The saccharolytic, proteolytic and toxigenic potentials of the organisms are useful in identification.

Clostridium perfringens

Habitat and transmission

Spores are found in the soil, and vegetative cells are normal flora of the colon and vagina. This bacterium causes two discrete diseases, due either to exogenous or endogenous infection:

- **gas gangrene** (myonecrosis) resulting from infection of dirty ischaemic wounds (e.g. war injuries)
- **food poisoning** due to ingestion of food contaminated with enterotoxin producing strains.

Characteristics

A short, fat bacillus. Spores are not usually found as they are formed under nutritionally deficient conditions. More tolerant of oxygen than other clostridia.

Table 13.1 Common *Clostridium* species associated with human disease

Clostridium spp.	Disease
C. perfringens	Gas gangrene, food poisoning, bacteraemia, soft-tissue infections
C. tetani	Tetanus
C. botulinum	Botulism (food-borne, infant, wound)
C. difficile	Pseudomembranous colitis, antibiotic-associated diarrhoea
Other species (e.g. C. septicum, C. ramosum, C. novyi, C. bifermentans)	Bacteraemia, gas gangrene, soft-tissue infections

Toxins. A variety of toxins (at least 12), including collagenase, proteinase and hyaluronidase, are formed, the most notable of which is the α-toxin, which lyses the phospholipids of eukaryotic cell membranes (i.e. a phospholipase). *Clostridium perfringens* is divided into five types (A–E) on the basis of toxins formed; type A is the human pathogen.

Culture and identification

Grows well on blood agar under anaerobic conditions, producing β-haemolytic colonies; some are non-haemolytic. The saccharolytic characteristic is used for identification purposes as it ferments litmus milk, producing acids and gases responsible for the so-called 'stormy clot' reaction.

Nagler's reaction. The neutralization of the α-toxin of the organism growing on agar plates by a specific antitoxin is useful in identification. In this test the organism is streaked on an agar plate containing egg yolk (which contains high concentrations of phospholipase), half of the plate having been spread with antitoxin; an opaque reaction develops, surrounding the growth of *C. perfringens* in the untreated half of the plate, while in the other half no such reaction occurs as the toxin is neutralized by the antitoxin (Fig. 13.3).

Pathogenicity

Causes gas gangrene and food poisoning.

Gas gangrene (myonecrosis). Wounds associated with traumatized tissue (especially muscle) may become infected with *C. perfringens* and other clostridia, with severe, life-threatening spreading infection. Activity of the bacillus in injured tissue results in toxin and enzyme production, allowing the organism to establish and multiply in the wound. Characteristic signs and symptoms include **pain, oedema** and **crepitation** produced by gas in tissues.

Food poisoning. Some strains of *C. perfringens* produce an **enterotoxin** which induces food poisoning. This is due to the ingestion of large numbers of vegetative cells from contaminated food, which then sporulate in the gut and release enterotoxin. The disease is characterized by watery diarrhoea with little vomiting.

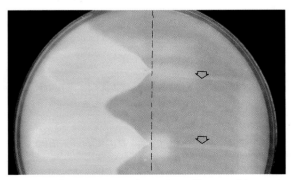

Fig. 13.3 Nagler's reaction: when *Clostridium perfringens* is grown in a medium containing egg yolk (lecithin) the enzyme (lecithinase) activity can be detected as opacity around the line of growth. On the right of the plate no opacity develops, as antitoxin previously applied to this half of the plate has neutralized the toxin. A positive control (top arrow) and a test sample which is also positive (bottom) are shown.

Treatment and prevention

Gas gangrene. Rapid intervention with:
(1) extensive debridement of the wound
(2) antibiotics (penicillin or metronidazole)
(3) anti-α-toxin administration.

Food poisoning. Symptomatic therapy only; no specific treatment.

Clostridium tetani

Habitat and transmission

Clostridium tetani is present in the intestinal tract of herbivores, and spores are widespread in soil. Germination of spores is promoted by poor blood supply and necrotic tissue and debris in wounds.

Characteristics

Long, thin bacilli with terminal spores giving the characteristic 'drumstick' appearance. Produces an extremely potent neurotoxin, **tetanospasmin**, by vegetative cells at the wound site. Another less powerful toxin, **tetanolysin**, is haemolytic in nature.

Culture and identification

Grows on blood agar, anaerobically, as a fine spreading colony. Identification in vitro is by a toxin neutralization test on blood agar, or in vivo by inoculation of culture filtrate into mice. The 'two-mouse model' is used: one animal is protected with antitoxin and the other is unprotected; the latter dies with typical tetanic spasms.

Pathogenicity

The agent of **tetanus** (lockjaw), which is a typical toxin-mediated disease. The powerful, heat-labile neurotoxin (tetanospasmin) is produced at the wound site and released during cell lysis (Fig. 13.4). It is retrogradely carried via the peripheral nerves (intra-axonally) to the central nervous system where it blocks inhibitory mediators at spinal synapses. This causes sustained muscle spasm and the characteristic signs of spasm of jaw muscles (lockjaw, **trismus**) and facial muscles (**risus sardonicus**), and arching of the body (**opisthotonos**). Toxin genes are plasmid-coded. *Clostridium tetani* also produces an oxygen-labile haemolysin (tetanolysin); the clinical significance of this enzyme is not clear.

Treatment and prevention

Antitoxin (hyperimmune human α-globulin) administered with or without toxoid, depending on the immunization history of patient. Prevention is by tetanus toxoid (a component of the DTP vaccine) with boosters every 10 years (see Ch. 37).

Clostridium difficile

Found in the faeces of 3–6% adults and almost all healthy infants, *Clostridium difficile* is the agent of antibiotic-associated colitis which may lead to sometimes lethal pseudomembranous colitis. It multiplies in the gut under the selective pressure of antibiotics. Although clindamycin was

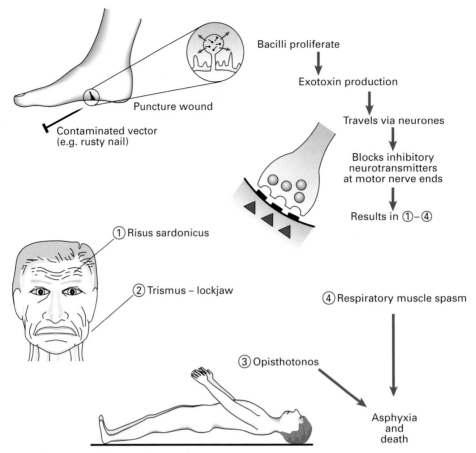

Fig. 13.4 Pathogenesis of tetanus and its sequelae.

earlier singled out as the main cause of colitis, it is now known that common drugs such as ampicillin may occasionally precipitate the disease. Treatment is to withhold the offending antibiotic and administer oral vancomycin or metronidazole.

BACILLUS SPECIES

The genus *Bacillus* comprises nearly 50 species of sporing, Gram-positive, chain-forming bacilli. Most are soil saprophytes. Two species, *B. anthracis* and *B. cereus*, cause significant morbidity.

Bacillus anthracis

Spores of *Bacillus anthracis* can survive in soil for years. Humans are accidental hosts, and infection (anthrax) is acquired when spores enter abrasions on the skin or are inhaled. Infection causes septicaemia and death; pulmonary anthrax (woolsorters' disease) is a life-threatening pneumonia caused by inhalation of spores. The polyglutamic acid capsule of the organism is antiphagocytic.

Bacillus cereus

Bacillus cereus causes food poisoning, especially when reheated, contaminated rice is eaten (particularly in restaurants serving rice-based dishes).

Bacillus stearothermophilus and Bacillus subtilis

These are used as biological indicators to test the sterilization efficacy of autoclaves, ethylene oxide and ionizing radiation (see Ch. 37).

KEY FACTS

- *Actinomyces* spp. are **potentially pathogenic commensals,** and are frequent isolates from dental plaque
- *They cause cervicofacial (most common), ileocaecal and thoracic actinomycoses, which are essentially chronic, granulomatous infections*
- **'Sulphur granule'** production (a tangled mass of filamentous organisms and debris) is a hallmark of actinomycosis
- *A prolonged course of antibiotics (up to 6 weeks) may be necessary to manage chronic actinomycosis*

- **Clostridia** are Gram-positive, anaerobic, spore-forming bacilli, though spores are not found in infected tissues
- *Pathogenic clostridia produce powerful exotoxins that are responsible for most disease symptoms*
- Spore-bearing *C. tetani* cells are characterized by their **drumstick shape**
- *Tetanospasmin and tetanolysin are toxins produced by* C. tetani, *the agent of tetanus*

KEY FACTS *(continued)*

- *Tetanus causes sustained muscle spasm (including the masticatory muscles) resulting in lockjaw (trismus), risus sardonicus and arching of the body (opisthotonos)*

- *Tetanus toxin (tetanospasmin) can be attenuated to form a toxoid. The latter is a component of the DTP (diphtheria–tetanus–pertussis) vaccine*

- *The spores of* Bacillus stearothermophilus *and* Bacillus subtilis *are used as biological indicators to test the sterilization efficacy of autoclaves, ethylene oxide and ionizing radiation*

FURTHER READING

Drobniewski, FA (1993). *Bacillus cereus* and related species. *Clinical Microbiology Reviews* 6, 324–338.

Greenwood, D, Slack, R, and Peutherer, J (eds) (1997). *Medical microbiology* (15th edn), Chs 21–23. Churchill Livingstone, Edinburgh.

Hatheway, CL (1990). Toxigenic clostridia. *Clinical Microbiology Reviews* 3, 66–98.

Schaal, KP, and Lee, HJ (1995). Actinomycete infections in humans — a review. *Gene* 115, 201–211.

14 Neisseriaceae, *Veillonella*, parvobacteria and *Capnocytophaga*

NEISSERIACEAE

The Neisseriaceae includes the genera *Neisseria* and *Moraxella*. Two species of *Neisseria* are human pathogens:
- *N. gonorrhoeae* (the gonococcus)
- *N. meningitidis* (the meningococcus).

There are a number of non-pathogenic species, such as *N. sicca*, *N. mucosa* and *N. lactamica*, which are members of the indigenous flora, including the oral mucosa. Hence it is important to differentiate these from the pathogenic species from oral samples.

Neisseria gonorrhoeae is the agent of **gonorrhoea**, the most frequently diagnosed venereal disease in western Europe and the USA. Gonococci frequently cause **pelvic inflammatory disease** (PID) and sterility in women, in addition to arthritis and sometimes septicaemia. *Neisseria meningitidis* is the aetiologic agent of meningococcal meningitis, a highly contagious disease associated with a mortality rate approximating 80% when untreated.

General characteristics

Non-motile, Gram-negative cocci ranging from 0.6 μm to 1.0 μm in diameter. On microscopy the cocci are seen as pairs with concave adjacent sides (bean-shaped); tetrads, short chains and clusters are occasionally seen but all show the characteristic pairing.

Pathogenic *Neisseria* species are nutritionally fastidious, especially on initial isolation from clinical specimens; the non-pathogenic species are less so. Though aerobic, most strains of *N. gonorrhoeae* are **capnophilic** (they require increased carbon dioxide for growth); haemolysed blood and solubilized starch enhance growth.

Members of this genus grow optimally at 36–39°C, although the non-pathogenic species can grow at temperatures below 24°C.

Neisseria gonorrhoeae

Habitat and transmission

The human urogenital tract is the usual habitat; oral, nasopharyngeal and rectal carriage in healthy individuals is not uncommon. Spread is by both homosexual and heterosexual intercourse or intimate contact.

Characteristics

Non-motile, Gram-negative, non-capsulate diplococci.

Culture and identification

Specimens are usually inoculated on to an enriched medium (lysed blood or chocolate agar normally) and incubated under 5–10% carbon dioxide (as the species is capnophilic). Small, grey, oxidase-positive colonies initially become large and opaque on prolonged incubation. Subsequent staining by fluorescent antibody techniques, and the production of acid from glucose but not from maltose or sucrose, confirms the identification. Gram-stained smears (of urethral exudate from men and the cervix in women) usually reveal Gram-negative, kidney-shaped intracellular cocci in pairs.

Pathogenicity

Gonococci possess a number of virulent attributes:
- **pili** allow gonococci to adhere and colonize epithelial surfaces and thus cause infection
- **IgA proteases** produced by some gonococci break the heavy chain of immunoglobulin A (IgA) thereby inactivating it (IgA is a major defence factor universally present on mucosal surfaces)
- some isolates of *N. gonorrhoeae* produce β-**lactamase**, which is plasmid-mediated
- a **tracheal cytotoxin** damages the ciliated cells of the fallopian tube, leading to scarring and sterility.

Treatment and prevention

The majority of gonococci are resistant to β-lactam drugs and hence the choice is β-lactamase-stable cephalosporins. Prevention of gonorrhoea requires the practice of 'safe sex', health education and contact tracing.

Neisseria meningitidis

Habitat and transmission

The main reservoir is the nasopharynx of normal people (10–25%). Droplet spread is the most common transmission mode.

Characteristics

This organism resembles the gonococcus but *N. meningitidis* cells are capsulate.

Culture and identification

As for *N. gonorrhoeae*. Presumptive identification is made by observing Gram-negative cocci in pairs in nasopharyngeal discharge, cerebrospinal fluid or blood smears. Selective media are not required as the organism is found pure in cerebrospinal fluid. Identified by the carbohydrate utilization test: produces acid from the oxidation of glucose and maltose. Serology is useful.

Pathogenicity

In susceptible individuals meningococci spread from the nasopharynx into the bloodstream (septicaemia), and then to the meninges. Septicaemia is accompanied by a rash. Eventual death may be due to meningitis or adrenal haemorrhage (Waterhouse–Friderichsen syndrome). The antiphagocytic properties of the capsule help dissemination, while the toxic effects are mainly due to the meningococcal endotoxin.

Treatment and prevention

Penicillin or cefotaxime (or equivalent cephalosporin).

Commensal *Neisseria* species

Commensal *Neisseria* species are common in the oral cavity, nose and pharynx, and sometimes in the female genital tract. The taxonomy of the group is confused. The three main species are *N. subflava*, *N. mucosa* and *N. sicca*. The main difference between these and the pathogenic *Neisseria* species is the ability of the commensal species to grow on ordinary agar at room temperature in the absence of carbon dioxide supplements.

These organisms are essentially non-pathogenic and are almost always found in oral specimens contaminated with saliva or mucosa. *Neisseria* species are among the earliest colonizers of a clean tooth surface. They consume oxygen during the early plaque formation and facilitate subsequent growth of facultative and obligate anaerobic late colonizers.

Moraxella

Moraxella (formerly *Branhamella*) are Gram-negative cocci closely related to the non-pathogenic *Neisseria* species, but asaccharolytic and non-pigmented. They are commensals of the human respiratory tract and are recognized opportunist pathogens causing meningitis, endocarditis, otitis media, maxillary sinusitis and chronic obstructive airways disease. As the majority of strains produce β-lactamase they may indirectly 'protect' other pathogens and thus complicate antibiotic therapy.

VEILLONELLA

Veillonella species are obligate anaerobic, Gram-negative cocci frequently isolated from oral samples. Three oral species are recognized: *Veillonella parvula* (the type species), *V. dispar* and *V. atypica*.

Veillonella parvula

Gram-negative, small anaerobic cocci. Found in the human oral cavity, mostly in dental plaque, they are considered as 'benevolent organisms' in relation to dental caries as they metabolize the lactic acid produced by cariogenic bacteria into weaker acids (acetic and propionic) with a reduced ability to solubilize enamel. No known pathogenic potential.

PARVOBACTERIA

Parvobacteria are so called because of their size (L. *parvus*, small). They are a miscellaneous, heterogeneous group of small, Gram-negative bacilli which cause a number of different diseases. They include the following genera:

- *Haemophilus*
- *Brucella*
- *Bordetella*
- *Pasteurella*
- *Francisella*
- *Actinobacillus*
- *Gardnerella*
- *Eikenella*.

Of these, *Haemophilus* and *Bordetella* spp. are of particular interest, as the former causes significant morbidity in the general population and the latter is the agent of whooping cough. Additionally, *Haemophilus* spp. and *Actinobacillus* spp. are common inhabitants of the oral cavity; the latter being an important periodontopathogen.

Haemophilus spp.

The genus *Haemophilus* is composed of tiny, non-motile, aerobic, Gram-negative coccobacilli; some are capsulated. One of its major distinguishing features is the requirement of two growth factors:

- **X factor** — haematin present in blood
- **V factor** — nicotinamide adenine dinucleotide (NAD) or NAD phosphate (NADP), a vitamin obtained from yeast and vegetable extracts or a metabolic product of most bacteria, including *Staphylococcus aureus*.

Haemophilus species cause a variety of diseases, as shown in Table 14.1.

Haemophilus influenzae

Habitat and transmission

An upper respiratory tract commensal of humans and associated animals, *Haemophilus influenzae* is a major aetiological agent of upper respiratory tract infections and acute exacerbations of chronic bronchitis. Although not the cause, *H. influenzae* is a common secondary colonizer of the respiratory tract after a bout of influenza (the agent of which is the influenza virus).

Characteristics

Small, Gram-negative, non-sporing, non-motile rods; predominantly coccobacillary in nature with a few long bacilli and filamentous forms. Virulent strains (for instance isolated from the cerebrospinal fluid in meningitis) are capsulated.

Culture and identification

Requires both V factor (NADP) and X factor (haematin) for growth on nutrient agar, but grows on blood-enriched media

Table 14.1 Some characteristics of *Haemophilus* spp.

Species	Factor requirement	Diseases caused
H. influenzae	X and V	Acute exacerbation of chronic bronchitis, epiglottitis, meningitis, sinusitis, otitis media, osteomyelitis, arthritis
H. parainfluenzae	V	Commensals of the oral cavity and upper respiratory tract; rarely cause disease
H. parahaemolyticus	V	
H. haemolyticus	X and V	
H. aphrophilus	X	
H. aegyptius	X and V	Conjunctivitis
H. ducreyi	X	Chancroid (a sexually transmitted disease — a soft sore)

containing these nutrients. Typically forms large colonies around colonies of other organisms that secrete the V factor — a phenomenon called '**satellitism**'. For example, if a blood agar plate (containing the X factor) seeded with *H. influenzae* is streaked with *Staphylococcus aureus* (which secretes the V factor) and incubated overnight at 37°C, the former will grow as large colonies adjacent to the streak of *S. aureus* (Fig. 14.1).

Pathogenicity

Haemophilus influenzae causes four major infections, often accompanied by septicaemia, especially in children and the elderly:
* meningitis
* acute epiglottitis
* osteomyelitis
* arthritis.

The most important virulence factor of *H. influenzae* is the **polysaccharide capsule**. An **IgA protease** and a factor that causes slowing and incoordination of (respiratory tract) ciliary beating are produced; the outer membrane and **endotoxin** may contribute to the pathogenesis; there are no known exotoxins. Non-capsulated strains cause exacerbation of chronic bronchitis.

Treatment and prevention

Ampicillin is given for β-lactamase negative strains. There are many other alternative antibiotics. Prevention by vacci-

nation (Hib) against invasive *H. influenzae* type b infection has been introduced in some countries. Close contacts of meningitis cases should be given rifampicin as a prophylactic measure.

Bordetella

There are three species in the genus *Bordetella*, of which *B. pertussis*, the agent of whooping cough, is the most important.

Bordetella pertussis

Habitat and transmission

Found in the human respiratory tract in diseased individuals; healthy carriage is not known. Spread is by the airborne route.

Characteristics

Short, sometimes oval, Gram-negative rods; fresh isolates may be capsulated. Fastidious growth requirements.

Culture and identification

Requires a special enriched medium for growth, i.e. Bordet–Gengou medium or blood–charcoal agar supplemented with antibiotics. On incubation for 3–5 days at 35°C, under high humidity, iridescent colonies resembling mercury drops appear on Bordet–Gengou medium. Identification is confirmed serologically.

Pathogenicity

Causes whooping cough, especially in preschool children (severe in those under 12 months). The characteristic symptom is the bout of **paroxysmal coughs** followed by the 'whoop' of rapid inhalation after coughing. Virulence factors identified are: tracheal cytotoxin, fimbrial antigen and endotoxin.

Treatment and prevention

Erythromycin is the drug of choice for patients and close contacts but antibiotics have little effect on the course of infection, although they may reduce spread and minimize superinfection.

Prevention is by immunization with whole-cell inactivated vaccine, a component of the diphtheria–tetanus–pertussis (DTP) vaccine of childhood. New acellular, subunit vaccines appear effective.

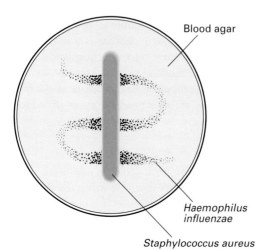

Fig. 14.1 Satellitism of *Haemophilus influenzae* (zigzag streak); enhanced growth adjacent to *Staphylococcus aureus* (vertical streak) which supplies the V factor.

Actinobacillus actinomycetemcomitans

The genus *Actinobacillus* includes species isolated from humans and mammals. The only species routinely isolated from the oral cavity is *Actinobacillus actinomycetemcomitans*, so named because it is frequently isolated with *Actinomyces* spp. from actinomycotic lesions. The reason for this association is unknown. Multiple biotypes and five serotypes (*a–e*) have been described. This species is a major infective agent in particularly · aggressive forms of periodontal disease in adolescents (localized aggressive periodontitis) and rapidly destructive periodontal disease in adults.

Habitat and transmission

Primary habitat is unknown, but is likely to be subgingival sites of humans and mammals. Infection is endogenous.

Characteristics

Small, short (0.4–1 μm), straight or curved rods with rounded ends. Electron microscopic studies have revealed bleb-like structures on the cell surface, which appear to be released from the cells. Fresh isolates possess fimbriae (lost on subculture).

Culture and identification

Grows as white, translucent, smooth, non-haemolytic colonies on blood agar; grows best aerobically with 5–10% carbon dioxide. Selective media are available for identification; the tryptone–soy–serum–bacitracin–vancomycin agar yields white, translucent colonies with a star-shaped internal structure, but this is not a consistent finding (Fig. 14.2). Identified by sugar fermentation and assimilation reactions and acid end-products of carbohydrate metabolism.

Pathogenicity

A number of virulence factors including lipopolysaccharide (endotoxin), a **leucotoxin, collagenase** and a **protease**

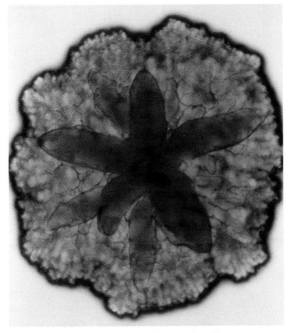

Fig. 14.2 A star-shaped colony of *Actinobacillus actinomycetemcomitans*.

cleaving IgG have all been isolated from *A. actinomycetemcomitans*. The leucotoxin, in particular, is thought to play a significant role in subverting the host immune response in the gingival crevice. Together with other coagents *A. actinomycetemcomitans* is involved in localized aggressive periodontitis and destructive periodontal disease in adults. Also isolated from cases of infective endocarditis, and from brain and subcutaneous abscesses.

Treatment

This species is sensitive to tetracycline.

Eikenella

Members of the genus *Eikenella* resemble *Haemophilus* spp., and are commensals of the human oral cavity and the intestine. Although in the past their presence was linked to periodontal diseases, this has now been disproved. The type species is *Eikenella corrodens*. These organisms are capnophilic, Gram-negative, short coccobacillary forms which are asaccharolytic. When grown on non-selective media they corrode the agar surface (hence the name *corrodens*). Human infection usually results from predisposing factors, such as trauma to a mucosal surface, which allow the organism access to the surrounding tissues; thus they may cause extraoral infections, including brain and abdominal abscesses, peritonitis, endocarditis, osteomyelitis and meningitis. Also associated with human bites or fist-fight injuries.

CAPNOCYTOPHAGA

The genus *Capnocytophaga* was created for fusiform species isolated from periodontal pockets, which, unlike *Fusobacterium* and *Bacteroides* spp., grow under capnophilic conditions. They have a characteristic ability to glide over routine blood agar (compare 'swarming' of *Proteus* spp.). Species recognized include *Capnocytophaga ochracea* (type species), *C. sputigena*, *C. gingivalis*, *C. granulosa* and *C. haemolytica*.

Habitat

The primary ecological niche is the subgingival area.

Characteristics

Long, thin fusiform organisms that demonstrate gliding motility seen on bright-field microscopy.

Culture and identification

Facultative anaerobes, but most strains require carbon dioxide for growth. Colonies spread over the agar surface with uneven edges and may be pink, yellow or white. Identification is by gliding characteristic, cell morphology, biochemical reactions and acid end-products.

Pathogenicity

Opportunist pathogens, sometimes associated with gingivitis and other systemic infections in immunocompromised patients; some strains produce an IgA1 protease.

KEY FACTS

- All *Neisseria* species are kidney-shaped, **Gram-negative cocci** usually arranged in pairs, and are **oxidase-positive**

- Pathogenic *Neisseria* have fastidious growth requirements, unlike the non-pathogenic species which are often part of the normal flora

- *Neisseria gonorrhoeae* (the gonococcus) is the agent of the common sexually transmitted disease, **gonorrhoea** and its complications

- *Neisseria meningitidis* (the meningococcus) is an important cause of **meningitis** in children and young adults

- *Veillonella* spp. present in plaque are considered **'benevolent organisms' in relation to dental caries** as they metabolize lactic acid produced by cariogenic bacteria into weaker acids

- The generic name *Haemophilus* is derived from their requirement of blood or blood products to support growth

- **Haemophilus influenzae** *causes meningitis, acute epiglottitis, osteomyelitis and arthritis, often accompanied by septicaemia, especially in children and the elderly*

- Bordetella pertussis *is the agent of whooping cough (pertussis); prevented by the whole-cell vaccine incorporated in the childhood DTP vaccination programme*

- **Actinobacillus actinomycetemcomitans** *is a coagent of localized aggressive periodontitis (formerly localized juvenile periodontitis) and destructive periodontal disease in adults (also an agent of infective endocarditis, and brain and subcutaneous abscesses)*

- *Eikenellae* and *Capnocytophaga* species are **oral commensals** and their role in oral disease is unclear

FURTHER READING

Duerden, BI, and Drasar, BS (eds) (1991). *Anaerobes in human disease.* Edward Arnold, London.

Greenwood, D, Slack, R, and Peutherer, J (eds) (1997). *Medical microbiology* (15th edn), Chs 24 and 37. Churchill Livingstone, Edinburgh.

15 Enterobacteria

Most of the commensal Gram-negative rods that inhabit the normal gastrointestinal tract, and sometimes cause disease, belong to the family Enterobacteriaceae. All species belonging to this family are **Gram-negative, facultative anaerobes that ferment glucose**. The major medically important species are listed in Table 15.1.

GENERAL CHARACTERISTICS OF ENTEROBACTERIA

Habitat

Found in the human gut, at a density of approximately 10^9 cells per gram of faeces. However, the predominant species in the gut is *Bacteroides*.

Characteristics

Rapidly growing cells $2\,\mu m \times 0.4\,\mu m$ in size; may appear coccobacillary. Many species are motile and possess a capsule, especially on initial isolation. All species are endotoxigenic because of the lipopolysaccharide outer cell wall. They also possess **pili** and **flagella**, which mediate adhesion and locomotion, respectively (Fig. 15.1).

Culture and identification

Grow well on ordinary media (e.g. blood agar, MacConkey's agar), producing characteristic circular, convex and glistening/mucoid colonies. Some motile species form swarming patterns on agar cultures. Most species are non-pigmented; a few produce red, pink, yellow or blue pigments.

Enterobacteriaceae ferment a large number of carbohydrates. This property, together with other biochemical tests, is used to identify and differentiate species:

Lactose fermentation. Growth on indicator media is used for the initial categorization of Enterobacteriaceae into two groups: **lactose fermenters** and **lactose non-fermenters**. Several selective media, such as MacConkey's and CLED (cystine–lactose–electrolyte-deficient) media, are available for this purpose. On MacConkey's agar the lactose fermenters appear as pink colonies, while on CLED medium the colour of lactose fermentation is yellow.

Other biochemical tests. Commercially available kit systems are routinely used to identify species of enterobacteria.

The commonly available test systems are based on 10 (API 10E) or 20 (API 20E, Rapid E) biochemical tests (Fig. 15.2).

Serological tests. These are based on the antigens of the organisms. All species have the somatic (O) antigen, and most have the flagellar (H) antigen. The capsular (K) antigen is seen in some species. The antigens are useful in the classification of species and invaluable for epidemiological investigation of outbreaks of disease. Identification of strains within a species can also be done by **bacteriophage typing, bacteriocin typing, plasmid analysis** and **polypeptide analysis**.

Pathogenicity

All Enterobacteriaceae are potentially pathogenic. Patients who are immunosuppressed, undergoing mechanical or medical manipulation, and have underlying disease are most susceptible to infection.

Endotoxin shock. This can be precipitated in humans by the **lipopolysaccharide** which all Enterobacteriaceae release when they are destroyed. **Toxic lipopolysaccharide** comprises lipid A, the core polysaccharide, and the O antigen; the lipid A is responsible for most of the symptoms associated with endotoxic shock. The toxic effects of lipopolysaccharide are many and include **fever, hypotension, intravascular coagulation** and effects on the **immune system**. Large doses of endotoxin may cause death.

Treatment

The antibiotic sensitivity patterns of enterobacteria are complex as they readily acquire resistance-coding plasmids. A spectrum of antibiotics are used, including ampicillin/amoxycillin, cephalosporins, aminoglycosides, trimethoprim, chloramphenicol and ciprofloxacin.

ESCHERICHIEAE

The tribe Escherichieae includes five genera: *Escherichia, Salmonella, Shigella, Edwardsiella* and *Citrobacter*. The most important human pathogens in this group, *Escherichia coli* and the *Salmonella* and *Shigella* species, are described here.

Table 15.1 Enterobacteria commonly causing human disease

Genus	Representative species (no. of species)	Disease
Escherichia	E. coli (5)	Gastroenteritis, wound and urinary tract infection
Shigella	S. dysenteriae S. flexneri S. boydii S. sonnei	Dysentery
Salmonella	S. typhi S. typhimurium (7 subgroups)	Enteric fever (typhoid) Food poisoning
Klebsiella	K. pneumoniae (7)	
Morganella Proteus Providencia	M. morganii (2) P. mirabilis (4) P. stuartii (5)	Urinary tract infection and other types of sepsis
Yersinia	Y. pestis (11)	Plague, septicaemia, enteritis, etc.
Citrobacter Enterobacter Serratia	C. freundii (4) E. cloacae (13) S. marcescens (10)	Low pathogenicity, opportunistic infections

Escherichia coli

Habitat and transmission

Indigenous commensal of the human intestinal tract; transmission is either endogenous or exogenous.

Characteristics

Gram-negative rods, motile, sometimes capsulate, facultative anaerobe, bile-tolerant

Culture and identification

Grows well on blood agar; ferments lactose (hence pink colonies on MacConkey's agar and yellow on CLED agar). Commercial kits, such as API 20E, are used in identification (Fig. 15.2). Biotyping systems are useful for strain delineation.

Pathogenicity

Escherichia coli is a major agent of sepsis; it causes the following diseases.

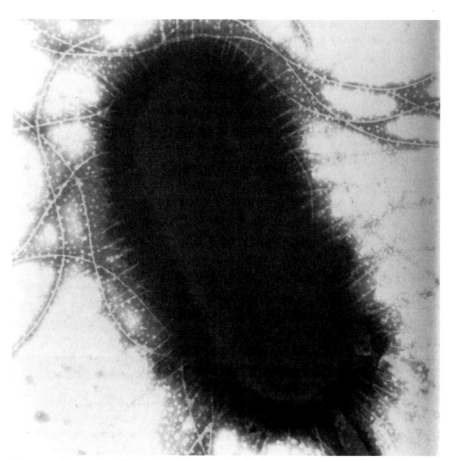

Fig. 15.1   A scanning electron micrograph of *Escherichia coli* showing fimbriae and flagella (×10 000).

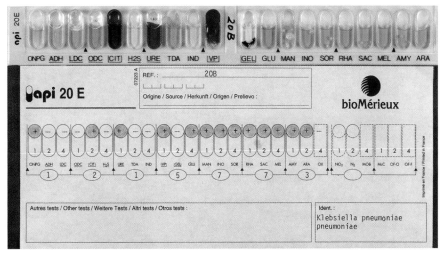

Fig. 15.2 Commercial identification kit for Enterobacteriaceae. This plate illustrates a colour reaction profile obtained after overnight incubation of the organism. The identity of the organism is *Klebsiella pneumoniae*.

Urinary tract infection. Young women and elderly adults are the most susceptible. The disease varies from simple urethritis to serious pyelonephritis.

Diarrhoeal diseases. These range from simple diarrhoea to severe disease leading to excessive fluid loss and dehydration, which may be fatal in malnourished infants and elderly debilitated adults. Many strains of **enteropathogenic** *E. coli* have powerful toxins and other mechanisms by which they cause diarrhoea:

- **enterotoxins**: mainly two types, both coded by plasmids, one is **heat-labile** (LT) and is similar in action to the cholera toxin, and the other is **heat-stable** (ST)
- **enteroinvasiveness**: some strains have the ability to invade intestinal epithelial cells and cause inflammation
- **adhesive factors** are produced by some strains enabling adhesion to mucosae; termed 'colonization factor antigens', these are mediated by plasmid-coded pili
- **Vero cytotoxicity** is caused by strains that have the ability to induce cytopathic effects on Vero cells (grown in tissue culture). Verotoxin (VT) producers can cause diarrhoea with haemorrhagic symptoms (e.g. *E. coli* O157).

Based on the above, diarrhoea-producing *E. coli* can be divided into four types:

- **enteropathogenic** *E. coli* (EPEC)
- **enteroinvasive** *E. coli* (EIEC)
- **enterotoxigenic** *E. coli* (ETEC)
- **enterohaemorrhagic** *E. coli* (EHEC).

Neonatal meningitis and septicaemia. Other infections *E. coli* may cause include neonatal meningitis, septicaemia, and wound infection, particularly after surgery of the lower intestinal tract.

SALMONELLAE

The genus *Salmonella* has a bewildering spectrum of more than 2000 species living in the intestinal tract of humans, domesticated animals and poultry. *Salmonella typhi* and *S. paratyphi* differ from others in that humans are the only known natural host.

Salmonella spp.

Habitat and transmission

Leading sources of salmonella infection are poultry products (i.e. flesh and eggs) and pet turtles (in the USA). **Occupational salmonellosis** affects veterinary and slaughterhouse workers. Infection is by ingestion of contaminated food, or person-to-person via the faecal–oral route. The carrier state, which develops in some after infection, is an important source of organisms.

Characteristics

Gram-negative, motile, non-sporing rods. All except *S. typhi* are non-capsulate; facultative anaerobes.

Culture and identification

Culture on MacConkey's medium or desoxycholate–citrate agar yields non-lactose-fermenting colonies. A combination of biochemical tests and serotyping is required for full identification. The latter is complex as salmonellae have a variety of antigens; notable are the **O** (**somatic**) and the **H** (**flagellar**) antigens; virulent strains, notably *S. typhi*, have a capsular polysaccharide antigen designated the **Vi** (**virulence**) antigen. There are more than 1700 serotypes of *S. enteritidis*.

Pathogenicity

The major types of salmonellosis (diseases due to *Salmonella*) are enteric fever, gastroenteritis and septicaemia.

Enteric fever (typhoid fever). Caused by *S. typhi* or *S. paratyphi* A, B or C (see Ch. 26).

Gastroenteritis. The most common form of salmonellosis, and can be due to any of the *S. enteritidis* serotypes. Symptoms appear 10–24 hours after ingestion of highly contaminated food or beverage. Nausea, vomiting, abdominal cramps, headache and diarrhoea are common.

Septicaemia. Frequently caused by *S. dublin* or *S. choleraesuis*; a fulminant, sometimes fatal, disease independent of intestinal symptoms. Pneumonia, meningitis and osteomyelitis may result from haematogenous spread of the bacteria.

Treatment and prevention

Proper cooking of foods derived from animal sources. Typhoid vaccine, a killed suspension of *S. typhi*, is available for those travelling to or living in areas where typhoid fever is endemic.

SHIGELLAE

Shigella species cause bacillary dysentery. The genus is divided into four species (*S. dysenteriae*, *S. sonnei*, *S. flexneri* and *S. boydii*) and a variety of serotypes.

Shigella spp.

Habitat and transmission

The only reservoir is the human intestine. Infection is spread by the faecal–oral route under crowded conditions. A minute dose of the organisms is adequate to cause disease.

Characteristics

Gram-negative, non-motile rods (compare salmonellae); non-capsulate.

Culture and identification

All species grow well on ordinary media and are non-lactose fermenters (except *S. sonnei*, a slow lactose fermenter). Commercial kits are used in identification.

Pathogenicity

Although shigellae do not invade systemically like salmonellae, they locally invade the intestinal epithelium (ileum and colon). The resultant intense inflammatory response is characterized by bloody, mucopurulent diarrhoea (dysentery). Although no enterotoxin is produced, the exotoxin of *Shigella* species is neurotoxic.

Treatment and prevention

Severe dysentery is managed by fluid and electrolyte replacement. Antibiotics should be avoided as many strains are resistant to multiple antibiotics. Spread can be controlled by improving sanitation and personal hygiene to interrupt faecal–oral transmission; hand hygiene is critical.

KLEBSIELLEAE

A number of species belonging to this tribe, namely *Klebsiella*, *Enterobacter* and *Serratia*, are indigenous to the human intestinal and respiratory tracts. They are also occasionally isolated from the oral cavity and hence are considered transient oral commensals. They cause serious disease in immunocompromised patients, especially in hospital environments (**nosocomial infection**).

Klebsiella pneumoniae

As the name indicates, *Klebsiella pneumoniae* may sometimes cause a severe destructive pneumonia. It also causes nosocomial urinary tract infection. The virulence of the organism is mainly due to its large antiphagocytic capsule. This species is isolated from the oropharynx or gastrointestinal tract of about 5% of healthy people, and the isolation rate is higher in the hospitalized.

Enterobacter spp.

Enterobacter species are indigenous to the intestinal tract, but can be found on plants and as free-living saprophytes. They may cause nosocomial urinary tract infection, and very rarely a primary infection. *Enterobacter cloacae* and *E. aerogenes* are the most frequently isolated as transients in the oral cavity.

Serratia spp.

Serratia marcescens grows as characteristic magenta-coloured colonies. It may occasionally cause fatal disease in neonates, and in immunosuppressed and debilitated individuals.

PSEUDOMONADS

Pseudomonas species are not enterobacteria but they are included in this chapter for convenience as they are Gram-negative rods with somewhat similar properties. The genus contains a large number of species, but only a few are human pathogens. They are widely distributed in the environment and may cause disease, especially in hospital settings. *Pseudomonas aeruginosa* is the most important species to cause such infection and is a special problem in burn patients.

Pseudomonas aeruginosa

Habitat and transmission

Colonizes the human intestine in a few healthy individuals and in a large proportion of hospitalized patients. Colonizes environmental surfaces, especially under moist conditions.

Characteristics

Aerobic, Gram-negative rods, motile by means of polar flagella. Grow over a very wide temperature range, including room temperature.

Culture and identification

Grows easily on routine media, producing irregular, moist, iridescent colonies with a characteristic 'fishy' aroma. Identified using commercial kits.

Pathogenicity

Virulence factors identified include lipopolysaccharide endotoxin, an exotoxin, extracellular proteases and elastases, and an extracellular 'slime' which prevents phagocytosis.

Treatment and prevention

Although this species is resistant to most antimicrobials, it is sensitive to aminoglycosides and certain β-lactams (e.g. acylureidopenicillins), cephalosporins and polymixin. Prevention is by good asepsis in hospitals and rational antibiotic therapy (to prevent emergence of resistant isolates).

KEY FACTS

- Enterobacteria are **Gram-negative, facultative anaerobes** that ferment glucose and usually **live in the intestinal tract**

- This extensive group of bacteria are **classified** according to their **somatic (O) antigen, flagellar (H) antigen** and **capsular (K) antigen**

- Most if not all possess **pili; capsules** and **flagella** may be present

- **All** produce **endotoxin** and **some produce** powerful **exotoxins**

- *Escherichia coli is the predominant facultative inhabitant of the human intestinal tract*

- *Diarrhoea-producing E. coli can be divided into enteropathogenic (EPEC), enteroinvasive (EIEC), enterotoxigenic (ETEC) and enterohaemorrhagic (EHEC) types*

- *Salmonellae and shigellae are responsible for a variety of gastrointestinal disorders*

- *Shigella is the cause of most dysentery in the West*

- *Hundreds of species of Salmonella have been identified; they are the agents of typhoid fever, gastroenteritis and septicaemia*

- *Klebsiella, Enterobacter* and *Serratia*, together with *E. coli*, are indigenous to the human intestinal and respiratory tracts but are also occasionally isolated from the oral cavity; hence they are considered to be **transient oral commensals**

- *The latter groups may cause serious disease in compromised patients, especially in hospital environments (nosocomial infection)*

FURTHER READING

Christie, AN (1987). *Infectious diseases* (4th edn), vol. 2, Chs 4–6. Churchill Livingstone, Edinburgh.

Greenwood, D, Slack, R, and Peutherer, J (eds) (1997). *Medical microbiology* (15th edn), Chs 25–28. Churchill Livingstone, Edinburgh.

Sedgley, C, and Samaranayake, LP (1994). Oropharyngeal prevalence of *Enterobacteriaceae* in humans: a review. *Journal of Oral Medicine and Oral Pathology* 23, 104–113.

16 Vibrios, campylobacters and *Wolinella*

Bacteria belonging to these three genera (together with others such as the genus *Helicobacter*) are morphologically similar, being Gram-negative curved bacilli. They are enteric pathogens of humans or part of the normal flora. Because of their unusual growth requirements (formate and fumarate needed) they have to be cultured in special media.

VIBRIOS

The genus *Vibrio* includes two important human pathogens but their natural habitat is water. *Vibrio cholerae* causes cholera, while *V. parahaemolyticus* causes a less severe diarrhoea. The main symptom of cholera is watery diarrhoea that can be fatal as a result of severe dehydration, water and electrolyte loss.

Vibrio cholerae

Habitat and transmission

Water contaminated with faeces of patients or carriers; no animal reservoir. A life-threatening, watery diarrhoea (rice-water stools) is the characteristic disease.

Characteristics

Gram-negative slender bacilli, comma-shaped with pointed ends. Highly motile by means of a single polar flagellum. May be seen directly in stool samples by dark-field microscopy.

Culture and identification

Grows in alkaline conditions (pH 8.5–9.2 approximately): selective media for culture such as TCBS (thiosulphate–citrate–bile–sucrose) medium are based on this property. This, together with biochemical tests and serology, helps identification. Serotyping is based on the somatic O antigens. All diarrhoea-producing strains of *V. cholerae* are designated as O1 and are subdivided into three major serotypes — the Ogawa, Inaba and El Tor strains.

Pathogenicity

Vibrio cholerae has the ability to colonize the intestinal tract in very high numbers and about 10^8 cells per millilitre are seen in patients' faeces. The cells attach to but do not invade the intestinal mucosa. Pathogenicity is due to secretion of an enterotoxin, which binds to ganglioside receptors on mucosal cells. After a lag period of 15–45 minutes, adenylate cyclase is activated and the cAMP concentration inside the intestinal cells increases. This in turn leads to excretion of electrolytes and water and subsequent diarrhoea, leading to severe dehydration.

Treatment and prevention

Intravenous administration of fluids and electrolytes is essential for recovery. Oral administration of a solution containing glucose and electrolytes (oral rehydration therapy) is successful, but the patient must be capable of consuming the liquid by mouth. Severely ill patients are generally too weak to ingest fluids. Antibiotics (usually tetracycline) do not affect the disease outcome once the enterotoxin attaches to the intestinal cells but they prevent subsequent attacks by reducing the number of toxin-producing *V. cholerae* cells in the intestine.

Immunization with a whole-cell vaccine is of limited use. New vaccines are under development.

Vibrio parahaemolyticus

This vibrio requires a relatively high salt concentration for growth, and is distributed worldwide in marine environments, for example in South-East Asia. A common agent of acute enteritis associated with the consumption of improperly cooked seafood; it accounts for about half of all cases of food poisoning in Japan.

There is no specific treatment for diarrhoea. The best control measure is the consumption of only thoroughly cooked seafood.

CAMPYLOBACTERS

The genus *Campylobacter* contains medically important species that are important human pathogens, once classified as vibrios. *Campylobacter jejuni* is the major human pathogenic species; *C. rectus* has been isolated from active periodontal disease sites and has been implicated as a periodontopathogen.

Campylobacter spp.

Habitat and transmission

The natural reservoir is animals. Organisms are acquired from contaminated food and milk.

120

Characteristics

Curved, seagull-shaped, Gram-negative rods; mobile with a single polar flagellum.

Culture and identification

Campylobacter jejuni grows best under microaerophilic (i.e. an environment of 10% oxygen and 10% carbon dioxide) and thermophilic (a temperature of 43°C) conditions in an enriched medium. Further identification is by biochemical tests and antibiotic susceptibility patterns.

Pathogenicity

Gastroenteritis, especially in children, is the most common human infection caused by *Campylobacter* species. It resembles dysentery and is usually self-limiting, but may last for several days. The heat-labile enterotoxin of *C. fetus* is implicated. Campylobacters may occasionally cause bacteraemia, meningitis, endocarditis, arthritis and urinary tract infection. Some strains of *C. rectus* isolated from periodontal disease sites produce a cytotoxin somewhat similar to that of *Actinobacillus actinomycetemcomitans*.

Treatment and prevention

No specific therapy is necessary for the mild diarrhoea. Good food and hand hygiene is important.

Helicobacter pylori

This organism (previously classified as a campylobacter) causes a significant proportion of gastritis and duodenal ulcers in humans; it may play a role in gastric cancer. Antimicrobial therapy eradicates the bacteria from the stomach and resolves many of the ulcers that were formerly thought to be due to gastric acidity. A few studies have demonstrated the presence of this organism, albeit in small numbers, in human supragingival plaque.

WOLINELLA

Members of the genus *Wolinella* are curved or helical Gram-negative motile rods. Motility is due to a polar flagellum; anaerobes and require formate and fumarate for growth. The main species is *Wolinella succinogenes*.

Habitat

These organisms are frequently isolated from the oral cavity, especially the gingival sulcus.

Culture and identification

A selective medium is available for culturing the organism from plaque samples. Identification is by colonial characteristics (dry, spreading or corroding colonies), whole-cell protein profiles and serology.

Pathogenicity

Although some studies have shown a high correlation between periodontal disease activity and isolation of *Wolinella* spp., the pathogenic role is not clear. The organisms can induce alveolar bone loss in gnotobiotic rats. A possible periodontal pathogen.

KEY FACTS

- **Vibrios** are small, **comma-shaped, Gram-negative, oxidase-positive** bacteria that prefer an alkaline growth environment
- **Vibrio cholerae** *is the major pathogen in the genus and is responsible for cholera epidemics, especially in the developing world*
- **Campylobacter jejuni** *is a thermophilic, microaerophilic vibrio that causes human diarrhoeal illness*
- **Helicobacter pylori** *causes a significant proportion of gastritis and duodenal ulcers in humans, and may play a role in gastric cancer*

FURTHER READING

Greenwood, D, Slack, R, and Peutherer, J (eds) (1997). *Medical microbiology* (15th edn), Chs 30, 31. Churchill Livingstone, Edinburgh.

Bacteroides, Porphyromonas and *Prevotella*

The genera described in this chapter are obligately anaerobic, short Gram-negative rods or coccobacilli. Historically only the *Bacteroides* genus was known, but the application of new taxonomic techniques has resulted in the definition of two additional genera: *Porphyromonas* and *Prevotella*. Together they comprise a substantial proportion of the microflora of the dental plaque, intestine and the female genital tract.

- *Bacteroides* spp. are mainly restricted to species found **predominantly in the gut** and are the most common agents of serious anaerobic infections; *B. fragilis* is the main pathogen.
- *Porphyromonas* spp. are asaccharolytic pigmented species and form part of the normal oral flora. They are agents of periodontal disease and hence considered as **periodontopathic** organisms.
- *Prevotella* spp. include saccharolytic oral and genitourinary species; some species are periodontopathic.

Collectively, *Porphyromonas* and *Prevotella* species are referred to as **black-pigmented anaerobes**, as some organisms from these genera form a characteristic brown or black pigment on blood agar (Fig. 17.1). This pigment, a metabolic end-product of (blood) haemin, is thought to act as a defence barrier protecting the cells from the toxic effects of oxygen. Some species belonging to these genera are listed in Table 17.1.

BACTEROIDES

Bacteroides fragilis

Habitat and transmission

Bacteroides species are the most predominant flora in the intestine (10^{11} cells per gram of faeces), far outnumbering *Escherichia coli*. They cause serious anaerobic infections such as intra-abdominal sepsis, peritonitis, liver and brain abscesses, and wound infection.

Characteristics

Strictly anaerobic, Gram-negative, non-motile, non-sporing bacilli, but may appear pleomorphic. The polysaccharide capsule is an important virulence factor.

Culture and identification

These organisms have stringent growth requirements; they demonstrate slow growth on blood agar and appear as grey to opaque, translucent colonies. They grow well in Robertson's cooked meat medium supplemented with yeast extract.

Identified by biochemical tests, growth inhibition by bile salts, antibiotic resistance tests and gas–liquid chromatographic analysis of fatty acid end-products of glucose metabolism.

Pathogenicity

Mainly the result of its endotoxin and proteases. No exotoxin has been reported. Other organisms, such as coliforms, are commonly associated with sepsis. The latter facultative anaerobes utilize oxygen in the infective focus and facilitate the growth of the anaerobic *Bacteroides* strains. Consequently many *Bacteroides* infections are **polymicrobial** in nature.

Treatment and prevention

Sensitive to metronidazole and clindamycin. Resistant to penicillins, first-generation cephalosporins and aminoglycosides. Penicillin resistance is due to β-lactamase production. As *Bacteroides* spp. are normal gut commensals, infections are **endogenous** and diseases are virtually impossible to prevent.

PORPHYROMONAS

Porphyromonas gingivalis

Habitat and transmission

Found almost solely at subgingival sites, particularly in advanced periodontal disease. Sometimes recovered from the tongue and tonsils.

Characteristics

Non-motile, short, pleomorphic, Gram-negative rods.

Culture and identification

Grows anaerobically, with dark pigmentation, on media containing lysed blood (Fig. 17.1); identified by biochemical characteristics using commercially available kits (e.g. AnIdent); DNA and molecular probes are now used to identify these organisms directly from plaque samples.

Pathogenicity

An aggressive periodontal pathogen in both humans and animals (e.g. guinea-pig, monkey, beagle dogs); its fimbriae

Fig. 17.1 Black-pigmented colonies of periodontopathogen *Porphyromonas gingivalis* on blood agar. The pigment is thought to be related to breakdown products of the blood.

mediate adhesion and the capsule defends against phagocytosis. Produces a range of virulence factors including many proteases that destroy immunoglobulins, complement and haem-sequestering proteins, a haemolysin and a collagenase.

PREVOTELLAE

This genus includes a number of pigmented as well as non-pigmented species that are moderately saccharolytic; all produce acetic and succinic acid from glucose. *Prevotella melaninogenica* is the type species (Table 17.1).

Prevotella spp.

Habitat and transmission

The predominant ecological niche of all *Prevotella* species appears to be the human oral cavity. Strains of *P. intermedia* are associated more with periodontal disease, while *P. nigrescens* is isolated more often from healthy gingival sites.

Table 17.1 Anaerobic Gram-negative bacilli of clinical interest

Organism	Main colonization sites
Bacteroides	
B. fragilis group:	Colon
B. fragilis	
B. ovatus	
B. vulgatus	
B. distasonis	
B. capillosus	Colon, oropharynx
B. ureolyticus	Oropharynx, intestine, genitourinary tract
Porphyromonas	
P. gingivalis	Oropharynx
P. endodontalis	Oropharynx
Prevotella	
P. intermedia	Oropharynx
P. nigrescens	
P. melaninogenica	Oropharynx
P. loescheii	Oropharynx
P. pallens	Vagina, oropharynx
P. corporis	Vagina, oropharynx

Culture and identification

Non-motile, Gram-negative rods; brown-black colonies on blood agar (when pigmented). Molecular techniques are required to differentiate some species.

Pathogenicity

Prevotella intermedia is a true periodontopathogen. The pathogenicity of other subdivided species awaits clarification. Oral non-pigmented species such as *P. buccae*, *P. oralis* and *P. dentalis* are isolated on occasion from healthy subgingival plaque. Some of the latter are associated with disease, and increase in numbers and proportions during periodontal disease.

KEY FACTS

- *Bacteroides*, *Porphyromonas* and *Prevotella* form a substantial proportion of the microflora of the **dental plaque, colon** and the **female genital tract**
- *Bacteroides* spp. are the **predominant** flora **in the intestine**
- Collectively *Porphyromonas* and *Prevotella* species are referred to as **black-pigmented anaerobes**
- *Porphyromonas gingivalis* is found almost **solely at subgingival sites**, and is a key periodontopathic organism (i.e. a **periodontopathogen**)

- The **virulence** of *Porphyromonas gingivalis* is partly due to its many **proteases** (which destroy immunoglobulins, complement and haeme-sequestering proteins), a **haemolysin** and a **collagenase**
- Strains of *Prevotella intermedia* are associated more with **periodontal disease**, while *P. nigrescens* is isolated more often from **healthy gingival sites**

FURTHER READING

Duerden, BI, and Drasar, BS (eds) (1991). *Anaerobes in human disease.* Edward Arnold, London.

Greenwood, D, Slack, R, and Peutherer, J (eds) (1997). *Medical microbiology* (15th edn), Chs 15–17. Churchill Livingstone, Edinburgh.

Shah, HN, Mayrand, D, and Genco, RJ (eds) (1993). *Biology of the species* Porphyromonas gingivalis. CRC Press, Boca Raton.

18 Fusobacteria, *Leptotrichia* and spirochaetes

Fusobacteria are non-sporing, anaerobic, non-motile, non- or weakly fermentative, spindle-shaped bacilli (with fused ends: hence the name). They are normal inhabitants of the oral cavity, colon and female genital tract and are sometimes isolated from pulmonary and pelvic abscesses. Fusospirochaetal infections, which they cause in combination with spirochaetes, are noteworthy. *Fusobacterium nucleatum* (the type species) and *F. periodonticum* are isolated mainly from periodontal disease sites, and others such as *F. alocis* and *F. sulci* are sometimes found in the healthy gingival sulcus.

FUSOBACTERIA

Fusobacterium nucleatum

Habitat and transmission

Several subspecies of *F. nucleatum* have been identified, in different habitats. These include *F. nucleatum* subsp. *polymorphum* found in healthy gingival crevice, and *F. nucleatum* subsp. *nucleatum* recovered mainly from periodontal pockets. A third subspecies is *F. nucleatum* subsp. *vincenti*. Infections are almost invariably **endogenous**.

Characteristics

Gram-negative, strictly anaerobic, cigar-shaped bacilli with pointed ends (Fig. 18.1). Cells often have a central swelling. A Gram-stained smear of deep gingival debris obtained from a lesion of acute ulcerative gingivitis is a simple method of demonstrating the characteristic fusobacteria, together with spirochaetes and polymorphonuclear leucocytes (Fig. 18.2). These together with the clinical picture confirm a clinical diagnosis of acute ulcerative gingivitis.

Culture and identification

Grows on blood agar as dull, granular colonies with an irregular, rhizoid edge. Biochemical reactions and the acidic end-products of carbohydrate metabolism help identification. As fusobacteria can remove sulphur from cysteine and methionine to produce odoriferous hydrogen sulphide and methylmercaptan, they are thought to be associated with **halitosis**.

Pathogenicity

The endotoxin of the organism appears to be involved in the pathogenesis. *Fusobacterium nucleatum* is usually isolated from polymicrobial infections; it is rarely the sole pathogen. Thus in combination with oral spirochaetes (*Treponema vincentii* and others) it causes the classic **fusospirochaetal infections**. These are:

- **acute (necrotizing) ulcerative gingivitis** or trench mouth (see Ch. 33)
- **Vincent's angina**, an ulcerative tonsillitis causing tissue necrosis often due to extension of acute ulcerative gingivitis.
- **cancrum oris** or **noma**: a sequel of acute ulcerative gingivitis with resultant gross tissue loss of the facial region.

As fusobacteria coaggregate with most other oral bacteria they are believed to be important bridging organisms between early and late colonizers during plaque formation.

Antibiotic sensitivity and prevention

Fusobacteria are uniformly sensitive to penicillin, and being strict anaerobes are sensitive to metronidazole. Regular oral hygiene and antiseptic mouthwashes are the key to prevention of oral fusobacterial infections in susceptible individuals.

LEPTOTRICHIA

Leptotrichia spp. are oral commensals previously thought to belong to the genus *Fusobacterium*. They are Gram-negative, strictly anaerobic, slender, filamentous bacilli, usually with one pointed end. *Leptotrichia buccalis*, present in low proportions in dental plaque, is the sole representative of this genus.

SPIROCHAETES

Spirochaetes are a diverse group of spiral, motile organisms comprising five genera. Of these, three genera are human pathogens:

- *Treponema* causes syphilis, bejel, yaws, pinta and, in the oral cavity, acute necrotizing ulcerative gingivitis (together with fusobacteria)
- *Borrelia* causes relapsing fever and Lyme disease
- *Leptospira* causes leptospirosis.

Spirochaetes are helical organisms with a central protoplasmic cylinder surrounded by a cytoplasmic membrane (Fig. 18.3).

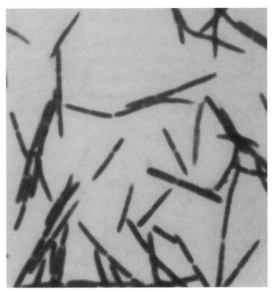

Fig. 18.1 Photomicrograph of fusobacteria showing characteristic cigar-shaped cells with pointed ends.

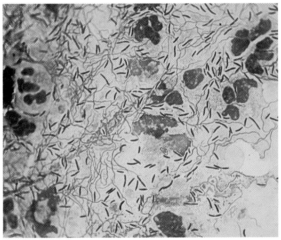

Fig. 18.2 A Gram-stained smear obtained from deep gingival plaque of a patient with acute ulcerative gingivitis (see also Fig. 33.6) showing the fusospirochaetal complex.

The cell wall is similar to Gram-negative bacteria but stains poorly with the Gram stain. Underneath the cell wall run three to five **axial filaments** which are fixed to the extremities of the organism. Contractions of these filaments distort the bacterial cell body to give it its helical shape. The organism moves either by rotation along the long axis or by flexion of cells. Because of their weak refractile nature, dark-ground microscopy is used to visualize these organisms in the laboratory, although immunofluorescence is more useful for identification purposes. All spirochaetes are strictly anaerobic or microaerophilic.

Treponema

The coils of *Treponema* are regular, with a longer wavelength than that of leptospires (Fig. 18.3). A number of species and subspecies are recognized, some of which are important systemic pathogens, while others are oral inhabitants implicated in periodontal disease.

Treponema pallidum

Habitat and transmission

Lesions of primary and secondary syphilis. Transmission is by direct contact with lesions, body secretions, blood, semen and saliva, usually during sexual contact; from mother to fetus by placental transfer.

Characteristics

Slender, corkscrew-shaped cells with 6 to 12 evenly spaced coils, $6–14\,\mu m \times 0.2\,\mu m$; too slender to visualize by light microscopy but can be seen by silver impregnation or immuno-fluorescent techniques; strictly anaerobic and extremely sensitive to drying and heat, hence dies rapidly outside the body.

Culture and identification

Cannot be cultured in vitro, but can be propagated in the testes of rabbits; *T. pallidum* thus harvested can be used as antigens to detect specific antibody in the patient's serum.

Dark-ground microscopy of tissue fluid from primary and secondary clinical lesions helps identification but serological tests are the mainstay of diagnosis.

Pathogenicity

Causes syphilis, a sexually transmitted disease with protean manifestations (see Ch. 27). The virulence factors of *T. pallidum* are not well characterized. Immunopathology plays a significant role in disease manifestations especially in the late (tertiary and quaternary) stages of the disease.

Antibiotic sensitivity and control

Penicillin is the drug of choice; for allergic patients tetracycline is an alternative. Prevention of syphilis is based on early detection, contact tracing and serological testing of pregnant women.

Treponema pallidum subsp. pertenue

The agent of yaws, characterized by chronic, ulcerative, granulomatous lesions of skin, mucosae and bone. The disease, widespread in the tropics, is spread by direct contact.

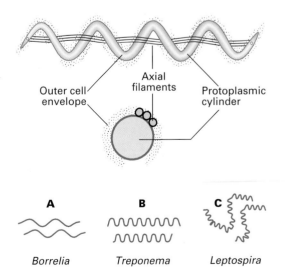

Fig. 18.3 Structure of a spirochaete (top) and the morphology of the three major genera of spirochaetes.

Treponema carateum

The agent of pinta; a non-venereal skin infection character-ized by depigmented and hyperkeratotic skin. The disease affects mainly dark-skinned natives of Central and South America and the West Indies.

Oral treponemes

All oral spirochaetes are classified in the genus *Treponema*. Although many species have been described, only four have been cultivated and maintained reliably: *T. denticola*, *T. vincentii*, *T. pectinovarum* and *T. socranskii*.

Habitat and transmission

Predominantly the oral cavity of humans and primates, at the gingival margin and crevice in particular. Transmission routes are unknown. Infections are endogenous.

Characteristics

Motile, helical rods, 5–15 µm × 0.5 µm, with irregular (three to eight) spirals which are less tightly coiled than, for instance, *T. pallidum* (Figs. 18.3 and 18.4). Cell walls are Gram-negative but stain poorly. The size is variable, and can be used as a basis for classification (large, medium or small).

Culture and identification

In contrast to *T. pallidum*, oral spirochaetes can be grown in vitro. They are strict anaerobes, slow-growing in oral treponema isolation (OTI) medium. Subspecies can be differentiated by fermentation reactions and serology (agglutination).

Suspect lesions of acute necrotizing ulcerative gingivitis or advanced periodontitis can be examined by obtaining a Gram-stained smear of deep gingival plaque and visualizing the characteristic fusospirochaetal complex under light microscopy (see Fig. 18.2); alternatively, dark-ground microscopy may be used.

Pathogenicity

These organisms are a component of the fusospirochaetal complex of acute necrotizing ulcerative gingivitis and Vincent's angina; a coagent of advanced periodontal disease. The ability to travel through viscous environments enables oral spirochaetes to migrate within the gingival crevicular fluid and to penetrate sulcular epithelial linings as well as gingival connective tissue. Virulence factors are little known; endotoxin is possibly contributory to disease. *Treponema denticola* is more proteolytic than other species and degrades collagen and dentine.

Antibiotic sensitivity and control

Sensitive to penicillin and metronidazole. Prevention of infection is achieved by good oral hygiene practices.

Borrelia burgdorferi

Habitat and transmission

Found in ticks and small mammals, particularly deer. Transmission is by a tick vector.

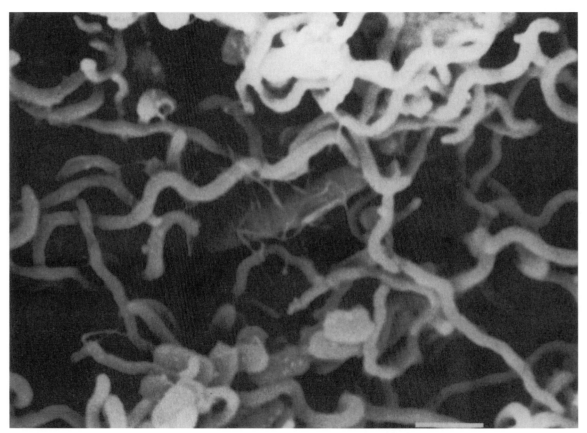

Fig. 18.4 Scanning electron micrograph of the radicular surface of a tooth affected by advanced periodontal disease showing the spirochaetes on the root surface.

Characteristics

This species is a helical spirochaete, 0.18–0.25 µm × 4.3 µm. Gram-negative, it grows under microaerophilic conditions at 34°C. Identification is by serology and immunofluorescence or enzyme-linked immunosorbent assay (ELISA).

Pathogenicity

The agent of **Lyme disease**, a generalized infection with neurological and cardiac manifestations and arthritis. One of the earliest and most common neurological manifestations is unilateral **facial palsy**.

Antibiotic sensitivity

Sensitive to tetracycline and amoxicillin (amoxycillin).

Other *Borrelia* species

These include *Borrelia recurrentis* and *B. duttonii*, agents of louse-borne and tick-borne relapsing fever seen in parts of Africa, Asia and South America.

Leptospira

Leptospira biflexa and *L. interrogans* are the recognized species, each of which comprises a number of serogroups.

These organisms are found in damp environments such as stagnant water and wet soil. The kidneys of some rodents and domestic animals act as a reservoir for *L. interrogans*. The urine of these animals serves as a vehicle of transmission of human leptospirosis, the symptoms of which vary from mild febrile illness to fatal attacks of jaundice and renal failure.

KEY FACTS

- **Fusobacteria are non-sporing, anaerobic,** spindle-shaped **bacilli** inhabiting the **oral cavity, colon** and **female genital tract**
- The type species *Fusobacterium nucleatum* and *F. periodonticum* are isolated mainly from periodontal disease sites and hence considered to be **periodontopathic bacteria**
- *Fusospirochaetal infections caused by fusobacteria in combination with spirochaetes are acute ulcerative gingivitis, Vincent's angina and cancrum oris (or noma)*

- **Spirochaetes are long, slender, coiled** and highly **mobile** bacteria that do not take up the Gram stain
- **Spirochaetes** comprise three genera: *Treponema*, *Borrelia* and *Leptospira*
- **Treponema pallidum,** *the agent of syphilis, cannot be cultivated in vitro and is uniformly sensitive to penicillin*
- All oral spirochaetes are classified in the genus *Treponema* (type strain *T. denticola*)
- **Treponema denticola** *is a coagent of fusospirochaetal infection and advanced periodontal disease*

FURTHER READING

Bolstad, AI, Jensen, HB, and Bakken, V (1996). Taxonomy, biology and periodontal aspects of *Fusobacterium nucleatum*. *Clinical Microbiology Reviews* 9, 55–71.

Duerden, BI, and Drasar, BS (eds) (1991). *Anaerobes in human disease*. Edward Arnold, London.

Greenwood, D, Slack, R, and Peutherer, J (eds) (1997). *Medical microbiology* (15th edn), Chs 37, 38. Churchill Livingstone, Edinburgh.

19 | Mycobacteria and legionellae

Mycobacteria are widespread both in the environment and in animals; they cause two major human diseases — tuberculosis and leprosy. They are aerobic, acid-fast bacilli (not stained by the Gram stain because of the high lipid component of the cell wall). The major medically important pathogens are:

- *Mycobacterium tuberculosis*, the agent of **tuberculosis**; one of the top three infectious diseases affecting humans globally
- *M. bovis* causes tuberculosis in humans as well as in cattle
- *M. africanum*, which also causes human tuberculosis
- *M. leprae*, the agent of **leprosy** — a disease affecting millions in Asia and Africa
- Mycobacteria other than tuberculosis bacilli (**MOTT**), such as *M. avium–intracellulare* complex and *M. kansasii*, which cause frequent disease in HIV-infected patients.

Mycobacterium tuberculosis

Habitat and transmission

Found in infected humans, mainly in the lungs; in the body it resides primarily in the cells of the reticuloendothelial system; transmission is by coughing (droplet spread).

Characteristics

Acid- and alcohol-fast, slender, beaded bacilli; non-sporing. As the organisms do not take up the Gram stain because of the long-chain fatty acids (mycolic acid) in the cell wall, a special stain (the **Ziehl–Neelsen stain**) is required to visualize them. However, fluorescent microscopy, with auramine stain, is now used commonly for this purpose.

Culture and identification

This species does not grow on ordinary media and requires **Löwenstein–Jensen medium** for growth (constituents: whole egg, asparagine, glycerol, malachite green). Slow-growing (2–3 weeks; sometimes up to 6 weeks), at 37°C. They grow as 'rough, tough and buff' colonies — rough due to dry, irregular growth, tough due to difficulty in lifting the colony from the surface, and buff due to the pale yellow colour (Fig. 19.1).

In general, identification of mycobacteria is based on their rate of growth, optimum temperature requirements, and pigment production in the presence or absence of light; bio-chemical tests are also helpful. These slow procedures are being supplanted by more efficient nucleic acid probe techniques.

Pathogenicity

This organism is the agent of tuberculosis, a chronic, granulomatous, slowly progressive infection, usually of the lungs; eventually many other organs and tissues may be affected. A pandemic disease, tuberculosis is especially common in the developing world owing to HIV infection (15–20% of individuals with HIV disease may have tuberculosis). The oral cavity is affected secondary to primary disease elsewhere (see Ch. 35). The hallmark of the disease is granuloma formation and caseation mediated by cellular immunity. No exotoxins or endotoxins.

Antibiotic sensitivity and control

Long-term therapy (6–9 months) with antituberculous drugs (isoniazid, rifampicin, pyrazinamide, ethambutol). As drug resistance is growing and a persistent problem, combination therapy should always be given. Tubercle bacilli resistant to a number of antituberculous drugs (**multidrug-resistant tuberculosis**, MDR-TB) is a growing problem.

Prevention is by **BCG** (bacille Calmette–Guérin) **vaccination** containing live attenuated organisms, in childhood. Pasteurization of milk and general improvement of living standards have played a valuable role in prevention.

Mycobacterium bovis

This organism infects cattle. Humans become infected by ingesting *M. bovis*-contaminated milk. Infection is rarely seen in the west owing to eradication of the disease in cattle. The organism specifically causes the childhood disease **scrofuloderma**, characterized by enlarged, caseous cervical lymph nodes. *Mycobacterium bovis* is similar in many respects to *M. tuberculosis*; in the laboratory it can be distinguished from the latter by its poor growth on Löwenstein–Jensen medium and ready infection of rabbits.

Mycobacterium leprae

Habitat and transmission

Humans are the only known hosts of *M. leprae*, which resides mainly in the skin and nerves. Prolonged contact is thought to be the mode of transmission.

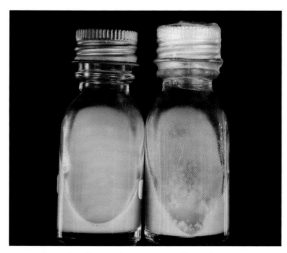

Fig. 19.1 Growth of *Mycobacterium tuberculosis* on Löwenstein–Jensen medium: the bottle on the left is uninoculated; the bottle on the right shows 'rough, tough and buff' colonies of the organism.

Table 19.1 Comparison of the different types of leprosy

	Tuberculoid	Lepromatous
Cell-mediated immunity	++	– or ±
Antibody response	–	++
Widespread lesions	–	+
Numbers of *Mycobacterium leprae* in lesions	±	++

Key: ++, predominant; +, common; ±, uncommon; –, absent.

Characteristics

Aerobic, acid-fast bacilli (they are not alcohol-fast, i.e. de-colorized by alcohol); no known toxins.

Culture and identification

Cannot be cultured in vitro but grows on the footpads of mice or armadillos, yielding chronic granulomas at the in-oculation site.

Pathogenicity

The leprosy bacillus causes a slow, progressive, chronic disease which mainly affects the skin and the nerves; the lesions are predominantly seen in the cooler parts of the body. Two forms of leprosy are recognized (Table 19.1).

Lepromatous leprosy. The cell-mediated immune response is depressed or absent; *M. leprae* bacilli are usually seen in large numbers in the lesions and in blood; commonly involves mucosae, especially the nose (Fig. 19.2); leads to much disfigurement.

Tuberculoid leprosy. Associated with an intense cell-mediated immune response to the organisms; principally involves the nerves, with resultant anaesthesia and paraes-

thesia. Hence damage to extremities is caused, with resultant loss of fingers, toes, etc. (see Ch. 35 for oral manifestations).

Antibiotic sensitivity and control

Antileprotic drugs are dapsone, rifampicin and clofazimine. As drug resistance is a growing problem, combination therapy is always given. No vaccine is available. Family contacts may be given dapsone.

MOTT

Mycobacteria other than tuberculosis bacilli (MOTT) is a collective name given to a group of mycobacteria of low human pathogenicity. These species include *M. avium*, *M. intracellulare*, *M. kansasii*, *M. marinum*, *M. fortuitum* and others.

Habitat and transmission

Isolated from soil, water, birds and animals.

Culture and identification

Grow on Löwenstein–Jensen medium but differ from 'pathogenic' mycobacteria in the colour of pigment pro-duced and temperature requirements. Some species pro-duce pigments in the dark (**scotochromogens**), others after exposure to light (**photochromogens**), and still others are non-chromogenic.

Pathogenicity and antibiotic sensitivity

In the main MOTT cause pulmonary infection, often with *M. tuberculosis*; infections are especially seen in compromised individuals (e.g. in HIV disease). These mycobacteria are thought to be passengers in the disease process. They are usually sensitive to the normal antituberculous drugs.

Mycobacterium marinum, associated with the keeping of tropical fish, causes skin ulcers.

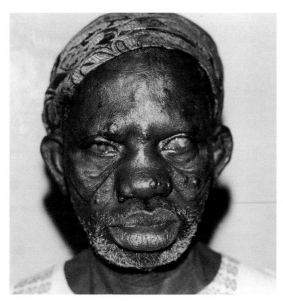

Fig. 19.2 A patient with lepromatous leprosy. Note the saddle nose and associated general disfigurement and blindness.

LEGIONELLA

There are currently some 39 recognized species belonging to the genus *Legionella*, but *L. pneumophila*, the species first described, is the most important human pathogen. They cause atypical pneumonia, both in community dwellers and hospitalized patients.

Legionella pneumophila

Habitat and transmission

Ubiquitous organism found in soil and water, including air-conditioning units, domestic and hospital water supplies, and sometimes in dental unit water systems. Spread is known to occur by contaminated aerosols.

Characteristics

Gram-negative slender rods, which stain faintly with the standard Gram stain.

Culture and identification

Does not grow on ordinary media; grows slowly (3 weeks) in a special medium (cysteine–charcoal–yeast extract agar) under 5% carbon dioxide. Identification is by direct immunofluorescence.

Pathogenicity

The portal of entry is the respiratory tract and infection results in **legionnaires' disease**, a severe form of pneumonia. Older men who smoke and drink alcohol in excess are typically affected. Other risk factors are cancer and immunosuppression. The clinical picture is variable, ranging from mild influenza-like illness to severe pneumonia with mental confusion, diarrhoea, haematuria and proteinuria. A less severe form of pneumonia (**Pontiac fever**) may be produced by some legionellae.

Antibiotic sensitivity and control

Erythromycin is the drug of choice and may be combined with rifampicin or ciprofloxacin.

It is impossible to eradicate the organism from water supplies as it is ubiquitous, but protective measures include increasing chlorine concentration and the temperature of hospital water supplies; aerosolization of water should be minimized.

KEY FACTS

- Mycobacteria are acid-fast, beaded bacilli and resist decolorization with strong acids (after mordanting in stain). Hence a special stain, the Ziehl–Neelsen stain, is used to visualize them
- The above property is due to the high lipid content (40–60%) of the cell wall (mycolic acid), which is also an effective defence mechanism resisting phagocytosis
- *Mycobacterial infections are chronic, granulomatous (leads to granuloma formation) and insidious*
- *Mycobacterium tuberculosis, the agent of tuberculosis, is a long, slender, non-sporing, beaded bacillus*
- It grows slowly (up to 6 weeks) in Löwenstein–Jensen medium as 'rough, tough and buff' colonies

- *Multidrug-resistant tuberculosis (MDR-TB) is becoming an increasingly common problem, especially in the developing world*
- *Leprosy, a disfiguring, chronic illness, is caused by* Mycobacterium leprae
- Up to 39 species belonging to the genus *Legionella* are recognized; *L. pneumophila* is the most important human pathogen
- Legionellae are Gram-negative slender rods, but stain faintly with the standard Gram stain
- Legionella pneumophila *causes legionnaires' disease, a condition that may range from a mild influenza-like illness to severe pneumonia with mental confusion, especially in the elderly*

FURTHER READING

Bagg, J (1996). Tuberculosis: a re-emerging problem for health care workers. *British Dental Journal* 180, 376–381.

Fallon, RJ (1996). *Legionellaceae*. In Collee, JG, Fraser, AG, Marmion, BP, and Simmons, A (eds) *Mackie and McCartney's Practical medical microbiology* (14th edn). Churchill Livingstone, Edinburgh.

Greenwood, D, Slack, R, and Peutherer, J (eds) (1997). *Medical microbiology* (15th edn). Chs 19, 34. Churchill Livingstone, Edinburgh.

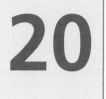

20 Chlamydiae, rickettsiae and mycoplasmas

Chlamydiae, rickettsiae and mycoplasmas are a miscellaneous group of organisms with properties common to both bacteria and viruses. Although they are categorized together in this chapter for the sake of convenience, they differ markedly from each other and cause divergent human diseases. A comparison of bacteria, chlamydiae, rickettsiae, mycoplasmas and viruses is given in Chapter 2, Table 2.1.

CHLAMYDIAE

The chlamydiae are a group of microorganisms related to Gram-negative bacteria. However, unlike bacteria they are unable to grow on inanimate culture media. They are therefore obligatory intracellular parasites. Their main characteristics include the following:
- larger than most viruses and hence visible by light microscopy
- both DNA and RNA are present
- obligate intracellular parasites with a complex growth cycle
- sensitive to tetracycline, erythromycin, sulphonamides.

There are three species in the genus *Chlamydia*:
- *Chlamydia trachomatis* is an agent of many diseases (see below)
- *Chlamydia pneumoniae* causes acute respiratory tract infection including sore throat, mild pneumonia, and fever in humans
- *Chlamydia psittaci* primarily causes disease (**psittacosis**) in birds such as pet parrots and budgerigars, from whom humans contract the infection. The human infection, also known as psittacosis, takes the form of a **primary atypical pneumonia**.

Chlamydia trachomatis

Causes a spectrum of diseases:
- **Ocular infections** — neonatal conjunctivitis (blennorrhoea), keratoconjunctivitis, blindness (trachoma). Trachoma is a major cause of blindness in the developing world.
- **Genital infections** — non-specific urethritis, the most common sexually transmitted disease in the UK. In the tropics it causes lymphogranuloma venereum.
- **Pneumonia** — in neonates.

Culture and diagnosis

Identified by **tissue culture** (e.g. HeLa cells), **serology** (complement fixation test) and **fluorescent antibody staining** of smears from the lesion.

Antibiotic sensitivity

Tetracycline is effective for all chlamydial infections.

RICKETTSIAE

Rickettsiae are pleomorphic organisms, smaller than bacteria but resembling them structurally and metabolically, including cell wall formation. They, like chlamydia and viruses, are obligate intracellular parasites. The best-known human rickettsial disease is **typhus**, which spreads wildly in conditions of malnutrition and poverty. Rickettsiae are:
- coccobacilli, with a multilayered outer cell wall resembling that of Gram-negative bacteria
- obligate intracellular parasites which replicate by binary fission
- visible by light microscope when special stains are used (e.g. Giemsa)
- able to infect many species, including arthropods, birds and mammals; members of the genus are transmitted to humans via bites of infected arthropods
- sensitive to tetracycline and chloramphenicol.

There are two genera within the Rickettsieae: *Rickettsia* and *Coxiella*.

Rickettsia

Rickettsial diseases include:
- **typhus**, an acute febrile illness, now rare, with a maculopapular rash transmitted by the rat flea; the fatality rate is frequently high as a result of haemorrhagic complications
- **spotted fevers** — Rocky Mountain spotted fever and other tick-borne fevers.

Coxiella

Coxiella burnetii, an organism closely resembling rickettsiae, causes **Q fever**, a typhus-like illness. Usually Q fever presents 131 as a 'non-bacterial' pneumonia, but lesions may be seen in the brain and other organs, including the heart, with resultant infective endocarditis.

Culture and diagnosis

- Guinea-pig inoculation
- Serology: rising titre of antibody in paired sera.

Antibiotic sensitivity

Tetracycline or chloramphenicol.

MYCOPLASMAS

Mycoplasmas are the smallest prokaryotes capable of binary fission, and they grow, albeit slowly, on inanimate media. Mycoplasmas are indeed wall-less bacteria, without the peptidoglycan cell wall but bound by a plasma membrane consisting of lipids and sterols (including cholesterol). Hence they are highly **pleomorphic**. The most important species of the genus *Mycoplasma* is *M. pneumoniae*, which causes:

- a common pneumonia, atypical pneumonia
- mucocutaneous eruptions, including the oral mucosa
- haemolytic anaemia.

Mycoplasma pneumoniae

Primary atypical pneumonia

Primary atypical pneumonia takes the form of fever, non productive cough, severe headache, weakness and tiredness. The acute illness lasts for about 2 weeks, but in a majority the symptoms last longer.

Mucocutaneous eruptions

Mycoplasma pneumoniae may cause skin rashes and ulcerations of both the oral and vaginal mucosa. These appear as maculopapular, vesicular or erythematous eruptions. The skin lesions, which often affect the extremities, have a target or iris appearance (target lesions). In the oral mucosa erythematous patches may appear first, quickly becoming bullous and erosive. This leads to extensive blood encrustations, especially the labial lesions. When the oral ulceration is associated with the skin rash and conjunctivitis it is called **Stevens–Johnson syndrome**.

Culture and diagnosis

Mycoplasma can be cultured in special media but is a slow grower (about 10 days); the colonies have a characteristic 'fried egg' appearance. Immunofluorescence of colonies transferred to glass slides is useful (as they do not take up the Gram stain well).

Serology is useful as the culture results are delayed. Complement fixation testing for *M. pneumoniae* antibodies is diagnostic.

Antibiotic sensitivity

Tetracycline for adults and erythromycin for children.

Oral mycoplasmas

Mycoplasmas have been isolated from saliva, oral mucosa and dental plaque but their significance is not clear. The oral species are poorly characterized and include *Mycoplasma buccale, M. orale* and *M. salivarium*. The latter two species have been isolated from salivary glands, and are thought to play a role in salivary gland hypofunction. Estimates of the oral carriage of mycoplasma vary from 6% to 32%.

KEY FACTS

- **Chlamydiae** are obligatory **intracellular parasites** related to Gram-negative bacteria
- **Chlamydia trachomatis** *causes ocular (neonatal conjunctivitis, keratoconjunctivitis, blindness — trachoma), genital (non-specific urethritis, lymphogranuloma venereum) and respiratory tract (pneumonia) infections*
- **Rickettsiae** are tiny **coccobacilli resembling Gram-negative bacteria**, and like chlamydiae are **obligatory intracellular parasites**
- All members of the genus *Rickettsia* are **transmitted** to humans by **bites** of infected **arthropods**
- *Rickettsial diseases include typhus, an acute febrile illness (frequently fatal) with a maculopapular rash*

- **Mycoplasmas** are the **smallest prokaryotes** capable of binary fission, and exist as **pleomorphic** morphologic forms (as they lack peptidoglycan cell wall)
- **Mycoplasma pneumoniae** *is an important human pathogen and causes atypical pneumonia, haemolytic anaemia and mucocutaneous eruptions*
- *Mucocutaneous eruptions often affect the extremities and have a target or iris appearance (**target lesions**)*
- *The oral mucosal lesions of* **M. pneumoniae** *appear erythematous at first and quickly become **bullous and erosive**, leading to extensive **blood encrustations***
- **Oral mycoplasmas** (*M. buccale, M. orale, M. salivarium*) have been **isolated from saliva, oral mucosa** and **dental plaque**, but their significance in either health or disease is unclear

---

FURTHER READING

Greenwood, D, Slack, R, and Peutherer, J (eds) (1997). *Medical microbiology* (15th edn), Chs 40–42. Churchill Livingstone, Edinburgh.

21 Viruses of relevance to dentistry

This chapter gives an outline of the viruses that are of special relevance to dentistry. The DNA viruses are described first, followed by the RNA viruses (see Table 4.1).

DNA VIRUSES

Papovaviruses

These DNA viruses infect both humans and animals; however, human disease is infrequent.

Human papillomavirus

Human papillomavirus (HPV) mainly causes skin warts (verrucae); also associated with a number of lesions including oral papillomas, oral verrucous carcinomas and focal epithelial hyperplasia. There are more than 70 serological types of HPV, some of which are more closely associated with lesions (both benign and cancerous) than others.

Skin warts
- **Clinical features**: warts typically are benign epithelial tumours. Specific serological types of HPV are associated with anogenital warts (condylomata acuminata) and are seen in all cervical biopsies that show precancerous change.
- **Epidemiology**: warts are generally more common in children than in adults. The virus is likely to be transmitted by direct contact or autoinoculation.

Oral infections with HPV. Over 40% of healthy individuals have HPV in the normal oral mucosa, suggesting that this is a reservoir of the virus.

Oral squamous papillomas and warts
- **Clinical features**: most are single, small (1 cm), pedunculated, exophytic lesions (Fig. 21.1). They rarely, if ever, progress to carcinomas.
- **Epidemiology**: occur mainly in the third to fifth decade of life, with a male preponderance.

Verrucous carcinoma. There is evidence to indicate that HPV is associated with human carcinomas, on the basis of:
- the frequent malignant change in virus-induced warts in **epidermodysplasia verruciformis**
- the frequent association of HPV-16, -18 and -33 with invasive cervical cancer

- development of cancer in vulvar warts in women with lymphoma.

Adenoviruses

These DNA viruses induce **latent infections** of the tonsils, adenoids and other lymphoid tissues of humans. However, most infections caused by adenoviruses are acute and self-limiting.

Adenoviral diseases

Acute respiratory disease is the most common adenovirus infection. It is an influenza-like illness seen commonly in military training camps. Clinically the main symptoms are pharyngitis and conjunctivitis. Although self-limiting, acute respiratory disease may be complicated by pneumonia in some cases. Other infections caused by these viruses include pharyngoconjunctival fever (a disease of infants and children), epidemic keratoconjunctivitis, pneumonia and gastroenteritis.

Epidemiology. Adenoviruses are ubiquitous and human beings are the only known reservoir for the human strains. The infections are spread from person to person by respiratory and ocular secretions. Adequate chlorination of pools may help decrease the spread of pharyngoconjunctival fever.

Herpesviruses

There are a range of different human herpesviruses, currently numbered 1 to 8 (see Table 4.3). All of them are structurally similar (enveloped, icosahedral with double-stranded DNA) and infect both humans and animals. They are the most common causes of human viral infections. All have the important property of remaining **latent**, with the ability to reinfect the host a variable period after the primary infection. Important human pathogens include herpes simplex virus types 1 and 2 (HSV-1 and HSV-2), varicella–zoster virus (VZV), cytomegalovirus (CMV) and Epstein–Barr virus (EBV) (see Ch. 4). Students of dentistry should be thoroughly conversant with the herpes group of viruses as the majority of them either cause oral infection or are intimately associated with orofacial tissues and saliva.

Structure

See Chapter 4.

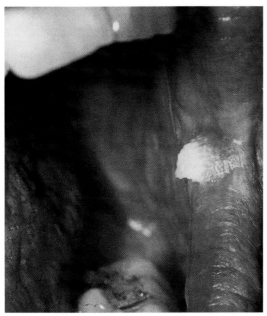

Fig. 21.1   A papilloma at the angle of the mouth.

Herpes simplex virus (human herpesviruses 1 and 2)

There are two types of herpes simplex virus: HSV-1 and HSV-2. They can be differentiated by serotyping, by DNA homology, and to some extent by clinical disease pattern.

Clinical disease

Disease due to HSV can be either a **primary infection**, due to first encounter with the virus, or a **reactivation** or **recurrent infection**, due to activation of the latent virus.

Primary infection. There is an **incubation period** of 2–20 days, depending upon the infected site and the infecting strain of virus. The lesions include:

- *primary gingivostomatitis* with lesions on the lips and mouth; very common (see Ch. 35)
- *genital herpes*: vesicular eruption of the genitalia, mostly due to HSV-2 (but up to a third of the cases may be due to HSV-1)
- *herpetic whitlow*: infection of the fingers, acquired by dentists and nurses as a result of contamination of the hands by virus-laced saliva or other secretions (Fig. 21.2)
- *conjunctivitis and keratitis*: less commonly, HSV infections involve the eyes, sometimes leading to blindness
- *encephalitis*: a result of either primary or recurrent infection; may lead to permanent defects or death.

Recurrent infections. Recurrence or reactivation of HSV entails activation of the non-infectious form of the latent virus residing in the neurons of either the trigeminal ganglion (Fig. 21.3) or the sacral ganglia. Reactivation is provoked by menstruation, stress, sunlight (possibly ultraviolet rays), local trauma, etc.; the lesions tend to recur at the site of the primary lesion. Herpes simplex virus has been implicated in Bell's palsy.

Epidemiology

Humans are the only known reservoir for HSV-1 and HSV-2; experimental infection can be induced in animals and cell cultures. As the virus is highly labile most primary infections are acquired through direct contact with a lesion or contaminated secretions. In general, HSV-1 causes orofacial lesions or lesions 'above the belt', while HSV-2 causes lesions 'below the belt', i.e. genital herpes (Fig. 21.4). However, because of sexual promiscuity or for other reasons this may not be always true. Type 1 HSV is acquired early in life, while HSV-2 appears after the onset of sexual activity.

As recurrent infection is common in the presence of high antibody titres, circulating antibodies appear to be unhelpful in controlling HSV infection. One reason for this may be the contiguous cell-to-cell spread of the virus, which cannot be prevented by antibody. Reactivation is not accompanied by a rise in herpes antibody titre.

Diagnosis

Diagnosis is usually achieved clinically; laboratory diagnosis is useful to confirm infection, especially in compromised patients. This entails:

- direct demonstration of viral antigens in vesicular fluid or scrapings by electron microscopy or immunofluorescence (Fig. 21.5)
- demonstration of characteristic multinuclear giant cells in scrapings from lesions; simple but not always successful
- propagation of virus in tissue culture.

Prevention

Control is difficult because of the high frequency of asymptomatic infection. It is important to avoid contact with acute herpetic lesions and contaminated body fluid (e.g. saliva) by routine wearing of gloves. No vaccine is available.

Treatment

The course of primary infection can be altered significantly with drugs that interfere with viral DNA synthesis, such as *aciclovir* and *vidarabine*, but these should be administered in the early prodromal phase of the disease for best results (see also Ch. 35).

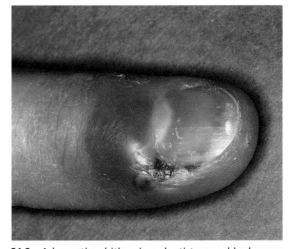

Fig. 21.2   A herpetic whitlow in a dentist caused by herpes simplex virus.

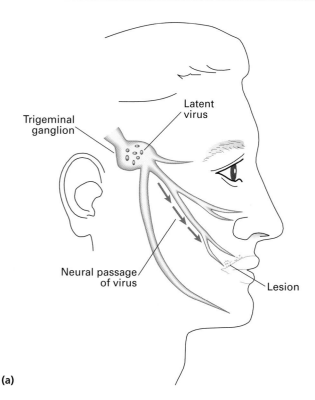

(a)

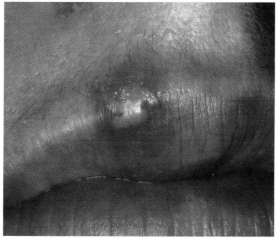

(b)

Fig. 21.3 Herpes labialis: (a) recurrence of facial herpes infection due to reactivation of the latent virus in the trigeminal ganglion; (b) clinical presentation of herpes labialis on the mucocutaneous junction of the upper lip.

Varicella–zoster virus (human herpesvirus 3)

This organism causes both **varicella** (chickenpox) and **herpes zoster** (shingles) — two different diseases due to an identical organism. Chickenpox is the primary infection, and zoster the reactivation of illness.

Clinical disease

Varicella. A common childhood fever, varicella is mild and self-limiting. The disease is more severe if contracted in adulthood. After a 2-week incubation period, fever develops, followed by a papular rash of the skin and mucous membranes, including the oral mucosa. The papules rapidly become vesicular and itchy but painless (in contrast to the rash in zoster).

Zoster (shingles). Occurs primarily as a reactivation of the virus in dorsal root or cranial nerve (usually trigeminal) ganglia (Fig. 21.6). The disease usually affects adults, and

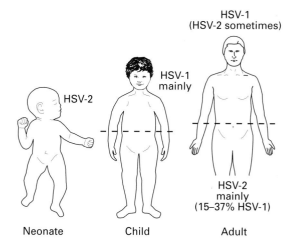

Fig. 21.4 Predominant distribution of infection with herpes simplex virus HSV-1 and HSV-2, in different age groups.

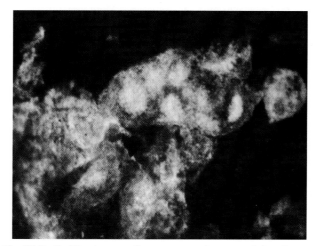

Fig. 21.5 Positive immunofluorescence of a smear taken from the lip lesion shown in Figure 21.3b (stained with anti-herpes antibody tagged to a fluorescing chemical) indicating that the patient has herpes labialis.

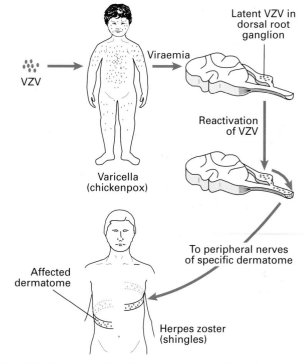

Fig. 21.6 Pathogenesis and sequelae of varicella–zoster virus (VSV) infection.

the virus is reactivated despite circulating antibodies. Zoster is triggered by trauma, drugs, neoplastic disease or immunosuppression.

The virus remains latent in ganglionic nerve cells and, after activation, travels back along the nerve fibre to the skin. Thoracic nerves supplying the chest wall are most often affected and the lesion presents as a unilateral, painful vesicular rash which extends in a horizontal strip from the middle of the back around the side of the chest wall ('belt of roses from hell'). Fever and malaise accompany the lesion. The rash may last for 2–4 weeks, with pain (**post-herpetic neuralgia**) persisting for weeks or months.

The trigeminal nerve is affected in about 15% of cases, with involvement of the ophthalmic, maxillary and mandibular divisions (in that order of precedence). Severe localized oral pain precedes the rash and may be easily confused with toothache (see Ch. 35). Involvement of the ophthalmic nerve may lead to eye lesions and sometimes blindness.

Ramsay Hunt syndrome is a rare manifestation of zoster, with a vesicular rash on the tympanic membrane and the external auditory canal, together with unilateral facial nerve palsy.

Epidemiology

Shingles is primarily a disease of older adults and immuno-compromised persons; it is rare in children. The incidence increases with advancing age, and with decreasing degree of immunocompetence. It is a highly contagious infection in a host not previously exposed to the virus. Transmission occurs by direct contact with skin lesions or droplet infection from infectious saliva.

Diagnosis

The clinical picture is pathognomonic, as the lesion distribution overlaps and accurately maps the distribution of the sensory nerve (Fig. 21.7). Serology, if needed, entails detecting a fourfold rise in antibody titre in paired sera (compare herpes simplex reactivation, where antibody rise is not significant).

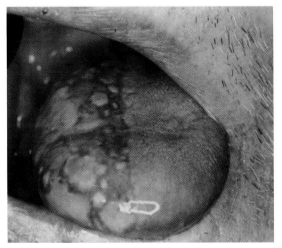

Fig. 21.7 Herpes zoster infection of the tongue: note the sharp midline demarcation of the lesion (due to reactivation of the virus travelling via the lingual branch of the right trigeminal nerve).

Treatment

Chickenpox is self-limiting and requires symptomatic treatment, if any. Disseminated zoster in immunocompromised patients requires antiviral drugs (e.g. aciclovir, vidarabine), which interfere with herpesvirus DNA replication. Varicella–zoster virus is less sensitive to aciclovir than is HSV and hence a higher dosage is required; therapy should start within 72 hours of onset. Systemic aciclovir may reduce the duration of the early infective phase and the associated pain. In addition it may reduce the prevalence of post-herpetic neuralgia.

Prevention

Passive immunization with varicella–zoster immune globulin (VZIG) may be indicated for persons at high risk of severe infection.

Epstein–Barr virus (human herpesvirus 4)

Epstein–Barr virus is widespread in humans, and most adults have antibody to the virus. The virus persists in latent form within lymphocytes after primary infection (lymphotrophic, unlike HSV and VZV which are neurotrophic). The genome resides in a latent form in B cells; latent EBV infection is common in the population. It is the aetiological agent of a number of diseases:
- infectious mononucleosis (glandular fever)
- Burkitt's lymphoma and other B-cell lymphomas
- nasopharyngeal carcinoma (especially in southern Chinese populations)
- oral hairy leukoplakia
- post-transplant lymphoproliferative diseases.

Infectious mononucleosis

An acute infection affecting lymphoid tissue throughout the body, infectious mononucleosis is commonly seen in teenagers, with a peak incidence at 15–20 years of age. The organism is present in saliva and is postulated to be transmitted during kissing — hence called '*kissing disease*'.

Incubation period. Incubation is 4–7 weeks; possibly shorter (10–40 days) in young children.

Signs and symptoms. Low-grade fever with generalized lymphadenopathy and abnormal lymphocytes in the blood (note that a similar illness, **glandular fever-like syndrome**, develops during the first fortnight after infection with HIV). Fever, tonsillitis and fatigue are common, and many patients have splenomegaly. Lymphocytosis is a characteristic feature, hence the term 'mononucleosis'; some 10% of the lymphocytes are atypical, with enlarged misshapen nuclei and increased cytoplasm (Fig. 21.8).

Chronic, persistent or reactivated EBV infection

This may take many clinical forms and is less common than acute mononucleosis, described above. The syndrome is characterized by persistent fatigue, with or without physical or laboratory findings.

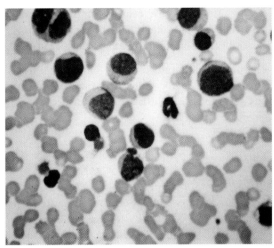

Fig. 21.8 Infectious mononucleosis: characteristic blood film with many mononuclear cells.

Epidemiology

The virus is ubiquitous and humans are its only known host. Spread of EBV is via respiratory secretions, primarily through oral contact. Those from lower socioeconomic classes are exposed to EBV at an early age and typically develop asymptomatic infections, while in higher socioeconomic classes, particularly in developed countries, primary infection is usually delayed to adolescence or young adulthood.

Diagnosis

As EBV cannot be easily propagated in culture, serological diagnosis is common:

- **indirect immunofluorescence** is used to detect EBV-specific IgM; the antibody is directed against both the capsid antigen and a non-capsid early antigen
- **haematology**: a blood film is useful for demonstrating atypical lymphocytosis in infectious mononucleosis
- **heterophile antibody** (non-specific): infectious mononucleosis is characterized by the appearance of heterophile (*hetero* other, *phile* liking) antibodies in the patient's serum, which agglutinate sheep or horse red blood cells. This property is made use of in the Paul–Bunnell diagnostic test.

Treatment

Infectious mononucleosis is generally mild and self-limiting, hence therapy is usually symptomatic.

Burkitt's lymphoma

Burkitt's lymphoma is a highly malignant tumour which spreads rapidly, with widespread metastases; it is particularly common in African children. The disease is especially common in areas of Africa with endemic malaria. Hence it is thought that the effect of the malarial parasite on the reticuloendothelial system could cause an abnormal response to infection with EBV. Under these conditions the EBV may become frankly **oncogenic**, producing a malignant transformation in lymphoid tissue (lymphoma) instead of the benign proliferation seen in infectious mononucleosis.

Nasopharyngeal carcinoma

A tumour with a remarkable geographic and probably racial distribution; it is particularly common among the southern Chinese. Epstein–Barr viral DNA is regularly present in the malignant epithelial cells of the tumour.

Hairy leukoplakia

The term 'hairy leukoplakia' is given to raised, white areas of thickening, particularly on the lateral border of the tongue (see Fig. 30.3). Although this new clinical entity was first described in HIV-infected patients, other immunosuppressed patients may develop the lesion, which is very closely associated with EBV. The DNA of EBV is present in the epithelial cells of hairy leukoplakia. The lesion is non-malignant but about a third of HIV-infected individuals who develop hairy leukoplakia may develop AIDS in 3–5 years. Demonstration of EBV in biopsy tissue of hairy leukoplakia is essential for a definitive diagnosis.

Cytomegalovirus (human herpesvirus 5)

Cytomegalovirus rarely causes disease unless other precipitating factors, such as immunocompromising states, are present. However, it can infect the fetus during pregnancy.

Clinical disease

Symptomless infection. The majority of infants show no signs of infection and diagnosis is made by serology. Although a large proportion of the infants are unharmed, a significant number of neonates with congenital infection show neurological sequelae, such as deafness and mental retardation, later in life. A minority develop a severe, often fatal illness associated with infection of the salivary glands, brain, kidneys, liver and lungs.

Postnatal infection. Later in life the virus may be activated by pregnancy, multiple blood transfusion or immunosuppression. Infection in immunocompromised patients can be severe and involve many organs, such as the lungs, liver, gastrointestinal tract and eyes.

Epidemiology

Infection appears to increase during the perinatal period and during early adulthood; patients with neoplastic disease or AIDS and transplant recipients often have local and disseminated CMV disease. The route of CMV transmission is not clear.

Diagnosis and treatment

Diagnosis is by viral isolation in human embryonic fibroblast tissue cultures; it is confirmed using immunofluorescence and DNA hybridization.

There are no proven regimens for therapy and prevention of CMV infections.

Human herpesvirus 6

A DNA virus closely related to CMV, human herpesvirus 6 (HHV-6) was isolated originally from peripheral blood cells of immunocompromised patients, such as those with AIDS. The virus shows affinity for T and B cells in particular. Infection with HHV-6 is common in childhood, and most primary infections are asymptomatic followed by latency. The pathogenicity of HHV-6 is unclear as yet.

Exanthem subitum (roseola infantum)

A common childhood disorder characterized by mild fever and a facial rash; appears to be associated with HHV-6 infection.

Mononucleosis with cervical lymphadenopathy

This is a febrile illness in adults with bilateral cervical lymphadenopathy, somewhat like glandular fever; thought to be a primary infection with HHV-6.

HHV-6 and the oral cavity

The virus is present in the saliva of most healthy adults, and it can also be demonstrated in ductal and alveolar epithelium of major salivary glands. There are no specific oral lesions reported for HHV-6, though erythematous papules seen in soft palate and uvula (Nagayama's spots) and in the pharynx are thought to be due to this organism. No occupational hazard from HHV-6 has been proved in dentistry but the virus may well be transmitted in saliva.

Human herpesviruses 7 and 8

These viruses have been recently identified: HHV-7 is a T-lymphotrophic virus and is implicated in rashes; HHV-8 is now known to be the agent responsible for Kaposi's sarcoma, a vascular endothelial tumour commonly seen in HIV disease; it is also implicated in sarcoidosis.

RNA VIRUSES

Orthomyxoviridae

These RNA viruses cause worldwide epidemics of influenza. They are subdivided as types A, B and C on the basis of the antigenic properties of their major **nucleocapsid protein** (NP) and viral envelope **matrix protein** (M protein). In addition to these antigenic differences they are characterized by a unique mechanism of frequent immunological variations within the subtypes. These variations are due to structural changes in the surface spike glycoproteins: **haemagglutinin** and **neuraminidase**. Influenza epidemics are due to the emergence of a new virus strain containing a haemagglutinin (and sometimes a neuraminidase) that differs from that of previously circulating viruses, so that the population has no (herd) immunity to the new haemagglutinin. Antigenic variation may occur due to:
- *Antigenic drift*, as a result of minor changes in the amino acid sequence of the haemagglutinin. These viruses survive because they are less susceptible to the antibodies most common in the population at the time.
- *Antigenic shift*, which constitutes the appearance of a new antigenic type unrelated or only distantly related to earlier types because of **genetic reassortment**. It occurs infrequently and has been identified only in influenza A (four major antigenic shifts have occurred since 1933).

These antigenic shifts are critically important in the production of vaccines for influenza: the vaccine used in previous years may have little or no effect because of these phenomena.

Influenza

Clinical features

Symptoms are sudden and appear 1–2 days after exposure. Major symptoms are high fever, accompanied by myalgia, sore throat, headache, cough and nasal congestion. Pneumonia is the most common serious complication of influenza; it is caused by secondary bacterial infection of the respiratory tract with weakened defences.

Epidemiology

Epidemic illness is common in non-immune or partially immune populations. Transmission occurs by aerosolization and subsequent inhalation of virus-laden respiratory secretions during sneezing and coughing (droplet spread). Rapid spread of illness may occur in confined populations (e.g. nursing homes, classrooms).

Treatment and prevention

Only symptomatic treatment is indicated. **Amantadine** is helpful for relieving symptoms and enhancing the effectiveness of immunization. The low success rate (about 70%) of the vaccination is mainly due to the difficulty of predicting the proper antigenic profile of the influenza strain; this unfortunately cannot be determined until the onset of the particular disease cycle.

Paramyxoviridae

The paramyxoviruses are enveloped, RNA viruses with an unsegmented genome, which cause major diseases of infancy and childhood. There are four groups of paramyxoviruses:
- parainfluenza virus
- mumps virus
- measles virus
- respiratory syncytial virus (RSV).

Parainfluenza and mumps viruses are antigenically related.

Parainfluenza viruses

The parainfluenza viruses cause human respiratory infections, especially in autumn and winter.

Clinical features

The major diseases caused by parainfluenza viruses, particularly in young children and infants, are laryngotracheobronchitis (croup), bronchiolitis and pneumonia. When adults are infected with any parainfluenza type the common cold is the usual result.

Epidemiology

Spread through respiratory/droplet secretions. Closed populations including young children are especially at risk.

Mumps virus

Mumps, measles, rubella and varicella (chickenpox) are the common childhood fevers. Mumps virus typically causes **parotitis** (mumps) of acute onset involving one or both parotid glands. The attenuated form of the mumps virus, incorporated in the combined **MMR** (measles, mumps, rubella) **vaccine**, leads to the development of antibody in 95% of vaccinees (see also Ch. 35).

Measles virus

Another agent of common childhood fever, measles virus causes one of the most highly infectious diseases known. Infection results in permanent immunity.

Clinical features

Measles is an acute febrile illness with a characteristic **exanthematous rash**. The virus enters through the respiratory tract and multiplies in the respiratory epithelium and regional lymphoid tissue for up to 12 days. In the next (viraemic) phase the virus spreads throughout the lymphoid tissues and skin. This stage is accompanied by prodromal symptoms: conjunctivitis, nasal discharge, headache, low-grade fever, sore throat and **Koplik's spots**. These are bluish-white, pinpoint spots surrounded by dark-red areolae which appear on the buccal mucosa opposite the molar teeth and sometimes near the orifice of the parotid duct. The measles rash appears to result from the interaction between virus-infected cells and either sensitized lymphocytes or antibody–complement complexes. The rash consists of fine, sparse, discrete macules. As the rash develops the Koplik's spots disappear.

Complications. The complication of measles virus infection are serious and could be:
- **Respiratory** complications (bronchopneumonia): the most serious; seen in 4% of patients, with or without secondary bacterial infection. **Otitis media** occurs in a smaller percentage.
- **Neurological** complications: include **encephalomyelitis** (with a mortality rate of some 10%) and **subacute sclerosing panencephalitis**. The latter is a rare, progressive, degenerative neurological disease of children and adolescents, causing mental and motor deterioration and death within a year.
- **Gangrenous stomatitis** and **noma**: seen in certain sub-Saharan African countries. A number of cofactors such as malnutrition, oral ulceration and acute necrotizing ulcerative gingivitis (ANUG) together with concurrent measles infection lead to progressive gangrene and gross destruction of the orofacial tissues, and consequent disfigurement.

Epidemiology

Measles is readily transmissible, usually via respiratory secretions and urine, especially during the prodromal phase and when the rash appears.

Prevention

The measles component of the MMR vaccine is a live attenuated virus which induces immunity for up to 10 years. However, in developing countries such as West Africa, where universal vaccination in childhood is not feasible, measles remains a severe disease and a major cause of death in childhood.

Respiratory syncytial virus

A major agent of lower respiratory tract disease, RSV causes worldwide epidemics of respiratory tract infection in infants and young children. Adults, although infected, develop only mild or non-apparent symptoms. The virus can cause colds, bronchiolitis and pneumonia, especially during the first 6 months of life. Approximately one-third of infants develop antibodies in the first year of life.

Picornaviridae

The Picornaviridae are non-enveloped, RNA viruses with an unsegmented genome. Four members of this family cause significant human disease: polioviruses, coxsackieviruses, echoviruses and rhinoviruses. The first three of these are enteroviruses.

Polioviruses

Polioviruses are agents of **paralytic poliomyelitis**.

Clinical features

Poliovirus infection is initiated by ingestion of infectious virions, after which primary replication occurs in oropharyngeal and intestinal mucosa. The virus drains into the cervical and mesenteric lymph nodes and then into the systemic circulation. Subsequent replication continues in a number of non-neural sites, leading to a persistent viraemia and spread into the central nervous system.

Paralytic poliomyelitis is unusual and depends on host factors that may predispose to neural infection. The incidence and severity of paralytic disease increase with age (e.g. teenagers are more likely than younger children to develop crippling disease).

Epidemiology

Polioviruses have a wide geographic distribution and spread rapidly, especially in densely populated areas with poor sewage control, such as in developing countries. Infection occurs mainly in the hot season and is spread in the faeces. Transmission is primarily by person-to-person contact through pharyngeal secretions, although the disease may spread by infected water.

Prevention

Spread of poliovirus disease has been successfully achieved through widespread immunization with either **killed** (Salk vaccine) or **live attenuated** virus (Sabin vaccine).

Coxsackieviruses

Coxsackieviruses are subdivided into two major groups, A and B, on the basis of the lesions they induce in suckling mice. Each group also has several serologically distinct subgroups. Most human coxsackievirus infections are mild and frequently asymptomatic. Serious infection, although rare, results in severe disease. Two diseases caused by group A coxsackieviruses are of particular dental interest: herpangina, and hand, foot and mouth disease.

Herpangina

Herpangina, caused by group A coxsackievirus, is common in children but may affect any age group.

Clinical features. The disease is characterized by fever, headache, sore throat, dysphagia, anorexia and occasionally a stiff neck. These symptoms are accompanied by herpes-like oropharyngitis, where the ulceration is predominantly on the tonsil, soft palate and uvula. The small, papulovesicular lesions are about 1–2 mm in diameter, with a greyish-white surface surrounded by red areolae. The disease is self-limiting and lasts for 3–4 days (see also Ch. 35).

Hand, foot and mouth disease

Hand, foot and mouth disease, also caused by group A coxsackievirus, is a relatively common infection in children. It is easily diagnosed because of its classic distribution in the hands, feet and mouth. The incubation period is about 3–5 days and resolution occurs within a week.

Clinical features. The disease may begin with facial pain, with tenderness along the course of the parotid duct and a few vesicles around the duct orifice. The onset of the oral and skin eruptions is accompanied by headache, malaise and sore throat, but in many there is little systemic upset. The oral lesions are generally bright-red macules which later form oval or grey vesicles with red areolae (see Ch. 35). The plantar surface of the feet and the palmar surface of the hands and sometimes the buttocks may be affected. These skin lesions are bright-red macules with pale centres which develop into thin-walled bullae or small ulcers with surrounding erythema. The lesions in the mouth, and on the hands and feet, are not always seen.

All serotypes of coxsackievirus have a worldwide distribution. They are highly infectious within families and closed communities and the greatest epidemic spread occurs in the summer and autumn. Viral transmission is by the faecal–oral route and from nasal and pharyngeal secretions. They enter through the mouth and nose, multiply locally and spread viraemically (compare polioviruses).

Rhinoviruses

The aetiological agents of the 'common cold' and a group of acute, afebrile upper respiratory diseases, rhinoviruses are readily inactivated at low pH conditions and require an incubation temperature of 33°C for maximal replication; hence they multiply well in the upper respiratory tract where the incoming air provides low temperature conditions suited to the virus.

Antigenicity

There is a vast array (more than 100) of immunologically distinct groups of rhinoviruses based on a single type-specific antigen. Hence the reason for recurrent colds, as the succeeding infective virus is likely to be antigenically different from the virus which caused the previous episode (i.e. immunity is effective only against **homologous challenge**).

Epidemiology

In a family unit rhinovirus transmission is usually initiated when a child introduces the virus, which spreads rapidly via nasal secretions. The disease is most common in the autumn, winter and early spring. Note, however, that rhinoviruses are not the only agents of the common cold, although they are the major culprits.

Togaviridae

Rubella

The agent of rubella (German measles) is a togavirus. Rubella is a childhood fever resembling measles, except that it has a milder clinical course and shorter duration. If rubella is contracted in early pregnancy the virus can cause severe congenital abnormalities and may cause the death of the fetus.

Epidemiology

Rubella is a highly contagious disease spread by nasal secretions. Because of its mild clinical symptoms the infection is often non-apparent and viral dissemination may be widespread before it is recognized. The disease may spread in the dental clinic environment. Females (especially of child-bearing age) should be immunized against the virus: the rubella component of the combined **MMR vaccine** contains a **live attenuated virus** which confers adequate protection.

Other RNA viruses

Other RNA virus families which have not been discussed here include the Arenaviridae, Bunyaviridae, Coronaviridae, Reoviridae, Rhabdoviridae and Retroviridae. Human immunodeficiency virus, which is in the latter family, is discussed in detail in Chapter 30 because of its major relevance to dentistry.

VIRUSES AND CANCER

Viruses that have the ability to cause cancer are called **oncogenic** viruses. A number of DNA viruses are oncogenic, but only one RNA virus is known to have this potential. The virus groups and the cancers they cause are summarized below.

Papovaviruses

The human **papillomaviruses** (HPV) cause benign warts, malignant carcinomas, and cervical cancers.

The **polyomavirus** and the **simian virus 40** (SV40) are oncogenic in laboratory animals.

Adenoviruses

Adenoviruses are oncogenic in newborn hamsters, but not in humans.

Herpesviruses

These are implicated in human cancers (see also above):
- **herpes simplex virus type 2** is a likely coagent of certain variants of **cervical cancer**
- **Epstein–Barr virus** is associated with **Burkitt's lymphoma** and **nasopharyngeal carcinoma**
- **human herpesvirus 8** is closely associated with the aetiology of *Kaposi's sarcoma* (an endothelial tumour) which is a well-recognized oral manifestation of HIV infection.

Hepadnaviruses

Hepatitis B virus is a well-known agent of human **hepatocellular carcinoma** (Ch. 29).

Retroviruses

Retroviruses include the human T-cell leukaemia viruses (HTLVs):
- **HTLV-I** is the agent of **adult T-cell leukaemia**, which is endemic in south-western Japan and the Caribbean region.
- **HTLV-II** is associated with human **lymphomas**.

KEY FACTS

DNA Viruses
- *Human papillomaviruses (HPV) are associated with benign epithelial tumours*
- *Adenoviruses cause acute respiratory disease, are ubiquitous, and humans are the only known reservoir*
- Up to **eight different types** of human **herpesviruses** (HHV) are described; they are **neurotrophic** and **epitheliotrophic**
- *Herpes simplex and zoster viruses cause primary and reactivation infection (post-primary infection)*
- *In general, herpes simplex viruses (HSV) types 1 and 2 cause infections 'above' and 'below the belt', respectively (i.e. oral and genital infections)*
- *Herpetic gingivostomatitis is the primary infection and herpes labialis the reactivation infection caused by HSV-1*
- *Varicella–zoster (HSV-3) causes chickenpox (primary) and zoster/shingles (reactivation) affecting well-defined dermatomes ('belt of roses from hell')*
- *Epstein–Barr virus (human herpesvirus 4) causes infectious mononucleosis or glandular fever, oral hairy leukoplakia, nasopharyngeal carcinoma, Burkitt's lymphoma and post-transplant lymphoproliferative diseases*
- *Cytomegalovirus (human herpesvirus 5) causes asymptomatic infection in adults; if infection occurs during pregnancy, transplacental passage of the virus may cause serious congenital defects or abortion*
- *Human herpesvirus 6 causes 'sixth disease' (or roseola infantum, exanthem subitum), a rash seen in young children*
- **Human herpesvirus 7** is isolated from lymphocytes carrying CD4; **not yet associated with disease**
- *Human herpesvirus 8 is the agent of Kaposi's sarcoma, a vascular endothelial tumour common in HIV disease*

RNA viruses
- *Orthomyxoviruses cause pandemics of influenza*
- Their success is due to the ability to undergo rapid antigenic changes (**antigenic shifts** and **antigenic drifts**) of haemagglutinin component of the outer surface spikes of the virus
- **Paramyxoviruses** include **parainfluenza** virus, **mumps** virus, **measles** virus and **respiratory syncytial virus**
- *Mumps virus is the major agent of parotitis (mumps)*
- *Measles is an acute febrile infection with an exanthematous rash; prodromal symptoms of measles include Koplik's spots on the buccal mucosa*
- *Complications of measles include bronchopneumonia, neurologic complications and gangrenous stomatitis or noma*
- *The MMR vaccine prevents measles, mumps and rubella*
- *Group A coxsackieviruses cause hand, foot and mouth disease of children and herpangina; oral lesions are papulovesicular, small and greyish-white*
- *Rhinoviruses are the agents of the common cold*
- **Oncogenic or cancer-causing viruses** include papillomaviruses, polyomavirus, simian virus, Epstein–Barr virus and HHV-8, human T-cell leukaemia viruses (retroviruses) and hepadnaviruses (causing hepatitis B)

FURTHER READING

Bagg, J (1994). Virology and the mouth. *Reviews in Medical Microbiology* 5, 209–216.

Cleator, GM, and Klapper, PE (1994). The Herpesviridae. In Zuckerman, AJ, Banatvala, JE, and Pattison, JR (eds) *Principles and practice of clinical virology* (3rd edn). John Wiley, Chichester.

Greenberg, MD (1996). Herpesvirus infections. *Dental Clinics of North America* 40, 359–368.

Scully, C, and Samaranayake, LP (1992). *Clinical virology in oral medicine and dentistry*. Cambridge University Press, Cambridge.

22 Fungi of relevance to dentistry

The study of fungi is called **mycology**. Fungi are **eukaryotic** microorganisms, as opposed to bacteria, which are **prokaryotic**. By far the most important fungus of relevance in dentistry is a yeast belonging to the genus *Candida*. It is an oral commensal in about half of the general population. In this chapter the general characteristics of some medically important fungi will be given, but the emphasis will be on fungal infections of the oral cavity — the **oral mycoses**, especially those caused by *Candida* species.

MORPHOLOGY

Fungi exhibit two basic structural forms: the **yeast** form (Fig. 22.1) and the **mould form**. While some fungi are capable of existing as both forms (**dimorphic**) at different times, others exist in one form only. This morphological switching depends on factors such as the environment and nutrient supply. Generally, dimorphic fungi exist as moulds in the natural environment (and in laboratory culture) and as yeasts in tissue.

- **Yeasts** are unicellular with spherical or ovoid bodies; all yeasts are similar morphologically on light microscopic examination.
- **Moulds** are multicellular with a variety of specialized structures which perform specific functions. The size and nature of these structures vary with different genera. **Hyphae** (singular: *hypha or hyphum*) are thread-like tubes containing the fungal cytoplasm and its organelles. They can be considered as the structural units of the mould. The hyphae are divided into unit cells by cross-walls called **septa**. The septa have pores that allow the movement of cytoplasm, and even organelles, between cells. The term **mycelium** is given to the mass of hyphae that forms the mould colony.

REPRODUCTION

Both asexual and sexual modes of reproduction are seen in fungi. It is believed that the sexual forms of fungi are not found in clinical material.

CLASSIFICATION

Taxonomy of fungi is a complex subject not dealt with here. Most of the medically important fungi are classified as **fungi imperfecti** as their sexual forms have not been identified. Fungi of medical importance are classified into:
- **yeasts**
- **filamentous fungi**
- **dimorphic fungi**.

The following methods are used in classification of fungi:
1. Yeasts are identified by biochemical reactions based on the fermentation and assimilation of carbohydrates, utilization of enzyme substrates and other metabolic activities.
2. Moulds are identified by their colour, texture and colonial and microscopic morphology. The specialized asexual reproductive structures of moulds are useful in differentiating various species of moulds.

CULTURAL REQUIREMENTS

Medically important fungi require different cultural and growth conditions when compared with bacteria:
1. The vast majority of medically important fungi grow aerobically.
2. **Sabouraud dextrose agar** (SAB) and variations of it, such as SAB plus antibacterial agents, and **potato dextrose agar** (PDA) are commonly used for laboratory culture of pathogenic fungi.

These mycological media differ from conventional bacteriological media in having a high carbohydrate content (SAB usually contains 3% dextrose or sucrose) and an acidic pH (approximately 4.0). Both these conditions are inhibitory to most bacteria. The SAB medium may also be supplemented with antibiotics to suppress bacterial growth.

PATHOGENICITY

In general, medically important fungi do not possess the virulent attributes of bacteria such as exotoxins and endotoxins (an exception is the **aflatoxin** produced by *Aspergillus* species); hence they cause slowly progressive chronic infections rather than the acute disease commonly seen in bacterial or viral diseases. However, they may cause life-threatening acute infections in immunocompromised patients (e.g. those with AIDS). The oral fungal pathogen *Candida* possesses a number of virulent attributes, including:

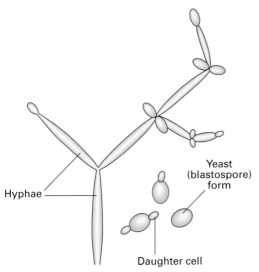

Fig. 22.1 The yeast (blastospore) and hyphal forms of *Candida albicans*.

- the ability to **adhere** to host tissues and prostheses (e.g. dentures)
- the potential to **switch** (e.g. rough to smooth colony formation) and modify the surface antigens
- the ability to form **hyphae** that helps in tissue invasion
- extracellular **phospholipase** and **proteinases** which appear to break down physical defence barriers of the host.

HUMAN MYCOSES

Human infections caused by fungi can be divided into:
- superficial mycoses
- subcutaneous mycoses
- systemic mycoses.

Superficial mycoses

Superficial mycoses involve the mucosal surfaces and keratin-containing structures of the body (skin, nails and hair). These infections, relatively common in Western countries, are in general cosmetic problems and are not life-threatening. Superficial mycoses include:

1. Yeast infections of mucosae which lead to **thrush** and similar manifestations (see Ch. 35).
2. **Dermatophyte** infection of skin, hair, etc., leading to ringworm or similar diseases.

Subcutaneous mycoses

Subcutaneous mycoses involve the subcutaneous tissue and rarely disseminate. They are the result of traumatic implantation of environmental fungi leading to chronic progressive disease, tissue destruction and sinus formation. Examples include sporotrichosis and mycetoma (Madura foot) which are common in the tropics and rare in the West.

Systemic mycoses (deep mycoses)

By far the most serious, and often fatal, systemic mycoses involve the internal organ systems of the body. The organisms are generally acquired through the respiratory tract and spread haematogenously. In the developed world they are increasingly seen in compromised patients with impaired defence systems when the organisms behave as opportunistic pathogens. In the developing world systemic mycoses (e.g. histoplasmosis, blastomycosis and coccidioidomycosis) occur in otherwise healthy individuals.

Opportunistic fungal infections

When fungi (such as *Candida albicans*) that are generally innocuous for healthy humans cause disease in compromised patient groups, they are called **opportunistic pathogens**. Such opportunistic mycoses are increasingly common owing to a global rise in compromised individuals such as HIV-infected patients, organ transplant recipients on immunosuppressive therapy, and cancer patients on cytotoxic and radiation therapy.

YEASTS

Yeasts are unicellular, oval or spherical organisms, 2–5 µm in diameter, and stain positively by the Gram method (Fig. 22.2). They are commonly seen to have lateral projections or buds called **daughter cells**. These gradually enlarge in size until they split off from the parent or mother cell to produce the next generation. Most yeasts develop pseudohyphae (chains of elongated budding cells devoid of septae) but only a few form true hyphae. Yeasts of the genus *Candida*, the most important fungal pathogen in the oral cavity, also form pseudohyphae. It is a common yeast which lives in the oral cavity of about half of the population and is also a resident commensal of the gut. It can cause either **superficial** or **systemic candidiasis** (candidosis). The superficial disease affects:
- the mucosa — mucosal candidiasis
- the skin — cutaneous candidiasis
- both the skin and the mucosa — mucocutaneous candidiasis.

The infection is usually **endogenous** in origin. Several species in the genus *Candida* are found in humans, including *C. albicans*, *C. glabrata*, *C. krusei* and *C. tropicalis* (Fig. 22.3),

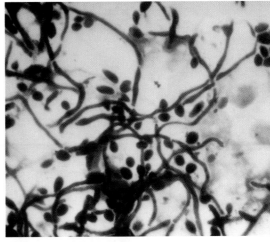

Fig. 22.2 A Gram-stained film of a smear from the fitting surface of the denture of a patient with *Candida*-associated denture stomatitis showing the blastospore and hyphal forms of the organism.

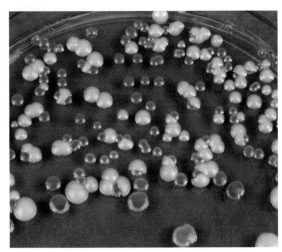

Fig. 22.3 *Candida albicans* and *Candida tropicalis* growing side by side on a special medium (Pagano–Levin agar) which elicits differential colour reactions. Mixed oral candidal infections are not uncommon.

but *C. albicans* is responsible for the vast majority of infections (> 90%). *Candida dubliniensis* is a newly recognized species of *Candida* very similar to *C. albicans*. First isolated from the oral cavity of HIV-infected patients, *C. dubliniensis* is now known to be a relatively common oral inhabitant both in health and disease.

Candida albicans

Habitat and transmission

Candida albicans is indigenous to the oral cavity, gastrointestinal tract, female genital tract and sometimes the skin; hence infection is usually endogenous, although cross-infection may occur, e.g. from mother to baby, and among infant siblings.

Characteristics

Candida albicans typically grows as spherical to oval budding yeast cells 3–5 μm × 5–10 μm in size. These are also called

blastospores (Fig. 22.4), but should not be confused with bacterial spores. **Pseudohyphae** (elongated filamentous cells joined end to end) are seen, especially at lower incubation temperatures and on nutritionally poor media.

Culture and identification

Cultures grow on Sabouraud medium as creamy-white colonies, flat or hemispherical in shape with a beer-like aroma. *Candida albicans* and *C. dubliniensis* may be differentiated from other *Candida* species by their ability to produce germ tubes and chlamydospores:

- When yeast cells are incubated for 3 hours at 37°C in serum, *C. albicans* and *C. dubliniensis* form **germ tubes** (incipient hyphae) whereas other *Candida* species do not (see Fig. 6.15).
- Both *C. albicans* and *C. dubliniensis* form round, thick-walled, resting structures called **chlamydospores** when incubated at 22–25°C with decreased oxygen on a nutritionally poor medium (e.g. cornmeal agar).

However, definitive identification of the species is made on the basis of carbohydrate assimilation (aerobic metabolism) and fermentation (anaerobic metabolism) reactions and other biochemical tests.

Pathogenicity

Candida species rarely cause disease in the absence of predisposing factors, a vast number of which have been identified, both for superficial and systemic candidiasis (Table 22.1).

Superficial candidiasis

1. **Mucosal infection**: the characteristic mucosal lesion of *Candida* is **thrush**. This is classically a white pseudomembrane on buccal mucosa and vagina which can be easily removed by wiping. Other oral manifestations include erythematous and hyperplastic variants (see Ch. 35). Candidal vulvovaginitis is common in women using oral contraceptives and is accompanied by a thick, yeasty-smelling discharge, vaginal itching and discomfort.

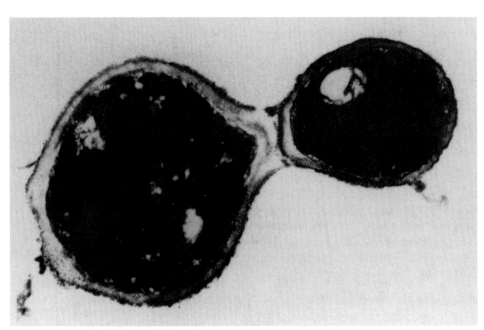

Fig. 22.4 A transmission electron micrograph of a blastospore of *Candida albicans* and a budding daughter cell.

Table 22.1 Factors predisposing to oral candidiasis

Chronic local irritants
Ill-fitting appliances
Inadequate care of appliances
Disturbed oral ecology or marked changes in the oral microbial flora by antibiotics, corticosteroids, xerostomia
Dietary factors
Immunological and endocrine disorders
Malignant and chronic diseases
Severe blood dyscrasias
Radiation to the head and neck
Abnormal nutrition
Age (e.g. very young or very old)
Hospitalization
Oral epithelial dysplasia
Heavy smoking

2. **Skin infection** is seen particularly on surfaces that are warm and moist. Candidal intertrigo consists of vesicular pustules that enlarge, rupture and cause fissures, especially seen in the obese.
3. **Nappy rash** in children may be caused by *C. albicans* derived from the lower gastrointestinal tract. Scaly macules or vesicles, associated with intense burning and pruritus, are common in nappy rash.
4. **Candidal paronychia** is a localized inflammation around and under the nails, caused by *Candida* when the hands are frequently immersed in water (e.g. in dishwashers and laundry workers).

Mucocutaneous candidiasis. Mucocutaneous candidiasis involves both the skin and the oral and/or vaginal mucosae. This rare disease is due to heritable or acquired defects in the host immune system or metabolism. Chronic mucocutaneous candidiasis is a rare condition associated with T-cell deficiency (see Ch. 35).

Systemic or deep candidiasis. This may involve the lower respiratory tract and urinary tract, with resultant **candidaemia** (*Candida* in blood); localization in endocardium, meninges, bone, kidney and eye is common. Untreated disseminated disease is fatal. Susceptible settings include organ transplantation, heart surgery, prosthetic implantation, and long-term steroid or immunosuppressive therapy. Rarely, a superficial infection is the cause of disseminated disease.

Diagnosis

1. Demonstration of yeasts in Gram-stained smear, followed by culture of specimen on Sabouraud agar.
2. Serology is helpful in the diagnosis of disseminated candidiasis.
3. Histopathological examination of a biopsy of the lesion; demonstration of tissue invasion by fungal hyphae helps establish a causal relationship.

Treatment

Candida infections can be treated by three groups of agents: the **polyenes**, the **azoles** and the **DNA analogues** (see Ch. 7). The agents used depend upon the type and severity of infection. Superficial infections can be treated topically with a polyene (nystatin or amphotericin) or an imidazole (miconazole, clotrimazole). Polyenes are also very effective for oral candidal infections. Systemic infections and disseminated candidiasis require intravenous amphotericin, either alone or in combination with flucytosine. The triazole agent fluconazole, effective for both superficial and systemic mycoses, is the drug of choice in treating *Candida* infections in HIV disease.

Prevention

Candidiasis is almost always endogenous in origin, therefore prevention entails correction of predisposing factors. Those who are compromised may require long-term prophylactic antifungal treatment, either continuously or intermittently.

Cryptococcus

Cryptococcus neoformans is a pathogenic yeast belonging to the *Cryptococcus* genus. It causes cryptococcosis, especially cryptococcal meningitis.

Habitat and transmission

This yeast is a ubiquitous saprophyte commonly isolated from soil enriched by pigeon droppings. Infection is initiated by inhalation of airborne yeast cells.

Characteristics

Cryptococcus neoformans is a budding yeast with a thick capsule, 5–15 μm in diameter.

Culture and identification

Identification is by sputum and spinal fluid culture on Sabouraud agar. Latex agglutination is used to detect the polysaccharide antigen in urine, blood or spinal fluid. Indian ink preparations of spinal fluid are used in the demonstration of the encapsulated yeast (Fig. 22.5).

Pathogenicity

Cryptococci cause an influenza-like syndrome or pneumonia. Subsequent fungaemia causes infection of the meninges. Reduced cell-mediated immunity exacerbates the infection; immunocompetent people may occasionally develop cryptococcal meningitis.

Treatment

Intravenous combination therapy with amphotericin and flucytosine.

FILAMENTOUS AND DIMORPHIC FUNGI AND ORAL DISEASE

The foregoing text describes one major group of fungi — yeasts — which are of dental and medical relevance. The

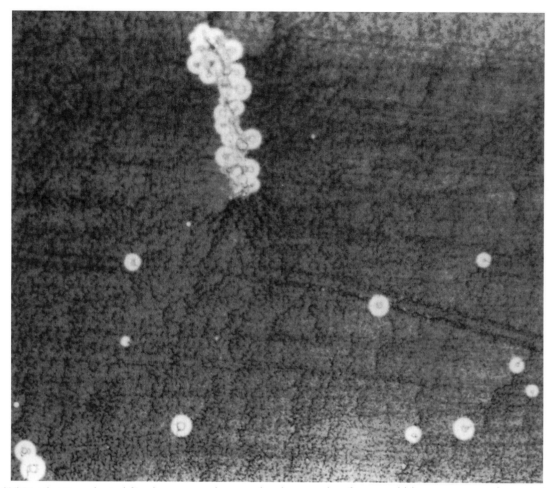

Fig. 22.5   Indian ink preparation of *Cryptococcus neoformans* showing capsules of yeasts which appear as translucent haloes.

other two main groups, **filamentous** and **dimorphic** fungi, usually do not cause oral disease except in immunocompromised groups. Organisms that are noteworthy and cause **oral ulceration** are *Penicillium marneffei*, *Histoplasma capsulatum*, *Histoplasma duboisii*, *Blastomyces dermatitidis* and *Coccidioides immitis* (Table 22.2).

Pathogenicity

In all these cases infection is usually acquired by inhalation, and the primary lesions are seen in the lungs. In a majority the initial lesion heals, often asymptomatically, and delayed hypersensitivity develops, with a positive skin test reaction to the appropriate antigen. Progressive disease may affect the lungs causing cavitation, and/or disseminate widely to involve the skin, oral and other mucous membranes and internal organs.

Diagnosis

Diagnosis may be by direct demonstration in exudate, sputum or biopsy specimens; isolation in appropriate culture media, and/or serology.

Treatment

Amphotericin is the drug of choice; itraconazole is an alternative.

Table 22.2   Dimorphic fungi that may cause oral ulceration, especially in immunocompromised patients

Fungus	Disease	Geographical distribution
Penicillium marneffei	Penicilliosis	South-East Asia
Blastomyces dermatitidis	North American blastomycosis	North America, especially Mississippi and Ohio valleys
Coccidioides immitis	Coccidioidomycosis	USA from California to Texas; South and Central America
Histoplasma capsulatum	Histoplasmosis	Eastern and central USA; occasionally other parts of the world
Histoplasma duboisii	African histoplasmosis	Equatorial Africa

KEY FACTS

- Fungi are **eukaryotic** microorganisms, as opposed to bacteria, which are **prokaryotes**
- Fungi exhibit two basic structural forms — the **yeast form** and **the mould form**: **yeasts** are unicellular with spherical/ovoid bodies while **moulds** are multicellular with a variety of specialized structures
- *Hyphae* (singular: *hypha* or *hyphum*) are thread-like tubes containing the fungal cytoplasm and its organelles (*mycelium*, a mass of hyphae)
- Fungi of medical importance are classified into **yeasts, filamentous fungi** and **dimorphic fungi**
- The vast majority of medically important fungi grow aerobically on **Sabouraud dextrose agar (SAB)** or its variations
- *Candida albicans* possesses a number of virulent attributes including the ability to **adhere** to host tissues/prostheses and form **hyphae**, colonial **switching** and the production of extracellular **phospholipase** and **proteinases**
- *Human infections caused by fungi can be broadly categorised as* **superficial, subcutaneous** *or* **systemic (deep)** *mycoses*
- *When fungi (such as* C. albicans) *that are generally innocuous in healthy humans cause disease in compromised patients they are called* **opportunistic infections**
- Candida, *a common yeast which lives in the oral cavity of some 50–60% of the population, can cause either* **superficial** *(mucosal, cutaneous or mucocutaneous) or* **systemic** *candidiasis*
- Species in the *Candida* genus found in humans include *C. albicans, C. glabrata, C. dubliniensis, C. krusei* and *C. tropicalis; C. albicans* is responsible for the vast majority of infections (> 90%)
- *C. albicans* is indigenous to the oral cavity, gastrointestinal tract, female genital tract and sometimes the skin; hence the infection is usually **endogenous**
- *C. albicans* and *C. dubliniensis* may be differentiated from other *Candida* species by their ability to produce **germ tubes** and **chlamydospores**
- *Candida* species rarely cause oral disease in the absence of predisposing factors, such as intraoral environmental changes (e.g. unhygienic prostheses, xerostomia) and/or systemic factors such as diabetes and immunodeficiency
- *The three major clinical manifestations of oral candidiasis are* **pseudomembranous, erythematous** *and* **hyperplastic** *variants (see Ch. 35)*
- *Demonstration of yeasts in* **Gram-stained smear,** *positive* **culture** *on Sabouraud agar and subsequent confirmation by biochemical or genetic techniques constitute a mycological diagnosis of candidiasis*
- *Candida* infections can be treated by three main groups of agents: the **polyenes,** the **azoles** and the **DNA analogues,** depending on the type and severity of infection
- *The triazole agent* **fluconazole** *is effective for both superficial and systemic mycoses, and is the drug of choice in treating* Candida *infections in HIV disease*
- *Resistance to azoles is seen in* Candida *species, usually following prolonged treatment, while resistance to DNA analogues and polyene group drugs is rare*
- *Treatment of candidiasis entails* **correction of predisposing factors,** *with or without oral or systemic* **antifungals**
- *Oral lesions due to fungi other than* Candida *are rare. These, such as* **cryptococcosis, histoplasmosis,** *and* **penicilliosis,** *may be seen in HIV disease and usually respond to intravenous amphotericin therapy*

FURTHER READING

Kibber, CC, MacKenzie, DWR, and Odds, FC (eds) (1996). *Principles and practice of clinical mycology.* Wiley, Chichester.

Odds, FC (1988). *Candida and candidosis* (2nd edn). Baillière Tindall, London.

Reichart, P, Samaranayake, LP, and Philipsen, HP (2000). Pathology and clinical correlates in oral candidiasis and its variants: a review. *Oral Diseases* 6, 85–91.

Samaranayake, LP, and MacFarlane, TW (eds) (1990). *Oral candidosis.* Wright, London.

Scully, C, El-Kabir, M, and Samaranayake, LP (1994). Candida and oral candidosis: a review. *Critical Reviews in Oral Biology and Medicine,* 5, 125–157.

Infections of relevance to dentistry

The aim of this section is to survey the major organ-related infections that are of particular interest in dentistry. Each infection in general is thematically organized, for the sake of convenience, according to its aetiology, clinical features, pathogenesis, laboratory diagnosis, and treatment and prevention.

- Infections of the respiratory tract
- Infections of the cardiovascular system
- Infections of the central nervous and locomotor systems
- Infections of the gastrointestinal tract
- Infections of the genitourinary tract
- Skin and wound infections
- Viral hepatitis
- Human immunodeficiency virus infection, AIDS, and infections in compromised patients

Infections of the respiratory tract

The human respiratory tract is highly susceptible to infectious diseases, and morbidity of this region accounts for the majority of general practitioner consultations and almost a quarter of all absence from work due to illness in the Western world. Most respiratory tract infections are mild, associated with cold, damp winter months when coughing and sneezing in enclosed spaces facilitate the spread of disease. Serious infections are seen in the very young and the very old, and in compromised patients, throughout the year.

Respiratory infections can be broadly classified into **upper** and **lower respiratory tract infections**, although both areas may be simultaneously affected by some agents, notably viruses. The throat, pharynx, middle ear and sinuses are involved in upper respiratory tract infections, while lower respiratory tract infections are confined to the trachea, bronchi and lungs.

NORMAL FLORA

In health the nose and the throat are colonized by commensal bacterial species, while the lower respiratory tract (the lower bronchi and alveoli) contain only a few, if any, organisms. The nose is the habitat of a variety of streptococci and staphylococci, the most significant of which is *Staphylococcus aureus*, especially prevalent in the anterior nares. Other commensal flora of the upper respiratory tract include corynebacteria, *Haemophilus* spp. and neisseriae. In health these endogenous (and other exogenous) organisms are unable to gain access to the tissues and cause disease because there is an effective array of defence mechanisms (Table 23.1).

IMPORTANT PATHOGENS OF THE RESPIRATORY TRACT

The major causative agents of bacterial and viral respiratory infections of both the upper and lower respiratory tract are illustrated in Figure 23.1.

INFECTIONS OF THE UPPER RESPIRATORY TRACT

The following infections of the upper respiratory tract of clinical relevance to dentistry are noteworthy:

- the sore throat syndrome
- streptococcal sore throat
  - rheumatic fever
  - acute glomerulonephritis
- diphtheria
- Vincent's angina
- infectious mononucleosis (Ch. 21)
- candidiasis (Ch. 22).

Sore throat syndrome

Clinical features

Sore throat is a very common symptom which may or may not be accompanied by constitutional changes. A number of agents may cause a sore throat but the majority (approximately two-thirds) of the infections are caused by viruses. The major bacterial pathogen involved is *Streptococcus pyogenes* (Lancefield group A). Sore throat is a frequent precursor of the common cold syndrome.

Streptococcal sore throat

Clinical features

Characteristic features are redness of pharynx and tonsils, possible oedema of fauces and soft palate with exudate (**acute follicular tonsillitis**). Children 5–8 years old are most commonly affected. Spread of infection may cause a **peritonsillar abscess** (quinsy throat); further spread may cause sinus infection (**sinusitis** — commonly maxillary sinusitis) or middle ear infection (**otitis media**). **Scarlet fever**, a childhood disease, is a complication of streptococcal upper respiratory tract infection and is accompanied by an erythematous rash and constitutional upset.

Pathogenesis and epidemiology

The condition is common, especially in winter, with the peak incidence in young schoolchildren with inadequate levels and range of antibodies. Transient streptococcal carriage for a few weeks is common after an acute episode. The rash in scarlet fever is due to the erythrogenic toxin produced by the aetiological agent (*Streptococcus pyogenes*).

Late sequelae of streptococcal infection

Immunologically mediated diseases can manifest in susceptible individuals as a late consequence of certain strains 151

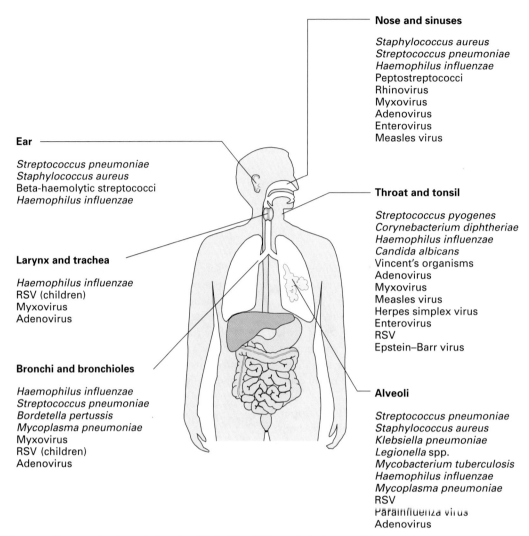

Fig. 23.1 Major causative agents of respiratory tract infection. RSV, respiratory syncytial virus.

Nose and sinuses

Staphylococcus aureus
Streptococcus pneumoniae
Haemophilus influenzae
Peptostreptococci
Rhinovirus
Myxovirus
Adenovirus
Enterovirus
Measles virus

Ear

Streptococcus pneumoniae
Staphylococcus aureus
Beta-haemolytic streptococci
Haemophilus influenzae

Throat and tonsil

Streptococcus pyogenes
Corynebacterium diphtheriae
Haemophilus influenzae
Candida albicans
Vincent's organisms
Adenovirus
Myxovirus
Measles virus
Herpes simplex virus
Enterovirus
RSV
Epstein–Barr virus

Larynx and trachea

Haemophilus influenzae
RSV (children)
Myxovirus
Adenovirus

Bronchi and bronchioles

Haemophilus influenzae
Streptococcus pneumoniae
Bordetella pertussis
Mycoplasma pneumoniae
Myxovirus
RSV (children)
Adenovirus

Alveoli

Streptococcus pneumoniae
Staphylococcus aureus
Klebsiella pneumoniae
Legionella spp.
Mycobacterium tuberculosis
Haemophilus influenzae
Mycoplasma pneumoniae
RSV
Parainfluenza virus
Adenovirus

of *Streptococcus pyogenes* (group A) infection. These are rheumatic fever and acute glomerulonephritis.

Rheumatic fever

Clinical features

Fever, pain, joint swelling and **pancarditis** (myocarditis, endocarditis and pericarditis) occur 2–5 weeks after strep-

tococcal sore throat. Cardiac manifestations may lead to **permanent heart damage**. In developed countries the incidence of rheumatic fever (and related heart disease) has declined markedly, possibly owing to changes in the virulence properties of the bacterium, improved affluence and social conditions, and effective antimicrobial therapy (e.g. penicillins). However, both rheumatic fever and consequent heart disease are still a major problem in the developing world.

The disease clears spontaneously but may lead to chronic valvular diseases of the heart such as stenosis or incompetence of the mitral or aortic valves in about 70% of patients. Affected individuals are **highly susceptible to bacterial endocarditis** later in life, when bacteraemias are created during **dental or surgical procedures** such as scaling. This complication can be prevented by prudent **antibiotic prophylaxis** prior to such procedures (see Ch. 24).

Pathogenesis

A number of theories have been proposed for rheumatic carditis:

- **rheumatic toxins**: extracellular products of group A streptococci reacting with heart tissue
- **autoimmunity**: induced by the localization of extracellular streptococcal products and antibodies in tissues
- **cross-reactivity**: the group A streptococcus cell-wall antigens and glycoproteins of human heart valves share the

Table 23.1 Natural antimicrobial defences of the respiratory tract

Mucociliary system
nasal vibrissae
action of cilia
mucous glands and goblet cells
Bronchoconstriction
Cough reflex
Non-specific mucosal defences
lactoferrin
lysozyme
α-antitrypsin
Alveolar macrophage system
Mucosal antibody (mainly secretory IgA)
Local cell-mediated immunity

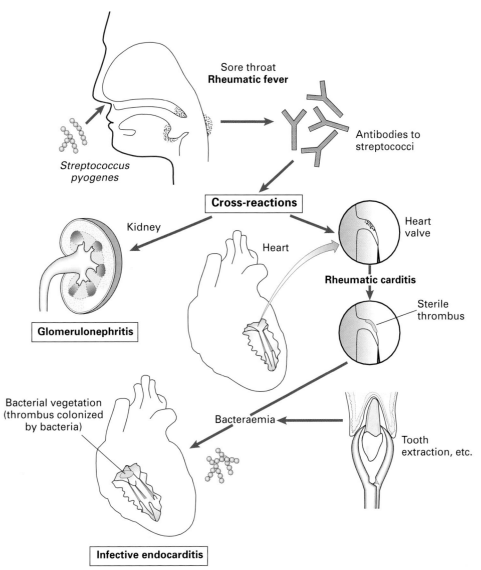

Fig. 23.2 Pathogenesis and sequelae of rheumatic carditis (events leading to infective endocarditis are also illustrated).

same antigenic determinants, thus the antibodies produced against the bacterial cell wall may cross-react with the heart valve components, with resultant cardiac complications (Fig. 23.2).

Laboratory diagnosis

Diagnosis is mainly clinical; throat swabs are useful to confirm the presence of *Streptococcus pyogenes*. Swabs cultured on blood agar aerobically and anaerobically yield characteristic β-haemolytic colonies, which can subsequently be identified by Lancefield grouping.

Infection can be proved by serological analysis of paired clotted blood samples. Evidence for **antibody to strep-tolysin O** should be sought (streptolysin O is a haemolysin produced by *Streptococcus pyogenes*). Antibodies to other streptococcal products such as hyaluronidase and DNAase may also be demonstrated immediately after an infection.

Treatment

Beta-haemolytic streptococci are universally sensitive to penicillin. Erythromycin is an alternative in cases of penicillin hypersensitivity. After eradication of *Streptococcus pyogenes*

with penicillin, reinfection must be prevented by long-term prophylaxis.

Acute glomerulonephritis

Acute glomerulonephritis is another immunological compli-cation that may follow streptococcal sore throat (and some-times skin infection). The latent period between infection and symptoms is shorter than in rheumatic fever.

Clinical features

The condition presents 1–3 weeks after the sore throat; char-acteristically there is haematuria, albuminuria and oedema, which manifests as a puffed face, especially on waking, and as the day wears on ankle oedema often develops. The disease spontaneously clears in the majority but in some residual kidney damage may progressively lead to renal failure.

Pathogenesis

Theories proposed include:
- **nephrotoxins**: production of toxic substances by nephritogenic streptococci, including streptolysin, cell-

wall extracts and uncharacterized diffusible substances released by the cells

- **immunological cross-reactivity**: between antigens of protoplasts of nephritogenic streptococci and soluble components of glomerular basement membrane
- **immune complexes**: thought to be formed by combinations of antistreptococcal antibody with either streptococcal antigens already circulating in the blood or deposited on the basement membranes.

Laboratory diagnosis

A clinical diagnosis is confirmed by past or present streptococcal infection.

Treatment

Penicillin is useful if the organism is still present at the infective focus.

Diphtheria

Diphtheria is caused by *Corynebacterium diphtheriae* (three main biotypes: gravis, intermedius and mitis).

Clinical features

After an incubation period of 2–5 days, a severe, acute inflammation of the upper respiratory tract, usually the throat, sets in. Severity of the disease is related to the infecting strain of the organism and the extent of the grey-white membrane which covers the fauces. The membrane is a product of a serocellular exudate. **Nasal diphtheria is often milder than laryngeal diphtheria**, which is serious because of the respiratory tract obstruction.

Pathogenesis

Corynebacteria produce a powerful **exotoxin** which is cardiotoxic and neurotoxic. This toxin diffuses throughout the body, affecting the myocardium, adrenal glands and nerve endings.

Epidemiology

The disease is rare in developed countries because of the successful immunization programme with the diphtheria–tetanus–pertussis vaccine. Outbreaks occur in non-immunized populations, especially in the developing world.

Treatment

Antitoxin must be used in addition to penicillin or erythromycin.

Vincent's angina

Vincent's angina is caused by the fusospirochaetal complex (fusobacteria and oral spirochaetes). These are normal commensals of the mouth and may overgrow, mainly as a result of poor oral hygiene superimposed on either nutritional deficiency, leucopenia or viral infections.

Treatment

Penicillin or metronidazole.

INFECTIONS OF THE PARANASAL SINUSES AND THE MIDDLE EAR

These can either be acute or chronic, and are often initiated as a secondary complication of a viral infection of the respiratory tract (e.g. a common cold). Some important examples are:
- acute infections:
  - otitis media
  - sinusitis
- chronic infections:
  - chronic suppurative otitis media
  - chronic sinusitis.

Acute infections

Otitis media

Inflammation of the middle ear may be caused by infection spreading via the eustachian tube, especially after a common cold. Mainly a childhood disease characterized by earache; recurrences are common.

Sinusitis

Inflammation frequently affecting frontal and/or maxillary sinuses is a familiar symptom of the common cold but resolves spontaneously. However, pain and tenderness with purulent discharge may indicate bacterial infection, in which case antibiotic therapy is indicated.

Aetiology

Both otitis media and sinusitis are due to endogenous infection (from reservoirs in the nasopharynx) by bacteria such as *Haemophilus influenzae*, *Streptococcus pneumoniae* and *S. pyogenes*.

Treatment

Amoxicillin (amoxycillin), ampicillin, erythromycin.

Chronic infections

Chronic suppurative otitis media

The term is given to chronic middle ear infection and suppuration (pus formation) associated with pathological changes. It can recur at intervals throughout childhood and also in adulthood; the main symptoms are profuse discharge and pain.

Chronic sinusitis

Chronic sinusitis is associated with headache, painful sinuses, nasal obstruction and mucopurulent discharge. Patients may also complain of toothache if the maxillary sinuses are affected.

Aetiology

The aetiology is the same as in acute infections, with endogenous spread of infection from the indigenous upper respiratory tract flora. However, in addition, other organisms such as *Staphylococcus aureus* and a range of enterobacteria and anaerobes (*Bacteroides* spp.) may be associated. The role of these organisms in the disease process is not clear.

Treatment

Antibiotic treatment is required, guided by antibiotic sensitivity testing of isolates. Nasal decongestants may be helpful.

INFECTIONS OF TRACHEA AND BRONCHI

Infection and consequent inflammation of the larynx (laryngitis), trachea (tracheitis) and bronchi (bronchitis) are common after viral infections of the upper respiratory tract. The following important diseases are outlined:
- bronchitis
- cystic fibrosis
- pertussis (whooping cough).

Bronchitis

Acute bronchitis in a patient with a healthy respiratory tract is usually a minor complaint possibly due to a viral infection. However, secondary bacterial infection of the damaged respiratory mucosa may result in severe attacks in those with a history of chronic bronchitis, bronchiectasis or asthma. Acute exacerbation of chronic bronchitis is a serious disease.

Aetiology

Two major agents are *Haemophilus influenzae* and *Streptococcus pneumoniae*. *Branhamella catarrhalis* and *Mycoplasma pneumoniae* may also be involved in some cases.

Clinical features

A dry cough which later turns productive with expectoration of yellow-green sputum; fever.

Pathogenesis and epidemiology

Bronchitis is primarily an endogenous infection due to the above-mentioned organisms. However, chronic bronchitis is the result of a vast number of additional aetiological factors including previous lung disease, smoking, poor housing, low socioeconomic class, urban dwelling, atmospheric pollution, and damp, cold and wintry weather conditions.

Diagnosis

The diagnosis is mainly clinical; sputum samples are cultured to isolate and to determine the antibiotic sensitivity profile of the aetiological agents.

Treatment

Ampicillin or amoxicillin, tetracycline, co-trimoxazole (combination of sulphamethoxazole and trimethoprim) and erythromycin are all used in the treatment, depending on the culture and sensitivity results. In chronic bronchitic patients antibiotic treatment should begin early in the infection to reduce severity.

Cystic fibrosis

Respiratory infection is a major problem in patients with cystic fibrosis. This inherited defect leads to production of abnormally thick mucus which blocks the respiratory 'tubes' and tubular structures in many different organs. However, the most disabling feature of this condition is chronic respiratory tract infection due to compromised natural defence mechanisms of the airways. The aetiological agents are usually *Staphylococcus aureus*, *Streptococcus pneumoniae* and *Pseudomonas aeruginosa*.

Pertussis (whooping cough)

Pertussis is caused by *Bordetella pertussis*.

Clinical features

An acute childhood disease (usually in the first year) with tracheobronchitis, the disease has an insidious onset. First stage is the **catarrhal stage** (about 2 weeks), which leads to a **paroxysmal stage** characterized by a cough and indrawing of breath which creates a 'whoop' — hence the name. There is a very low fatality rate but morbidity is high, leading to sequelae such as **bronchiectasis**.

Pathogenesis and epidemiology

Droplet spread; the attack rate in unprotected siblings may be as high as 90%. Whooping cough occurs in epidemic proportions every few years especially in unvaccinated populations.

Laboratory diagnosis

A **pernasal swab** or **cough plate** of charcoal–blood or Bordet–Gengou medium confirms the diagnosis. A pernasal swab is obtained by passing a swab along the floor of the nose to sample nasopharyngeal secretions; a cough plate is obtained by holding the culture plate in front of the mouth when coughing. The organisms grow as mercury drop colonies on charcoal–blood agar.

Treatment and prevention

Antibiotics are of little help; DTP vaccine is an effective preventive measure (see Ch. 37).

LUNG INFECTIONS

The following noteworthy infections are outlined:
- pneumonia
- legionnaires' disease
- respiratory tuberculosis
- empyema.

Pneumonia

Despite the diverse array of antibiotics available today, pneumonia remains a significant cause of morbidity and mortality in the very young, the very old and the immunocompromised. Pneumonia can be categorized into three main types:
1. **Lobar** (or **segmental**) pneumonia: consolidation is limited to only one lobe or segment of the lung.
2. **Bronchopneumonia**: usually bilateral, with consolidation scattered throughout the lung fields.
3. Primary **atypical** or **virus** pneumonia: with patchy consolidation of the lungs.

Table 23.2 Aetiological agents of pneumonia

Pneumonia	Main pathogens
Lobar pneumonia	Streptococcus pneumoniae
Bronchopneumonia	Streptococcus pneumoniae Haemophilus influenzae
Atypical pneumonia	Mycoplasma pneumoniae Coxiella burnetii Chlamydia psittaci
Legionnaires' disease	Legionella spp.

The aetiological agents of different types of pneumonia are given in Table 23.2.

Lobar and bronchopneumonia

Clinical features. These include fever, malaise, rapid arterial pulse and leucocytosis (in bacterial pneumonias); central cyanosis and breathlessness; cough and purulent sputum often laced with blood (in lobar pneumonias); herpes labialis of the lips; pleuritic chest pain may occur in pneumococcal pneumonias; and signs of lung consolidation on chest examination.

Pathogenesis and epidemiology. **Lobar pneumonia** is mainly caused by exogenous organisms, although the patient's own upper respiratory tract flora may sometimes be an endogenous cause. The major agent of disease is the **pneumococcus**. However, of some 80 serotypes of pneumococci only a few are implicated in the disease process. *Staphylococcus aureus* and *Haemophilus influenzae* are the other organisms involved.

The organisms invade the lung and deprive the alveolar cells of essential nutrients, thereby causing their destruction and death. This process is amplified in pneumococcal pneumonia by the resistance of the pneumococci to phagocytosis (due to the capsules) and the production of toxins such as **pneumolysins**.

The causative organisms of **bronchopneumonia** are similar to those of lobar pneumonia: pneumococci, *S. aureus* and *H. influenzae* are common; coliforms are sometimes implicated. Staphylococcal bronchopneumonia frequently follows influenza and bronchitis in the elderly and infirm and may lead to death.

Other notable organisms that cause pneumonia are *Mycoplasma pneumoniae*, *Coxiella burnetii* and *Chlamydia psittaci*.

Laboratory diagnosis. A properly taken, early-morning sample of sputum (as this is likely to be the most purulent) is essential for culture. Blood culture may be useful for diagnosing lobar pneumonia.

Treatment and prevention. Antibiotic therapy is dictated by sensitivity tests; penicillins are the first choice. For pneumococcal pneumonia, selective prophylaxis with pneumococcal vaccine is advised for high-risk groups (e.g. debilitated, institutionalized elderly people).

Primary atypical pneumonia

A pneumonia is atypical when its causative agent cannot be isolated in ordinary laboratory media and/or when its clinical picture does not resemble that of pneumococcal pneumonia. The major agent of primary atypical pneumonia is the virus-like organism *Mycoplasma pneumoniae* (see Ch. 20), although others such as *Legionella* may be involved (Table 23.2). Mycoplasmal pneumonia has an incubation period of 1–3 weeks and is endemic in the community.

Legionnaires' disease

Legionnaires' disease is caused by *Legionella pneumophila* and other *Legionella* species.

Clinical features, pathogenesis and epidemiology

An increasingly common cause of pneumonia with significant mortality, legionnaires' disease typically affects middle-aged smokers, often in poor general health. The illness resembles influenza and may lead to respiratory failure; associated symptoms are mental confusion, renal failure and gastrointestinal upsets.

The organism is a saprophyte that often exists in soil and stagnant water. Airborne spread is associated with cooling towers of air-conditioning systems and with complex modern plumbing systems; person-to-person airborne spread has not been documented. Concern has been expressed in the past that legionellae may multiply in stagnant water in dental unit water systems, and patients may be exposed to this health hazard when three-in-one syringes are used. Such fears appear to be unfounded.

Laboratory diagnosis, antibiotics and prevention

See Chapter 19.

Respiratory tuberculosis

Up to a third of the global population is thought to be infected by tuberculosis, which causes up to 3 million deaths each year. It is now the world's pre-eminent fatal disease. Caused by *Mycobacterium tuberculosis* and other atypical mycobacteria (Ch. 19) it is re-emerging as a result of both the HIV pandemic and the bacilli that are gradually acquiring resistance to the conventional antituberculous drugs — the so-called multi-drug-resistant tubercle bacilli (MDR-TB). Persons at increased risk of tuberculosis include dentists and their assistants, who are exposed to infectious droplet particles from their patients (Table 23.3).

Clinical features and pathogenesis

Respiratory tuberculosis is a chronic granulomatous disease with protean manifestations that mainly affects the lungs, although other organs and tissues are frequently involved. Infection is initiated after inhalation of contaminated aerosol droplets. The disease can be divided into **primary infection** and **post-primary infection**.

Primary infection. The primary focus of infection is the middle lower lung fields. This takes the form of a primary complex — the local lesion (**Ghon focus**) with enlargement of

Table 23.3 Groups at increased risk of tuberculosis

Children and young adults

Contacts of patients with active infection

Immunosuppressed individuals (e.g. HIV, drug therapy)

Health-care workers in close contact with patients

Socially disadvantaged poor, in crowded urban environments

Individuals with alcoholism, diabetes mellitus or silicosis

the regional hilar lymph nodes. Within 3–6 weeks the patient's cellular immunity is activated and replication of the bacilli will cease in most patients. The primary infection is entirely symptomless or sometimes associated with malaise, anorexia and weight loss. Cough is not a significant finding at this stage.

The primary infection is usually contained and the active focus may become walled-off and fibrotic. Antibiotic treatment at this stage may also resolve the infection. However, without such intervention the disease may progress in some, leading to death. The resultant systemic spread of disease may cause:

- tuberculous bronchopneumonia
- miliary tuberculosis: haematogenous spread of the bacilli with multiple infective foci throughout the body
- tuberculous meningitis
- bone and joint tuberculosis
- renal tuberculosis.

Post-primary infection. There may be a latent period of months or years before the tubercle bacilli initiate active disease after primary infection. Such post-primary infection commonly involves the lungs, leading to **caseous necrosis** and **fibrosis**. The symptoms of post-primary disease are loss of appetite and weight, tiredness, fever and night sweats, cough, sputum and haemoptysis. Breathlessness due to pleural effusion, pneumothorax and lung collapse may occur if not treated.

Treatment

Treatment of tuberculosis is complex, and depends on **combination drug therapy** to suppress the emergence of resistant bacilli. The recommended drugs in the UK are isoniazid, rifampicin, pyrazinamide and ethambutol. Treatment is usually initiated in hospital after which **directly observed treatment short term** (DOTS) is given for up to 8 months.

Prevention

Vaccination with a live, attenuated, bovine *Mycobacterium* strain **bacillus Calmette–Guérin** (BCG) provides immunity for most but not all. The vaccine is given to those that are Mantoux test negative.

The **Mantoux test** is an intradermal injection in the arm of purified protein derivative (PPD) from *M. tuberculosis* cultures. A hard lesion 10 mm or more in diameter 48–72 hours after injection indicates either active disease or past infection. Mantoux testing is not totally reliable as false negatives may occur.

The BCG vaccine is most effective in children and less so in adults. One disadvantage of the vaccine is that while it may or may not confer protection, it will yield a positive (Mantoux) skin test which eliminates the latter as a means of detecting early infection.

Other methods of preventing tuberculosis include improving social and living conditions and better nutrition.

Empyema

Empyema or pus in the pleural space is almost always caused by secondary bacterial spread entering the pleural space as a result of:

- tuberculosis, lung abscess or complication of pneumonia
- thoracic surgery or trauma
- hepatic or subphrenic abscess.

The organisms involved are similar to those that cause the primary infection; treatment depends on drainage and removal of the infected fluid and appropriate antibiotic therapy.

FUNGAL INFECTIONS OF THE LOWER RESPIRATORY TRACT

Inhalation of pathogenic spores or yeast cells may cause a number of fungal infections of the lower respiratory tract, especially in those who are immunocompromised. Such infections are becoming increasingly prevalent because of the pandemic HIV infection; they include blastomycosis, coccidioidomycosis, cryptococcosis and histoplasmosis. Pneumonias due to *Pneumocystis carinii* (PCP) are particularly common in AIDS patients and are the leading cause of death in HIV disease; they are treated with co-trimoxazole (sulphamethoxazole and trimethoprim) and aerosolized pentamidine.

RESPIRATORY INFECTIONS AND DENTISTRY

Respiratory infections are of special concern to dentists, as patients will regularly present for treatment during the prodromal period, the acute phase or the recovery stage of infections. The most common mode of transmission is the airborne route, although direct or indirect contact with contaminated **fomites** may spread some infections (see Ch. 36). The majority of infections that may spread in the dental clinic are thought to be caused by viruses, and it has been documented that dental personnel tend to suffer more from viral upper respiratory tract infections than the average individual. Such cross-infection may be minimized by wearing a face mask, and appropriate ventilation of the surgical suite. The transmission of more severe bacterial infections, such as diphtheria, pertussis and tuberculosis, can be prevented by immunization of the dental team as appropriate.

General anaesthesia should never be administered to patients with respiratory tract infection as this may cause reduced respiratory efficiency due to increased secretions and obstruction of the airways. Dental personnel suffering from acute respiratory infection should not attend work as they may transmit the infection to other staff and to their patients.

KEY FACTS

- *Human respiratory tract infections account for the majority of general practitioner consultations, and almost a quarter of all absence from work due to illness in the Western world*

- The **nose** is the **habitat of a variety of streptococci** and **staphylococci**, the most significant of which is *Staphylococcus aureus*, especially prevalent in the anterior nares

- *The major bacterial pathogen in the sore throat syndrome is* Streptococcus pyogenes *(Lancefield group A)*

- *Rheumatic fever and acute glomerulonephritis are immunologically mediated diseases that may manifest as a late consequence of* **Streptococcus pyogenes** *infection*

- *Rheumatic fever may lead to permanent endocardial damage, and these individuals are highly susceptible to bacterial endocarditis later in life, when bacteraemias are created during dental or surgical procedures*

- *Prudent antibiotic prophylaxis prior to such procedures in susceptible individuals prevents bacterial endocarditis*

- *Diphtheria, a severe, acute inflammation of the upper respiratory tract, usually the throat, is due to* **Corynebacterium diphtheriae**; *prevention is by the DTP vaccine*

- **Corynebacteria** produce a powerful **exotoxin** which is **cardiotoxic** and **neurotoxic**, affecting the myocardium, adrenal glands and nerve endings

- *Vincent's angina caused by the fusospirochaetal complex (fusobacteria and oral spirochaetes) can be treated by either penicillin or metronidazole*

- Both **otitis media and sinusitis** are due to endogenous infection with bacteria such as *Haemophilus influenzae, Streptococcus pneumoniae* and *S. pyogenes*

- *Pneumonia can be categorized into lobar (or segmental), bronchopneumonia and primary atypical or virus pneumonia*

- **Lobar pneumonia** is mainly caused by **exogenous organisms** (major agent: the *pneumococcus*) and sometimes by the patient's own upper respiratory tract flora

- The major agent of **primary atypical pneumonia** is *Mycoplasma pneumoniae*

- **Legionnaires' disease** is caused by *Legionella pneumophila* and other *Legionella* species that are saprophytic and exist in soil and stagnant water

- **Up to a third of the global population** is infected with *Mycobacterium* species that cause tuberculosis

- **Tuberculosis is re-emerging** as a result of both the **HIV pandemic** and the bacilli that are gradually acquiring **resistance to the conventional antituberculous drugs** — so-called multi-drug-resistant tubercle bacilli (MDR-TB)

- **Treatment of tuberculosis is complex**, and depends on combination drug therapy

- **Vaccination** with a live, attenuated, bovine *Mycobacterium* strain, **bacillus Calmette–Guérin (BCG)**, provides **immunity from tuberculosis**, for most but not all. The vaccine is given to those who are Mantoux test negative

- **Pneumonias** due to *Pneumocystis carinii* (PCP) are particularly common in AIDS patients and are the **leading cause of death in HIV disease**

FURTHER READING

Mims, C, Playfair, J, Roitt, I, Wakelin, D, and Williams, R (1998). Upper respiratory tract infections; Lower respiratory tract infections. In *Medical microbiology* (2nd edn), Chs 15, 17. Mosby, London.

Phelan, JA, Jimenez, V, and Tompkins, DC (1996). Tuberculosis. *Dental Clinics of North America* 40, 327–341.

Shanson, DC (1999). Infections of the lower respiratory tract. *Microbiology in clinical practice* (3rd edn), Ch. 14. Butterworth-Heinemann, Oxford.

Van-Arsdall, JA, et al (1983). The protean manifestations of Legionnaires' disease. *Journal of Infection*, 7, 51–62.

24 Infections of the cardiovascular system

In health the cardiovascular system is sterile, but a few organisms may enter the bloodstream (even in health) during routine procedures such as toothbrushing, especially in the presence of periodontitis. However, these bacteria have only a transient existence as the efficient defences of the blood quickly destroy them.

BACTERAEMIA, SEPTICAEMIA AND SEPSIS SYNDROME

Definitions

Bacteraemia: literally 'bacterial presence in the blood', where the bacterial burden in blood is usually very low and is clinically insignificant — i.e. bacteraemia is **asymptomatic**. Bacteraemia could be produced simply by brushing of teeth or chewing, especially in the presence of periodontitis.

Septicaemia: literally 'sepsis of the blood', seen when large numbers of organisms **enter** and/or **actively multiply** and persist in the bloodstream, producing clinical signs and symptoms such as hypotension, fever and rigors.

Sepsis syndrome: a systemic response to microbial products or constituents circulating in the blood mediated by inflammatory cytokines (see below).

Septicaemia and sepsis syndrome

Aetiology

Some common predisposing factors and agents that cause septicaemia are shown in Table 24.1.

Pathogenesis and clinical features

Once the bloodstream is invaded by microbes the host responds by activating its defence mechanisms, leading to the production of a cascade of **inflammatory cytokines** (e.g. interleukin-1, tumour necrosis factor; see Ch. 10). The cytokine release is orchestrated by endotoxins of Gram-negative bacteria, peptidoglycan of Gram-positive bacteria, and exotoxins from both these groups. Generally these cytokines are beneficial in eliminating the organisms but excessive production may lead to organ dysfunction and circulatory septic shock — the **sepsis syndrome**.

Some of these patients are said to develop the **systemic inflammatory response syndrome** (SIRS) depending on their clinical signs; these include hypotension, fever, rigors,

oliguria and renal failure. Sometimes the infection may trigger a pathological activation of the coagulation system (**disseminated intravascular coagulation**), and due to the resultant consumption of platelets and clotting factors, severe **bleeding disorders**.

Diagnosis

Blood should be cultured for a diagnosis of septicaemia. As the number of organisms circulating in the blood may vary from time to time, depending on the disease condition, more than one blood culture may be required; whenever possible this should be carried out before antibiotic therapy is instituted. Several positive cultures are required to ensure that the culture result is not due to contamination from the venepuncture site. Cultures from sites suspected to be causing the infection are useful (e.g. pus from an abscess) to establish and localize the infective focus.

Treatment

The principles of therapy are:
- aggressive bactericidal (rather than bacteriostatic) intravenous antimicrobial therapy in adequate dosage
- stabilization of the haemodynamic status (e.g. intravenous fluids, cardiogenic drugs, oxygen)
- identification of the focus of infection and appropriate action (e.g. removal of a foreign body, surgical intervention by draining an abscess).

INFECTIONS OF THE HEART

Important pathogens that cause pericarditis, myocarditis and endocarditis are shown in Figure 24.1. Of these, infective endocarditis is the most important disease of relevance to dentistry.

Infective endocarditis

Definition

Inflammation of the endocardium of the heart valves, and sometimes the endocardium around congenital defects, resulting from an infection.

Microbial aetiology

Bacteria are predominantly involved, although other organisms, such as fungi, rickettsiae and chlamydiae, may occasionally cause endocarditis (Table 24.2). More than 80% 159

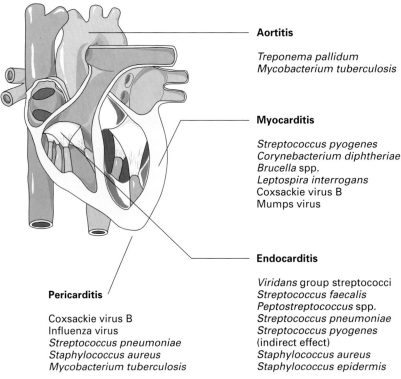

Aortitis

Treponema pallidum
Mycobacterium tuberculosis

Myocarditis

Streptococcus pyogenes
Corynebacterium diphtheriae
Brucella spp.
Leptospira interrogans
Coxsackie virus B
Mumps virus

Endocarditis

Viridans group streptococci
Streptococcus faecalis
Peptostreptococcus spp.
Streptococcus pneumoniae
Streptococcus pyogenes
(indirect effect)
Staphylococcus aureus
Staphylococcus epidermis

Pericarditis

Coxsackie virus B
Influenza virus
Streptococcus pneumoniae
Staphylococcus aureus
Mycobacterium tuberculosis

Fig. 24.1 Major infectious agents of aortitis, pericarditis, myocarditis and endocarditis.

of infective endocarditis is caused by streptococci and staphylococci. The position held by the *viridans* group of organisms in the league table indicates the major role played by the oral commensals in causing this life-threatening disease. It is noteworthy that nearly all patients with *viridans* endocarditis have a previous heart lesion, and about a quarter give a history of a recent dental procedure as a precipitating factor.

Clinical features

Although two clinical forms of the disease — **acute** and **subacute** — have been identified, the line of demarca-

tion between these forms is not often clear. The acute form is a rapidly progressive condition and is caused by bacteria such as *Streptococcus pneumoniae, Staphylococcus aureus* and *Streptococcus pyogenes*. The subacute form is more insidious, chronic, and progresses rather slowly. The agents of this form of the disease are less virulent bacteria, such as *viridans* streptococci, *Staphylococcus epidermidis, Streptococcus faecalis*, etc.

Signs and symptoms

The classic signs are fever, malaise, loss of weight, anaemia, splinter haemorrhages, petechiae, cardiac murmur, haematuria and splenomegaly.

Diagnosis

Clinical signs supported by positive blood culture are used to make the diagnosis. Repeated culture may be necessary to

Table 24.1 Some common predisposing factors and agents of septicaemia

Predisposing factor	Agent
Abdominal sepsis	Enterobacteria *Bacteroides fragilis* *Streptococcus faecalis*
Infected wounds, burns	*Staphylococcus aureus* *Streptococcus pyogenes* Enterobacteria
Osteomyelitis	*Staphylococcus aureus*
Pneumonia	*Streptococcus pneumoniae*
Intravascular devices	*Staphylococcus aureus* *Staphylococcus epidermidis* Enterobacteria
Food poisoning	*Salmonella* spp. *Campylobacter* spp.
Meningitis	*Streptococcus pneumoniae* *Neisseria meningitidis* *Haemophilus influenzae*
Immunosuppressed patients	Enterobacteria *Staphylococcus aureus*, etc.

Table 24.2 Causative microorganisms in infective endocarditis (cumulative data from several sources)

Microorganisms	Cases (%)
Total streptococci	60
Viridans group	35
S. faecalis	13
Microaerophilic streptococci	3
Anaerobic streptococci	2
Others	7
Total staphylococci	25
S. aureus	20
S. epidermidis	5
Miscellaneous	5
Culture negative	10

isolate the causal organism owing to the low-grade bacter-aemia. If possible, blood should be collected when the temperature of the patient rises, indicating fever due to bacteraemia. At least 10 ml of blood should be collected prior to antibiotic therapy and cultured under aerobic and anaerobic conditions (see Fig. 6.4). Any agent isolated from two different blood culture sets (on separate occasions) is considered significant. Identification and antibiotic sensitivity tests are then performed on the isolate.

Pathogenesis and epidemiology

Infective endocarditis normally occurs in patients with some pathological condition of the endocardium, although those with apparently normal heart valves may rarely be affected. The predisposing conditions include valve prostheses, septal defects, atheroma of the valve, congenital valve deformities and pre-existing rheumatic fever (Table 24.3). Infective endo-carditis is the end result of the sequential interaction of events shown in Figure 23.2:
1. A breach of the endocardium, or an abnormality of the endocardial surface *per se*, is the first event which makes the valvular surface finally succumb to infection. Such a breach may occur because of the acute inflammatory valvulitis of rheumatic fever (consequential to *Strepto-coccus pyogenes* infection; see Fig. 23.2); or, in congenital heart diseases such as aortic valve disease and ventricular septal defect, when alterations of the blood flow patterns (haemodynamic turbulence) may result in the deposition of fibrin and platelets at foci where high-velocity jets of blood hit the valvular surface.
2. The microscopic platelet aggregates which form on the breached endocardium detach and **embolize** harmlessly or stabilize and **consolidate** through fibrin deposition, forming a sterile **thrombus**. The latter is a potential trap for circulating microbes. Such sterile thrombus formation is called **non-bacterial thrombotic endocarditis**. Platelets also have the potential to adhere to other 'foreign' surfaces such as prosthetic valves.

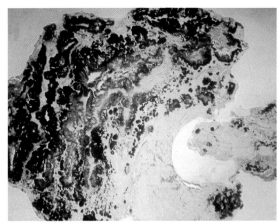

Fig. 24.2 Micrograph of an infected heart valve teeming with Gram-positive streptococci.

3. The next critical event occurs when organisms circulating in the blood (e.g. after a tooth extraction or scaling) attach to or become trapped in the thrombotic endocardium or the prosthetic device. The resultant platelet–fibrin–bacterial mass, now called the **bacterial vegetation**, constitutes the primary pathology of infective endocarditis (see Figs 23.2 and 24.2).
4. Once the organisms are attached to the lesion they multiply and colonize this niche in an exuberant manner. As a result, further aggregation of platelets and fibrin deposition ensues, protecting the organisms from the body defences. The organisms now reside in a sanctuary inaccessible to phagocytes by virtue of the **fibrin–platelet barrier**. Further, the bacteria may be sheltered from antibiotics and host antibodies as the vegetation is essentially **avascular** in nature. As a result it is necessary to use an intensive course of prolonged, high-dose antibiotic therapy to eradicate such an infective focus.
5. Even if endocarditis is successfully treated, the healed valve is permanently scarred and thickened and such residual abnormalities make the patient highly vulnerable to episodes of reinfection.

Treatment

High-dosage **single** or **combination antibiotic therapy**, guided by the microbiological findings from the blood culture, is necessary. The antibiotic regimen selected should be:
- bactericidal and not bacteriostatic
- delivered parenterally
- of several weeks' duration (usually up to 4 weeks).

The rationale behind management is:
1. To eradicate the organisms totally, without leaving residual pockets or reservoirs.
2. To administer high concentrations of antibiotic so that it may penetrate, by diffusion, into the focal aggregates of bacteria in the avascular cardiac vegetations.
3. To assess antibiotic levels in blood regularly, by **laboratory monitoring**, throughout the treatment period. Special sensitivity tests such as the **minimum inhibitory concentration** (MIC) and **minimum bactericidal concentration** (MBC) of the antibiotic (see Ch. 6) needs to be regularly performed to ascertain the **optimal level** of antibiotics that should be present in the

Table 24.3 Cardiac valvular disease predisposing to infective endocarditis

Disease	Degree of risk
Aortic valvular disease Prosthetic valves Mitral insufficiency Ventricular septal defect Patent ductus arteriosus Coarctation of aorta Previous infective endocarditis	High
Mitral valve prolapse and stenosis Pulmonary and tricuspid valve disease Degenerative (calcific) aortic valve disease Non-valvular intracardiac prosthetic implants	Intermediate
Atrial septal defect Coronary artery disease Cardiac pacemakers Arteriosclerotic plaques	Low/negligible

circulation to eradicate the organisms, and to avoid the **toxic effects** (e.g. nephrotoxicity, ototoxicity) of amino-glycosides such as gentamicin, which is commonly prescribed in combination with other drugs.

Infective endocarditis and dentistry

The oral cavity acts as a portal of entry for organisms causing bacteraemia, and dental manipulations may set in motion the disease process leading to infective endocarditis. Bacteraemia can occur after dental procedures such as **extractions**, **surgical** or **non-surgical endodontics**, **gingivectomy**, **root-planing**, **scaling** and **flossing**, **intraligamentary injections** and **reimplantation** of avulsed teeth. The frequency of bacteraemia is also related to the preoperative **oral sepsis** of the patient and the degree of **trauma** and **tissue injury**; toothbrushing may sometimes cause bacteraemia, depending on the degree of sepsis.

The real risk of development of infective endocarditis in a 'risk' patient following dental procedures is difficult to ascertain, and has been estimated to vary between 10% and 90%. A proportion of infections is likely to be associated with random transient bacteraemias which commonly follow mastication, and even toothbrushing, in patients with chronic periodontitis.

Infective endocarditis prophylaxis

As eventual development of endocarditis may well be the most common potentially fatal complication of dental treatment, all dentists must have a good working knowledge of the problem and the appropriate preventive measures. Procedures requiring prophylaxis are shown in Table 24.4.

Accurate identification of at-risk patients

The main risk conditions are shown in Table 24.3. Dentists usually identify patients at risk from their **medical history**. It is also important to obtain confirmatory and expert information from the patient's medical practitioner.

Patient awareness of risk status and dental involvement in cardiac clinics

Warning cards given to patients with cardiac disease increase their awareness of the disease. Dentists should be part of the medical team involved in the preoperative and postoperative management of patients undergoing cardiac surgery who are at risk.

Table 24.4 Procedures requiring antimicrobial prophylaxis in persons at risk from endocarditis

Tooth extraction

Oral surgery involving the periodontal tissues

Periodontal surgery

Subgingival procedures including scaling

Intraligamentary injections

Reimplantation of avulsed teeth

Preventive dental care

Susceptible patients should be exposed to risky operative procedures as rarely as possible; this can be best achieved by careful and intensive oral hygiene instruction, dietary advice and regular dental examinations. The aim should be to reduce the amount of treatment to the absolute minimum necessary for the maintenance of a healthy natural dentition for life. The need to administer prophylactic antibiotics for dental procedures that could produce a bacteraemia capable of initiating infective endocarditis must be weighed carefully in each susceptible patient. If there is reasonable doubt, prophylaxis should be given.

Antibiotic and antiseptic prophylaxis

The main source of microorganisms in significant dental bacteraemias is supragingival and subgingival plaque; hence, local reduction in the numbers of such organisms before the start of treament can be achieved by irrigating the gingival crevice area with antiseptics (e.g. chlorhexidine gluconate gel 1% or mouthwash 0.2%, used 5 minutes before the procedure). *Note*: such topical antiseptic treatment should not be regarded as replacing antibiotic prophylaxis; it is merely an adjunct.

Awareness of postoperative morbidity

Even when antibiotic cover has been provided, patients at risk should be instructed to report any unexplained illness because of the insidious origin of infective endocarditis.

Cardiac patients who need antibiotic prophylaxis

Almost any type of heart lesion is susceptible to infection, but antibiotic prophylaxis is imperative for patients with:
- congenital cardiac defects
- rheumatic heart disease
- prosthetic cardiac valves
- previous history of endocarditis
- hypertrophic cardiomyopathy
- aortic valve disease (bicuspid valve).

Recommendations on antibiotic prophylaxis

A number of recommendations on antibiotic prophylaxis have been promulgated. The current British recommendations (Working Party of the British Society for Antimicrobial Chemotherapy) are given below and outlined in Figure 24.3.
1. The majority of risk patients (i.e. those who are not allergic to penicillin) who have not received penicillin more than once during the previous month, and require only local anaesthesia, should be given 3 g amoxicillin orally 1 hour before the operation, taken under supervision.
2. Oral clindamycin (600 mg) should be given to patients unable to take penicillin because of allergy or those who have taken penicillin more than once during the previous month.
3. Vancomycin (intravenous) and erythromycin (peroral) are other alternatives. As vancomycin has to be given by slow intravenous infusion this is not practicable in routine dentistry. Erythromycin can be administered orally but is associated with severe gastrointestinal disturbances.
4. For patients requiring general anaesthesia, oral administration of drugs immediately before surgery is con-

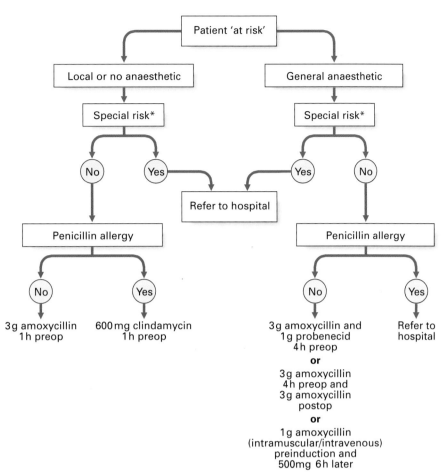

Fig. 24.3 Flowchart indicating the current British recommendations for antimicrobial prophylaxis against dentally induced infective endocarditis. These recommendations may vary slightly in other countries. (See text below for details.)

traindicated and prophylactic antibiotics need to be given by injection. Thus in high-risk patients (with the exception of those with prosthetic heart valves or individuals who are hypersensitive to penicillin) 1 g amoxicillin (amoxycillin) should be given intramuscularly or intravenously before induction, with a further 500 mg amoxicillin given by mouth 6 hours later. Alternative regimens include 3 g oral amoxicillin 4 hours before induction, then 3 g oral amoxicillin as soon as possible thereafter, or oral amoxicillin 3 g plus 1 g oral probenecid 4 hours before the procedure.

Some categories of at-risk patients need to receive prophylaxis in hospital and should be referred to the nearest consultant. Patients who should be referred include:

- patients who have received penicillin more than once in the previous month and require general anaesthesia
- patients who are allergic to penicillin and require general anaesthesia
- prosthetic valve patients requiring general anaesthesia
- patients who have had one or more attacks of infective endocarditis.

Details of prophylaxis for these patients are outside the competence of a general dental practitioner and will be found in the recommended texts.

The antibiotic recommendations of the American Heart Association (AHA) are slightly different. They recommend 2.0 g instead of 3.0 g amoxicillin (for those not allergic to penicillin), 500 mg of azithromycin or clarithromycin as alternatives to clindamycin (in penicillin-allergic patients).

Note: the antibiotic dosages given above are for **adults only** and should be appropriately adjusted for children (a rule of thumb is one-quarter of the adult dose for children under 5 years old and half the adult dose for children aged 5–10 years).

It is noteworthy that the recommendations of the AHA slightly differ from the foregoing British recommendations. Thus, the AHA recommends 500 mg of azithromycin or clarithromycin as alternatives to clindamycin. Other recommendations are 2.0 g of cefalexin or cefadroxil for those who do not have an immediate hypersensitivity reaction to penicillin (urticaria, angioedema or anaphylaxis).

Finally, it should be borne in mind that these recommendations are regularly reviewed by the authorities, and practitioners need to keep abreast of such developments.

PROSTHESES

Heart valve prostheses

The dental management of patients with replacement heart valves can be undertaken by dentists (as described above for other at-risk groups) as long as the patients require local anaesthesia, are not hypersensitive to penicillin and have not received penicillin within the past month. Otherwise the patient should be treated by the hospital service.

Hip joint replacements

There are few data on postoperative infection of hip prostheses to suggest that bacteria derived from the mouth are involved. The advice from the Working Party of the British Society for Antimicrobial Chemotherapy is that patients with prosthetic joint implants, including total hip replacements, do not require antibiotic prophylaxis, because the risks of prophylaxis outweigh the benefits. Nevertheless, it is important that the possible need for prophylactic cover should be discussed with the patient's doctor before dental treatment starts. Further, there should be liaison between orthopaedic surgeons and dentists to render patients dentally fit prior to insertion of replacements or implants.

KEY FACTS

- In health the cardiovascular system is sterile, but a few organisms may transiently enter the bloodstream during routines such as toothbrushing

- *Bacteraemia is asymptomatic and the bacterial burden in blood is very low, while in septicaemia large numbers of organisms enter and/or actively multiply and persist in the bloodstream producing clinical signs and symptoms such as hypotension, fever and rigors*

- *Bacteraemia can occur after dental procedures such as extractions, surgical or non-surgical endodontics, gingivectomy, root-planing and scaling, and flossing*

- *Sepsis syndrome is a systemic response to microbial products or constituents circulating in the blood mediated by inflammatory cytokines*

- Infective endocarditis is defined as the inflammation of the endocardium of the heart valves, and sometimes the endocardium around congenital defects, caused by an infection

- *More than 80% of infective endocarditis is caused by streptococci and staphylococci*

- *Infective endocarditis is diagnosed by positive blood culture; repeated culture may be necessary to isolate the causal organism*

- *The predisposing conditions for infective endocarditis include valve prostheses, septal defects, atheroma of the valve, congenital valve deformities and pre-existing rheumatic fever*

- *High-dose, single or combination antibiotic therapy, guided by the microbiological findings from the blood culture, is necessary to treat infective endocarditis*

- Infective endocarditis prophylaxis is based on accurate identification of patients at risk, patient awareness of risk status, dental involvement in cardiac clinics, preventive dental care, antibiotic and antiseptic prophylaxis, and awareness of postoperative morbidity

- Cardiac **patients who may need antibiotic cover** include those with congenital cardiac defects, rheumatic heart disease, prosthetic cardiac valves, previous history of endocarditis, hypertrophic cardiomyopathy, and aortic valve disease (bicuspid valve)

- *Drugs used in antibiotic prophylaxis of infective endocarditis include amoxicillin, clindamycin, vancomycin and erythromycin*

FURTHER READING

Dajani, AS, et al (1997). Prevention of bacterial endocarditis. Recommendations by the American Heart Association. *Journal of the American Medical Association*, 277, 1794–1801.

Durack, DT, et al (1994). New criteria for the diagnosis of infective endocarditis. *American Journal of Medicine*, 96, 200–209.

Editorial (1998). Sepsis. *Journal of Antimicrobial Chemotherapy*, suppl. A, vol. 41.

Shanson, DC (1999). Septicaemia; infections of the heart. In *Microbiology in clinical practice* (3rd edn), Ch. 19. Butterworth-Heinemann, Oxford.

Working Party of the British Society for Antimicrobial Chemotherapy (1992). Antibiotic prophylaxis and infective endocarditis. *Lancet* i, 1292–1293.

25 Infections of the central nervous and locomotor systems

As the cerebrospinal fluid is devoid of effective antimicrobial defences, generalized infection rapidly sets in when pyogenic organisms enter the subarachnoid space and the cerebrospinal fluid. This may be caused by:

- **direct spread** due to trauma and resultant breach of the integuments of the central nervous system
- **seeding** via blood from a peripheral infective focus.

Meningitis

Inflammation of the meninges, the membranes that cover the brain and spinal cord, is classified according to the aetiological agent, as:

- **bacterial meningitis** (also called pyogenic or polymorphonuclear meningitis)
- **viral meningitis** (also called aseptic or lymphocytic meningitis).

Bacterial meningitis

Bacterial meningitis is more severe than the viral type and remains a serious cause of morbidity and mortality despite antibiotic therapy. Prompt diagnosis is of the essence in preventing disabling sequelae of infection and death.

Clinical features. Symptoms include severe headache, fever, vomiting, photophobia and convulsions leading to drowsiness and unconsciousness. Signs are mainly those of meningeal irritation, i.e. neck and spinal stiffness, and **Kernig's sign** (pain and resistance on extending the knee when the thigh is flexed). These cardinal signs and symptoms may be absent in neonatal meningitis and meningitis in the elderly and the immunocompromised. Sequelae include encephalopathy (altered cerebral function), cranial nerve palsies, cerebral abscess, obstructive hydrocephalus and subdural effusion of sterile or infected fluid.

Aetiology. The common types of bacterial meningitis and the major agents are:

- meningococcal meningitis: *Neisseria meningitidis*
- *haemophilus* meningitis: *Haemophilus influenzae*, capsulated (Pittman type b)
- pneumococcal meningitis: *Streptococcus pneumoniae*
- tuberculous meningitis: *Mycobacterium tuberculosis* and other mycobacteria.

Epidemiology, treatment and prevention. Neisseria meningitidis (the meningococcus) is the main agent of meningitis in Britain and most infections are caused by group B strains. The disease is common in children and young adults. Penicillin is the drug of choice: cefotaxime and chloramphenicol are alternatives. *Haemophilus* meningitis is mostly seen in children between 1 month and 4 years old and is treated with chloramphenicol or cefotaxime. Pneumococcal infection, common in older patients and those without a functioning spleen, is treated with penicillin. Tuberculous infection is managed by 'triple therapy' as described in Chapter 23.

Meningitis may spread quickly in close household contacts. Avoiding overcrowding in living and working conditions is helpful. Chemoprophylaxis with antibiotics (e.g. rifampicin) in meningococcal infection can eliminate the carrier state, which may develop in some.

Meningitis due to other organisms. Rarely other organisms, such as *Listeria monocytogenes*, *Leptospira interrogans* and *Cryptococcus neoformans* (a fungus), may cause meningitis.

Laboratory diagnosis. Examination of the cerebrospinal fluid, usually obtained by a lumbar puncture, is essential. Changes that occur in the cerebrospinal fluid, depending on whether the aetiology is acute pyogenic, tuberculous or viral, dictate appropriate and timely therapy (Table 25.1). Cerebrospinal fluid should also be centrifuged and the deposit Gram-stained and cultured to isolate and identify the causative agent. Blood cultures are also useful in the diagnosis of bacterial meningitis.

Treatment. Treatment is dictated by the causative organism and its antibiotic sensitivity; because of the serious nature of the illness, empirical therapy with two or three antibiotic drugs is given immediately.

Viral meningitis

Viral or aseptic meningitis can be caused by many agents, as shown in Table 25.2.

Pathogenesis. The major routes of viral entry into the body are the respiratory and gastrointestinal tracts. From these portals they spread to the central nervous system by direct

Table 25.1 Cerebrospinal fluid in meningitis

	Normal	Acute pyogenic	Tuberculous	Aseptic
Appearance	Clear	Turbid	Clear or opalescent	Usually clear
Total protein	Normal	Greatly increased	Increased	Normal
Glucose	Normal	Greatly reduced or absent	Reduced	Normal
Lactate	Normal	Raised	Considerably raised	Normal
Cell count	Lymphocytes 0–3 × 10⁹/L	Greatly increased; polymorphs	Increased; mainly lymphocytes but some polymorphs	Increased lymphocytes

migration via the olfactory nerves or indirectly via blood. Cells involved in viral spread include capillary endothelial cells, epithelial cells of the choroid plexus and infected leucocytes.

Epidemiology. Children and young adults are the most affected.

Treatment. Viral meningitis is a benign, self-limiting condition and requires only symptomatic treatment. No antiviral drugs are indicated as the condition resolves in 1–2 weeks.

Encephalitis

Infection of the **brain substance** (as opposed to the meninges) is called encephalitis. This is a somewhat artificial division as patients often show signs and symptoms of meningitis and encephalitis at the same time.

Aetiology

The most frequently involved viruses are herpes simplex virus, mumps virus and arboviruses.

Pathogenesis

Encephalitis occurs after childhood illnesses such as measles, chickenpox and rubella, and rarely after immunization with vaccines such as pertussis. Affected patients often die or have debilitating sequelae.

Treatment

In contrast to viral meningitis, encephalitis is a very serious disease which needs prompt and specific antiviral therapy such as intravenous aciclovir.

Table 25.2 Major causes of viral meningitis and/or encephalitis in Great Britain

Echovirus
Mumps virus
Coxsackievirus
Herpes simplex virus
Adenovirus
Measles virus
Influenza virus
Varicella–zoster virus

Poliomyelitis

Poliomyelitis is caused by poliovirus types 1–3, belonging to the Picornaviridae.

Pathogenesis

The portal of infection is the mouth, and the virus multiplies in the lymphoid tissue of the pharynx and the intestine. It then enters the bloodstream and causes a viraemia, with resulting spread into the central nervous system causing neurological disease. The disease is an influenza-like illness, with meningitis and encephalitis. In some, damage to the anterior horn cells of the spinal cord leads to respiratory failure (requiring artificial ventilation) or permanent lower motor neuron weakness and paralytic poliomyelitis.

Epidemiology and prevention

Although epidemics of poliomyelitis were common in the past, it is now rare in the West owing to effective polio vaccine. However, the disease is still prevalent in developing countries, where universal vaccination programmes are difficult to implement, despite the goal of the World Health Organization to eradicate the disease by the year 2000. The polio vaccine is of two types: the killed (Salk) vaccine and the live attenuated (Sabin) vaccine (Ch. 37).

Cerebral abscess

Many bacteria may cause brain abscesses. These include streptococci (*Streptococcus milleri*, *S. faecalis*, *S. pneumoniae*), staphylococci, anaerobic cocci and coliforms. The infections are mostly **polymicrobial** in nature (i.e. mixed infections).

Pathogenesis

The infective agent may reach the brain in the blood or by direct extension. In the latter case, a brain abscess may result as a direct extension of sinus infection caused by oral bacteria or rarely, as a complication of acute or chronic dental infection. Infection may also follow traumatic injury to the maxillofacial region.

Treatment

Operative drainage and excision of the abscess (if well encapsulated) is supplemented by antibiotic therapy. Beta-lactam group antibiotics and gentamicin are very popular; metronidazole is also used because of its good penetration into abscesses, and as anaerobes are frequently involved.

Tetanus

Tetanus is caused by infection with *Clostridium tetani* (drumstick bacillus).

Clinical features

After an incubation period of 5–15 days the exotoxins produced by the organisms precipitate severe and painful muscle spasms:
- **lockjaw** — spasm of masseter muscles
- **risus sardonicus** — facial grimace due to spasm of facial muscles
- **Opisthotonos** — arched body due to spasm of the more powerful extensor muscles of the body (see Fig. 13.4).

Pathogenesis

Contamination of wounds with tetanus spores derived from dust, manured soil or rusty objects results in spore germination and release of the powerful exotoxins **tetanospasmin** and **tetanolysin** (see Chs 5 and 13). Although the bacteria remain localized at the site of infection, the exotoxins are absorbed at the motor nerve endings, and diffuse centripetally towards the anterior horn cells of the spinal cord, blocking the normal inhibitory impulses that control motor nerve function, with resultant sustained contraction of the muscles. Wounds of the face, neck and upper extremities are more dangerous than those of the lower extremities as they have a shorter incubation period and result in more severe disease.

Epidemiology

The main source of spores is animal faeces. The incidence is higher in the developing world because of lack of immunization and poor standards of wound care. Although tetanus is commonly associated with deep penetrating wounds, it can often result from superficial abrasions (e.g. thorn pricks). **Neonatal tetanus** due to infection of the umbilical stump is common in rural areas of developing countries.

Diagnosis

Diagnosis is mainly clinical as bacteriological confirmation frequently fails. Swab or exudate from the wound typically shows 'drumstick bacilli'; biochemical identification and confirmation by mouse pathogenicity is described in Chapter 13.

Treatment

1. **Supportive treatment**: muscle relaxants to control spasms, sedation, and artificial ventilation (for respiratory muscle paralysis).
2. **Antitoxin**: given intravenously in large doses to neutralize the toxin; it is of little use in the late stage of disease.
3. **Antibiotics**: penicillin or tetracycline to prevent further toxin production.
4. **Debridement**: excision and cleaning of the wound.

Prevention

Active immunization with adsorbed tetanus vaccine, also called **toxoid** (a component of diphtheria–tetanus–pertussis vaccine), should be given in childhood (during the first year of life and before school or nursery school entry).

Prophylaxis of wounded patients:
- if the patient is **immune**, a booster dose of toxoid or adsorbed tetanus vaccine if the primary course (or booster dose) was given more than 10 years previously, *and* human antitetanus immunoglobulin if the wound is dirty and more than 24 hours old
- if the patient is **non-immune**, human antitetanus immunoglobulin should be given, followed by a full course of tetanus toxoid by injection.

Penicillin may be given as prophylaxis, not only to prevent tetanus but also to avoid pyogenic infection.

Booster doses of toxoid 10 years after the primary course and again 10 years later maintain a satisfactory level of protection. Any adult who has received five doses is likely to have lifelong immunity.

INFECTIONS OF THE LOCOMOTOR SYSTEM

The two major infections associated with the locomotor system (i.e. bones and joints) are **acute septic arthritis** and **osteomyelitis**.

Natural defences in the locomotor system include:
- specialized macrophages in the synovial membranes of joints (highly phagocytic)
- a few mononuclear cells, complement and lysozyme of synovial fluid
- a rich vascular plexus traversing the medulla and cortex of bone with integral defences.

Important pathogens are listed in Figure 25.1.

Acute septic arthritis

Aetiology

Commonly associated bacteria are *Staphylococcus aureus*, *Haemophilus influenzae*, *Streptococcus pneumoniae* and other streptococci, *Neisseria gonorrhoeae* and non-sporing anaerobes such as *Bacteroides* spp. Other infrequent but notable agents are *Mycobacterium tuberculosis*, *Salmonella* spp. and *Brucella* spp.

Clinical features

Limitation of movement with swelling, redness and severe pain are the cardinal symptoms; usually only a single joint is involved. Crippling and permanent joint damage may result despite antibiotic therapy.

Pathogenesis

The condition may result from:
- traumatic injury through the joint capsule
- haematogenous spread, usually as a complication of septicaemia
- extension of osteomyelitis or spread of infection from an adjacent septic focus
- complication of rheumatoid arthritis
- infection of joint prosthesis.

Epidemiology

Acute septic arthritis occurs most commonly in children. Sources of infection are many and include sepsis of the skin,

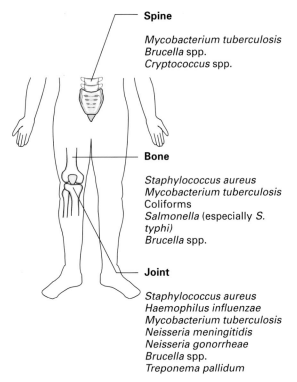

Spine

Mycobacterium tuberculosis
Brucella spp.
Cryptococcus spp.

Bone

Staphylococcus aureus
Mycobacterium tuberculosis
Coliforms
Salmonella (especially *S. typhi*)
Brucella spp.

Joint

Staphylococcus aureus
Haemophilus influenzae
Mycobacterium tuberculosis
Neisseria meningitidis
Neisseria gonorrheae
Brucella spp.
Treponema pallidum

Fig. 25.1 Major infectious agents of the locomotor system.

nasopharynx, sinuses, lung, peritoneum and genital tract. The source of infection of artificial joints could be the patient, the operating team or the theatre air.

Laboratory diagnosis

Diagnosis is by **direct film observation** and **culture** of aspirated joint fluid; **blood culture**; culture of specimens from the **suspected primary focus** of infection, e.g. throat, genital tract; and **serological tests** for salmonellosis and brucellosis, if suspected.

Treatment

Initial antibiotic therapy is given on an empirical or 'best guess' basis. Early administration of antibiotics, immediately after the specimen is taken, is essential to prevent chronic sequelae. Antibiotics may be injected directly into the joint or given systemically.

Reactive arthritis

Reactive arthritis is the term given to acute arthritis affecting one or more joints; it develops 1–4 weeks after infection of the genital (post-sexual reactive arthritis) or gastrointestinal tract (post-dysenteric reactive arthritis). The causative agent in post-sexual reactive arthritis is *Chlamydia trachomatis*; almost all patients are men. Post-dysenteric reactive arthritis may follow infections with *Salmonella*, *Shigella*, *Yersinia* or *Campylobacter*.

Reactive arthritis should be differentiated from septic arthritis as **it is not due to joint infection**. It is thought to be mediated by immunological mechanisms, and there is an apparent genetic predisposition to the disease.

Osteomyelitis

Osteomyelitis can be divided into acute and chronic forms. Acute infection usually occurs in children under 10 years old, whereas the chronic variety is more common in adults.

Aetiology

Acute. Mostly *Staphylococcus aureus* (some 75% of cases); other agents include *Haemophilus influenzae* (in preschool children), *Streptococcus pyogenes*, *S. pneumoniae* and other streptococci; *Salmonella*, *Brucella* and non-sporing anaerobes rarely.

Chronic. *Staphylococcus aureus* is most common; rarely *Mycobacterium tuberculosis*, *Pseudomonas aeruginosa*, *Salmonella* and *Brucella* spp.

Pathogenesis

Any septic lesion can be the source of the organism (e.g. a boil or pustule); spread to bone is usually haematogenous. Infection at all ages may be a result of major trauma (e.g. compound fracture) that exposes bone tissue to the environment.

Laboratory diagnosis

Diagnosis is by **blood culture** (a number of cultures may be required to isolate the infective agent(s), which circulate in the blood in very small numbers); **culture of pus** from the bony focus — pus may be obtained by needle aspiration or by open surgery; and by specimens from the **related infective focus**, e.g. 'cold abscess' pus in tuberculosis.

Treatment

Antibiotics alone are helpful if started early in the disease, by the parenteral route first and the oral route later. Penicillinase-resistant penicillin (such as flucloxacillin) should be given first if culture results are not available as *Staphylococcus aureus* is the predominant agent. Drugs that penetrate bone well (such as fusidic acid and clindamycin) are alternatives. Erythromycin is an alternative in patients hypersensitive to penicillin.

Surgery may be needed to drain pus and remove sequestra, if any.

Osteomyelitis of the jaws

Osteomyelitis of the jaws (see also Ch. 34) is uncommon owing to the relatively high vascularity of the jaws, especially the maxilla; therefore the mandible is more commonly affected than the maxilla. The following predisposing conditions are noteworthy:

- **bone disease**, such as Paget's disease or osteopetrosis, fibrous dysplasia, bone tumours
- **irradiation** of the jaws for cancer therapy (e.g. nasopharyngeal carcinoma)
- **trauma** superimposed on debilitating conditions such as malnutrition, and immunocompromised states.

KEY FACTS

- The cerebrospinal fluid is sterile and devoid of effective antimicrobial defences; it may be infected either directly from a contiguous focus (e.g. due to trauma) or indirectly via blood from a peripheral infective focus

- *Meningitis, defined as the inflammation of the meninges, can be broadly categorized as **bacterial meningitis** (also called pyogenic or polymorphonuclear meningitis) or **viral meningitis** (also called aseptic or lymphocytic meningitis)*

- The common types (and agents) of bacterial meningitis are: meningococcal meningitis (*Neisseria meningitidis*), haemophilus meningitis (*Haemophilus influenzae*), pneumococcal meningitis (*Streptococcus pneumoniae*) and tuberculous meningitis (*Mycobacterium tuberculosis* and others)

- *Examination of the cerebrospinal fluid, obtained by a lumbar puncture, is mandatory for diagnosis of the different types of bacterial meningitis*

- Viral or aseptic meningitis can be caused by many agents and the major routes of entry are the respiratory and gastrointestinal tracts

- *Viral meningitis is usually benign and self-limiting requiring only symptomatic treatment; no antiviral therapy is indicated*

- Polio vaccine is of two types: the **killed (Salk) vaccine** and the **live attenuated (Sabin) vaccine**; the latter given orally is the more popular.

- Contamination of wounds with *Clostridium tetani* spores derived from dust, manured soil or rusty objects results in spore germination and release of the powerful exotoxins **tetanospasmin** and **tetanolysin** to cause tetanus

- *Tetanus is **managed by supportive measures** (e.g. muscle relaxants, sedation and artificial ventilation), **antitoxin**, **antibiotics** (penicillin or tetracycline) and **wound debridement***

- *Tetanus preventive measures are: active immunization with **formol toxoid** (a component of DTP vaccine given in childhood), booster doses of toxoid once every 10 years for risk groups*

- Osteomyelitis can be divided into **acute** (seen in children under 10 years old) and **chronic osteomyelitis** (common in adults)

- The acute form is mostly caused by *Staphylococcus aureus* (some 75% of cases); in chronic osteomyelitis *S. aureus* is most common; rarely *M. tuberculosis*, *Salmonella*, *Brucella* spp., etc.

- *Osteomyelitis of the jaws is uncommon owing to their high vascularity (especially the maxilla)*

- *Predisposing conditions that result in osteomyelitis of jaws include bone disease (e.g. Paget's disease, osteopetrosis, fibrous dysplasia, bone tumours), irradiation and trauma superimposed on debilitating conditions such as malnutrition, and immunocompromised states*

FURTHER READING

Shanson, DC (1999). Infections of the central nervous system. *Microbiology in clinical practice* (3rd edn), Ch. 11. Butterworth-Heinemann, Oxford.

Shanson, DC (1999). Bone and joint infections. *Microbiology in clinical practice* (3rd edn), Ch. 18. Butterworth-Heinemann, Oxford.

26 Infections of the gastrointestinal tract

NORMAL FLORA

In healthy, fasting individuals the stomach is either sterile or may contain only a few organisms, because of its low pH and enzymes. The diet has a major effect on the gut flora. The small intestine may be colonized with streptococci, lactobacilli and yeasts (especially *Candida albicans*); the proportions of these and other organisms vary, depending on dietary habits. In the ileum a typical Gram-negative flora (e.g. *Bacteroides* spp. and Enterobacteriaceae) is seen, and the large intestine has a dense population of varied flora. These include members of the Enterobacteriaceae, *Streptococcus faecalis*, *Bacteroides* spp., *Clostridium* spp., bifidobacteria and anaerobic streptococci. The anaerobes outweigh the aerobes by far, and comprise the vast majority of the bacteria in the large intestine. Roughly 20% of the faeces contains bacteria, approximately 10^{11} organisms per gram.

Important pathogens

A diverse array of infections of the gastrointestinal tract is caused by an equally varied population of microbial agents (Fig. 26.1). The agents of diarrhoeal diseases including those that are considered common agents of **food poisoning** are listed in Table 26.1. The common bacterial diarrhoeal diseases in the developed world include those caused by:
- *Campylobacter* spp.
- *Shigella* spp.
- *Salmonella* spp.
- *Escherichia coli*
- *Staphylococcus aureus*
- *Clostridium perfringens*

Cholera caused by *Vibrio cholerae* is noteworthy as a common diarrhoeal disease in the developing world, together with the foregoing.

Less common diseases include infections caused by *Clostridium difficile* and *Bacillus cereus*.

COMMON DIARRHOEAL DISEASES

Campylobacter

Campylobacter coli and *C. jejuni* are among the most common diarrhoea-inducing agents in the Western world. They are curved, slender, Gram-negative bacilli present in the gut as well as in the oral cavity.

Pathogenesis and epidemiology

Symptoms vary from mild to severe, with any part of the small or large intestine affected. Dogs and cats are probable sources of infection but mass-produced poultry is the most common source. Eating contaminated food is a common cause of infection; note that campylobacters do not multiply in food. Patients may become symptomless carriers after recovery.

Diagnosis

A specimen of stool cultured on selective media will indicate the diagnosis.

Treatment

The infection is self-limiting; erythromycin is useful to relieve symptoms, ciprofloxacin is an alternative.

Prevention

Food and personal hygiene.

Shigella

Shigella causes bacillary dysentery, as opposed to amoebic dysentery caused by intestinal amoebae. It is an important cause of morbidity and death in young children, particularly in the developing world.

Aetiology

The genus *Shigella* contains four species: *S. dysenteriae*, *S. flexneri*, *S. boydii* and *S. sonnei*.

Pathogenesis and epidemiology

Infection is by ingestion of organisms. Once ingested, the bacteria attach to the mucosal villus epithelium, enter and multiply in these cells. The resultant death of the infected cells initiates an inflammatory reaction in the submucosa and lamina propria. Finally, necrosis and ulceration of the villus epithelium ensues, making the stools bloody and mucous. This

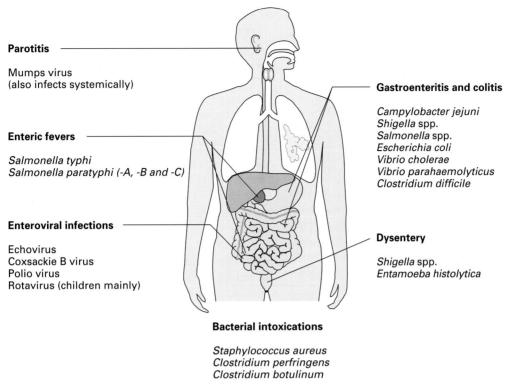

Parotitis

Mumps virus
(also infects systemically)

Gastroenteritis and colitis

Campylobacter jejuni
Shigella spp.
Salmonella spp.
Escherichia coli
Vibrio cholerae
Vibrio parahaemolyticus
Clostridium difficile

Enteric fevers

Salmonella typhi
Salmonella paratyphi (-A, -B and -C)

Enteroviral infections

Echovirus
Coxsackie B virus
Polio virus
Rotavirus (children mainly)

Dysentery

Shigella spp.
Entamoeba histolytica

Bacterial intoxications

Staphylococcus aureus
Clostridium perfringens
Clostridium botulinum

Fig. 26.1 Major infectious agents of the gastrointestinal tract.

type of severe reaction is usually due to *S. dysenteriae*, which is known to produce a potent **enterotoxin** and a **cytotoxin**. This infection may be life-threatening.

Dysentery due to other shigellae is generally milder and varies from asymptomatic excretion to a severe attack of diarrhoea with abdominal pain. *Shigella sonnei* is the usual agent of dysentery in Britain, while *S. boydii* is common in the Middle East and South-East Asia.

Spread of the disease is from hand to mouth. It occurs usually in nursery schools where the **index case** (i.e. the person with the disease) contaminates hands at toilet, and further contaminates lavatory handles and hand towels if personal hygiene is deficient. Subsequent handling of these bacteria-laden **fomites** (inanimate surfaces acting as vehicles of disease transfer), by healthy individuals results in hand-to-mouth transmission of the agents, leading to the

disease. Thus '**food, flies** and **fomites**' are classical means of spread.

Diagnosis

The diagnosis is made by examination of stool sample and culture on MacConkey's agar and selective media such as desoxycholate–citrate agar (DCA). Pale, non-lactose-fermenting colonies are then isolated and identified by biochemical tests; serological identification is performed subsequently.

Treatment

Antibiotics are of little use except in *S. dysenteriae* infection, where trimethoprim (first-line drug), ampicillin or tetracycline may be used.

Table 26.1 Aetiological agents of diarrhoeal diseases

Occurrence	Bacterial	Viral	Protozoal
Common	*Campylobacter* spp.[a] *Shigella* spp. *Salmonella* spp.[a] *Escherichia coli*[a] *Staphylococcus aureus*[a] *Clostridium perfringens*[a]	Rotavirus	*Entamoeba histolytica* (amoebic dysentery)
Uncommon	*Clostridium difficile* *Bacillus cereus*[a]	Adenovirus Astrovirus Norwalk virus, calicivirus[c]	*Giardia lamblia* (giardiasis)
Rare	*Vibrio cholerae*[b]		

[a] Common agents of 'food poisoning'.
[b] Rare in the developed world but very common in developing countries such as Bangladesh and India.
[c] Not discussed in text.

Prevention

Attention to personal hygiene, good sanitation with safe, pipe-borne water and adequate sewage disposal are important. All these measures are difficult to implement in conditions of poverty and poor housing.

Salmonella

A large number of different *Salmonella* species exist, together with an even more bewildering number (about 1500) of serotypes. Of these, about 14 are important pathogens. The common diarrhoea-causing organism is *S. typhimurium*. The other major pathogens of this group are *S. typhi* and *S. paratyphi-A*, *-B* and *-C*, which cause enteric fever, a septicaemic illness in which diarrhoea is a late feature of the disease.

Pathogenesis and epidemiology

The genesis of salmonella food poisoning is ill understood. Patients have mild gastrointestinal disturbances with an incubation period of about 1–2 days. Abdominal pain, diarrhoea (with or without fever) and vomiting are commonly present. Septicaemia is rare.

The organism is found in domestic animals and poultry and is spread via the faecal–oral route. On entering the gastrointestinal tract the salmonellae may either produce an enterotoxin (similar to toxigenic *Escherichia coli*) or invade the mucosa of small intestine (like shigellae).

Diagnosis

Examination of stool sample and culture on MacConkey (indicator) medium and selective media such as DCA or Wilson–Blair medium; pale, non-lactose fermenting (NLF) colonies on MacConkey medium and black, shiny colonies on Wilson–Blair medium. Subsequent identification is by biochemical tests and determination of serological status. The major antigens that are useful for the serotyping of salmonellae are the 'O' (somatic or body antigen) and the 'H' (flagellar) antigens.

Treatment

Treatment is rarely necessary. Antibiotics are contraindicated except in septicaemic cases; antibiotic therapy prolongs the carriage of the organism in the convalescent phase.

Prevention

Prevention includes control of animal food quality, good farming and abattoir practices, rigorous kitchen hygiene and good personal hygiene among food handlers, and exclusion of known human carriers ('excretors') from food handling. However, the best form of prevention is thorough cooking of food and avoidance of consumption of raw or partly cooked eggs and other animal-derived food.

Escherichia coli

Escherichia coli is a normal commensal of the gastrointestinal tract but certain strains, for some unknown reason, can behave as pathogens. As described in Chapter 15, they produce enterotoxins, and the enteroinvasive strains have the ability to invade the gut mucosa.

Pathogenesis and epidemiology

There are two types of *E. coli* diarrhoea:
- infantile gastroenteritis
- traveller's diarrhoea.

Infantile gastroenteritis. Accompanied by acute and profuse diarrhoea, this infection has an incubation period of 1–3 days. The disease is mainly caused by **enteropathogenic *E. coli*** (EPEC), but in a minority of cases **enterotoxigenic *E. coli*** (ETEC) strains contribute (Ch. 15). Common in the developing world because of poor sanitation and poverty; infection spreads direct from case to case and via fomites (see above for shigellae), and in some cases the mother may be the source of infection.

Traveller's diarrhoea. Accompanied by abdominal pain and vomiting, this infection is usually self-limiting, with a short incubation period of 1–2 days. The most frequent cause of diarrhoea in travellers (thus named 'Delhi belly', 'Tokyo two-step', etc.); it is usually spread by contaminated food.

Diagnosis

- **Infantile gastroenteritis**: faecal culture and identification of lactose-fermenting colonies in MacConkey's agar (compare salmonella and shigella above); confirmation by serology. (*Note*: viruses such as rotavirus may cause similar gastroenteritis and should be included in a differential diagnosis.)
- **Traveller's diarrhoea.** Owing to the self-limiting nature of the disease, diagnosis is usually made clinically.

Treatment

In **infantile diarrhoea**, treatment is by rehydration and correction of fluid loss and electrolyte balance. No antibiotics are necessary for either of the *E. coli* diarrhoeas. **Traveller's diarrhoea** is self-limiting.

Prevention

- **Infantile gastroenteritis**: scrupulous hygiene in neonatal units and personal hygiene of nursing staff is required; patients with diarrhoea should be screened. In the developing world, improved sanitation, housing, pipe-borne water supplies and antenatal health education will all help.
- **Traveller's diarrhoea**: public health measures.

Haemorrhagic syndromes

Though not diarrhoeogenic, two important haemorrhagic syndromes caused by *E. coli* are noteworthy here. **Haemorrhagic colitis** is seen in children and adults, while **haemolytic uraemic syndrome** is seen mainly in children — both produce outbreaks and sporadic infections; death may be the outcome in either. The agent is *E. coli* (mainly of the serotype O157) which produces **cytotoxins** VT1 and VT2 (demonstrated in the laboratory by their cytopathic effect on cultured monkey kidney cells called Vero cells); due to their verotoxigenicity these *E. coli* strains are known as **VTEC** (Ch. 15). These toxins are also called Shiga-like toxins. The main source of infection is beef.

Staphylococcus aureus

Staphylococcus aureus is a common cause of diarrhoea due to food poisoning. Symptoms ensue very quickly after the food intake, as the *S. aureus* enterotoxin is preformed in food.

Pathogenesis and epidemiology

The *S. aureus* enterotoxin has a local action on the gut mucosa, with resultant nausea and vomiting (and occasional diarrhoea) within a few hours after the food intake. Cooked food which is not stored at 4°C or frozen immediately but left at room temperature is the usual source of infection. The organism reaches the food from a staphylococcal lesion on the skin of a food handler and, if left at ambient or warm temperatures, may multiply in food and liberate the enterotoxin. The toxin is relatively heat-resistant; on heating contaminated food the *S. aureus* cells usually die, leaving the active toxin in the food which is ingested. Milk or milk products such as cream or custard may also act as sources of toxin.

Diagnosis

Diagnosis is by culture of faecal specimens, suspected food or vomitus (Ch. 11).

Treatment

The disease is self-limiting, hence no treatment is required.

Prevention

Prevention is by good food hygiene; quick refrigeration or freezing of leftover food; and exclusion of food handlers with septic lesions.

Clostridium perfringens

Clostridium perfringens, responsible for gas gangrene (see Ch. 13), also causes food poisoning.

Pathogenesis and epidemiology

Heat-resistant spores of *C. perfringens* survive in contaminated food during the heating procedure, and subsequently multiply in deep relatively anaerobic parts of the food (e.g. in meat pies). After the food is ingested, **sporulation** (spore formation) occurs in the gastrointestinal tract, and an enterotoxin is produced which alters the membrane permeability of the small intestine, causing diarrhoea.

Diagnosis

Diagnostic procedures are not usually performed. However, isolation of the same serotype of *C. perfringens* from the victim and the food is indicative of the disease source.

Treatment

Treatment is symptomatic; no antibiotics are necessary.

Prevention

Good food hygiene, including adequate cooking of food to kill the organisms, is required.

Cholera

Though rare in the West, cholera is a relatively common disease in some parts of the world especially in South-East Asia (e.g. Bangladesh). It is caused mainly by *Vibrio cholerae* O1.

Pathogenesis and epidemiology

Vibrio cholerae infects only humans and is transmitted via the faecal–oral route. Contaminated food and water are the main reservoirs of infection. Human carriers are frequently asymptomatic and may be incubating or convalescing from the disease. Once ingested, the organism colonizes the small intestine and secretes a protein exotoxin (an enterotoxin).

A large number of cholera vibrios (about 1 billion) need to be ingested for them to survive the acids of the stomach. They then adhere to the brush border of the intestine (by secreting a mucinase which dissolves the protective glycoprotein of the intestinal cells), multiply and secrete the enterotoxin (**choleragen**). The toxin stimulates the activity of the enzyme, adenyl cyclase, of the intestinal cells and increases the flow of water and electrolytes into the bowel lumen, leading to a massive, watery diarrhoea without inflammatory cells. Morbidity and death are due to dehydration and electrolyte imbalance. If fluid balance is adjusted promptly, the diarrhoea is self-limiting in about 7 days.

Clinical features

The hallmark of cholera is non-bloody, frothy and colourless diarrhoea: '**rice-water stools**'. The incubation period varies from 6 hours to 5 days. There is no abdominal pain, and symptoms are mainly due to dehydration, which also brings about cardiac and renal failure. The mortality rate is about 40% without treatment.

Diagnosis

Diagnosis is by culture of faeces on selective media, e.g. thiosulphate–citrate–bile salts (TCBS) agar.

Treatment

Prompt, adequate replacement of water and electrolytes (oral or intravenous). Tetracycline, although not essential, reduces the duration of symptoms and carriage of organisms in the faeces.

Prevention

Clean water supply, adequate sewage disposal and good personal hygiene are all important. A vaccine, made of killed organisms, is of limited use and does not interrupt transmission.

LESS COMMON AND UNCOMMON DIARRHOEAL DISEASES

Clostridium difficile

The agent of **antibiotic-associated pseudomembranous colitis**, a mild and self-limiting disease. Rarely, life-threatening fulminant infection may set in.

Pathogenesis and epidemiology

The organism is a normal commensal of the gut in some 3% of the population. Antibiotics (especially clindamycin, cephalosporins and less frequently ampicillin) suppress drug-sensitive normal flora, allowing *Clostridium difficile* to multiply and produce two toxins: an **enterotoxin** and a **cytotoxin**. These initiate the diarrhoea and the resultant **pseudomembranes** (yellow-white plaques) on the colon visualized by sigmoidoscopy.

Outbreaks are commonly reported in long-stay wards and hospitals.

Diagnosis

Clinical diagnosis is by proctosigmoidoscopy to detect the pseudomembranes. The toxin in stool samples can be detected by its toxic effect on cultured cells.

Treatment

Withdraw the offending antibiotic and replace fluids. Oral vancomycin, which is active against anaerobes, should be given.

Prevention

No specific preventive measure, but **prescribe antibiotics only when necessary**.

Bacillus cereus

Bacillus cereus is an aerobic, spore-forming Gram-positive bacillus commonly found in soil, air and dust.

Pathogenesis and epidemiology

The organisms can contaminate rice and soups, or survive cooking by **sporulation**. When the food is stored at room temperature, reheated or fried quickly, the spores germinate into vegetative forms, multiply and liberate **an enterotoxin**. The latter, when ingested with contaminated food, causes diarrhoea either within 1–2 hours (short incubation) or within 6–18 hours (long incubation). The disease is commonly associated with Chinese restaurants because of their bulk use of rice.

Diagnosis

Laboratory diagnosis is not usually done.

Treatment

Symptomatic treatment only is required, as the disease is self-limiting.

Prevention

Prevention is by adequate food hygiene and correct storage of food.

Enteric fever

The term 'enteric fever' is given to **typhoid** and **paratyphoid** infections caused by *Salmonella typhi* and *S. paratyphi-A*, *-B* and *-C*, respectively; *S. paratyphi-A* and *-C* are common

in the tropics while the type *B* is common in Europe. Both diseases are due to salmonellae that are significantly more virulent and hence invasive than those responsible for food poisoning.

Clinical features

Typhoid fever. The onset of typhoid fever is slow with fever and constipation (compare diarrhoea and vomiting of *S. enteritidis*). After the first week (following the 2–3 week incubation period), the bacteria enter the bloodstream (i.e. bacteraemia), with resultant high fever, delirium and tender abdomen with '**rose spots**' (rose-coloured papules on the abdomen). The disease begins to resolve by the third week, but severe complications such as intestinal haemorrhage or perforations may occur if the disease is not promptly treated. About 3% of typhoid patients become chronic carriers of the organism, a favourite reservoir of which is the gall bladder.

Paratyphoid fever. Paratyphoid fever is a milder febrile illness than typhoid fever. It is of short duration with transient diarrhoea or symptomless infection.

Pathogenesis and epidemiology

In typhoid fever the organism takes a complicated route inside the body after entering the alimentary tract (Fig. 26.2). The pathogenicity of salmonellae appears to depend both on their ability to survive and grow inside macrophages and on the potency of their endotoxin (O antigen of the lipopolysaccharide). Further, the typhoid bacilli possess a glycolipid, the virulence (Vi) antigen, that protects the organism from phagocytosis.

The reservoir of infection is the human gut, during both the **acute** and the **carrier** phases of the infection (which may last up to 2 months after the acute illness). Spread occurs via water, food or the faecal–oral route. Small numbers of *S. typhi* can cause typhoid fever, whereas large doses of *S. paratyphi* are required to initiate paratyphoid fever.

Diagnosis

Diagnosis is by isolation of the organisms from blood (first week of disease), stools and urine (second and third weeks) in selective media such as MacConkey's agar, DCA or bismuth sulphite agar or in fluid enrichment media. Identification is by biochemical tests (e.g. API test) and **serology** (screening for H and O antigens by appropriate antisera). Further typing with bacteriophages (**phage typing**) can be performed.

Widal test. When *S. typhi* cannot be isolated, the diagnosis can be made serologically by demonstrating a rise in antibody titre in the patient's serum. This classic test, called the Widal test, consists of demonstrating antibodies to flagellar H antigen (using formalized bacteria) and somatic O antigen (using boiled bacteria) of *S. typhi* and *S. paratyphi-A* and *-B*. Interpretation of the test is difficult if the patient has been immunized with typhoid vaccine.

Treatment

Chloramphenicol, co-trimoxazole and ciprofloxacin are useful drugs, both in the treatment of acute typhoid fever and of the carrier state.

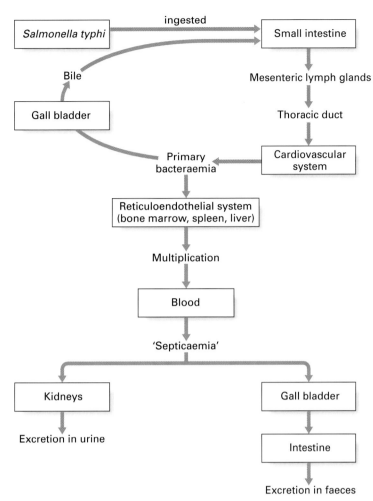

Fig. 26.2 Pathogenesis of typhoid fever.

Prevention

Good personal hygiene and public health measures, i.e. safe water supplies, adequate sewage disposal and supervision of food processing and handling, are of great importance. Carriers of the organism should not be employed in the food industry. Immunization is useful. Two types of vaccine are available for travellers to — or those living in — endemic areas:
- heat-killed *S. typhi*, given as two doses (4–6 weeks apart), subcutaneously
- live attenuated *S. typhi* (Ty 21a) given orally, in three doses, on alternate days.

NON-BACTERIAL CAUSES OF DIARRHOEA

The foregoing lists the major causes of bacterial diarrhoea. It is important to realise that there are a number of **viral** and **protozoal** agents that may cause diarrhoea. These major non-bacterial causes of diarrhoea are briefly outlined below (and see Table 26.1).

Infantile gastroenteritis due to rotavirus

Apart from *E. coli* diarrhoea in children, the major cause of infantile gastroenteritis is rotavirus infection. This infec-

tion, seen mainly in older children and sometimes in adults, may be accompanied by respiratory illness. Laboratory diagnosis is by electron microscopy of stools for viral particles or enzyme-linked immunosorbent assay (ELISA) for antigen in stools.

Protozoal diarrhoeal diseases

Amoebiasis (amoebic dysentery)

Caused by *Entamoeba histolytica*, the symptoms of amoebic dysentery vary from fulminating colitis to absence of symptoms. The disease is common in the tropics and is usually acquired via food contaminated by the cysts of the organism.

The drug of choice is metronidazole.

Giardiasis

Infection with *Giardia lamblia*, a flagellate protozoan with a pear-shaped body, gives rise to symptoms of abdominal discomfort, flatulence and diarrhoea; malabsorption and steatorrhoea may develop in chronic infection. Both children and adults are affected, and it is a common bowel pathogen in countries throughout the world.

The drug of choice is metronidazole.

KEY FACTS

- The usual method of spread of gastrointestinal pathogens is the faecal–oral route
- The common bacterial causes of diarrhoea are *Campylobacter* spp., *Shigella* spp., *Salmonella* spp., *Escherichia coli*, *Staphylococcus aureus*, *Clostridium perfringens* and *Vibrio cholerae*
- These organisms may **invade** the gut causing systemic disease (e.g. typhoid) or proliferate to produce locally acting toxins that **focally damage** the gastrointestinal tract (e.g. cholera)
- The genus *Shigella* contains four species: *S. dysenteriae*, *S. flexneri*, *S. boydii* and *S. sonnei*
- A large number of different *Salmonella* species exist (together with about 1500 serotypes), of which about 14 are important pathogens. The common **diarrhoeogenic** organism is *S. typhimurium*

- The term 'enteric fever' is given to **typhoid** and **paratyphoid** infections caused by *Salmonella typhi* and *S. paratyphi-A*, *-B* and *-C*, respectively
- *Escherichia coli* is a normal commensal of the gastrointestinal tract but certain strains cause infantile gastroenteritis and traveller's diarrhoea
- Distinct groups within the *E. coli* species such as EPEC and ETEC exhibit different pathogenic mechanisms — some are invasive, others toxigenic
- Cholera, a relatively common disease especially in South-East Asia, is caused mainly by *Vibrio cholerae* O1
- *The hallmark of cholera is non-bloody, frothy and colourless diarrhoea ('rice-water stools'); morbidity and death are due to dehydration and electrolyte imbalance*

FURTHER READING

Mims, C, Playfair, J, Roitt, I, Wakelin, D, and Williams, R (1998). Gastrointestinal tract infections. In *Medical microbiology* (2nd edn), Ch. 20. Mosby, London.

Shanson, DC (1999). Infections of the gastro-intestinal tract. In *Microbiology in clinical practice* (3rd edn), Ch. 15. Butterworth-Heinemann, Oxford.

27 Infections of the genitourinary tract

NORMAL FLORA AND THE NATURAL DEFENCES OF THE GENITOURINARY TRACT

The predominant vaginal flora in adult women consists of lactobacilli. They keep the vaginal pH low and appear to prevent the growth of potential pathogens. For instance, their suppression by antibiotics may lead to overgrowth of the yeast *Candida albicans* found in relatively low numbers in the healthy vagina. Other common groups of vaginal organisms include diphtheroids, streptococci, anaerobes and coliforms. Most of these organisms may behave as opportunistic pathogens when appropriate conditions supervene. Approximately 20% of women of childbearing age carry group B β-haemolytic streptococci in the vagina. These may be acquired by a baby during its passage through the birth canal, resulting in serious infections such as meningitis and sepsis.

The urine in the bladder is normally sterile, but the voided urine often becomes contaminated by flora from the distal portions of the urethra, such as *Staphylococcus epidermidis*, coliforms, diphtheroids and streptococci. Additionally, in females, the organisms present in the distal part of the urethra may include contaminants from the gut flora such as enterobacteria and lactobacilli. The flushing action of the urine is arguably the most important defence factor of the urethra in both males and females. Bactericidal mechanisms in the bladder mucosa, including local antibody response and lysozyme, play an important role in preventing ascending infection of the urinary tract.

Important pathogens

Important pathogens are listed in Figure 27.1 and Table 27.1.

SEXUALLY TRANSMITTED DISEASES

A large group of infections are essentially transmitted by sexual intercourse; they may affect both heterosexual and homosexual partners. Varying patterns of sexual behaviour can result in such infections manifesting in the oral cavity, oropharynx and the rectum; sexually transmitted diseases frequently — but not invariably — produce genital lesions; several produce severe systemic disease that may even lead to death, such as human immunodeficiency virus (HIV) infection and hepatitis B.

Gonorrhoea

Gonorrhoea is caused by *Neisseria gonorrhoeae* (the gonococcus).

Clinical features

In women: acute **urethritis**, increased vaginal secretions with purulent discharge. In men: acute gonococcal urethritis with severe **dysuria** and purulent discharge. The disease may involve the **rectum** and **oropharynx**. Pharyngitis, sore throat, tonsillitis and gingivitis may occur as a result of gonococcal infection, especially from orogenital contact in homosexual men. **Asymptomatic infection** is common in both men and women. Complications include prostatitis, salpingitis and occasionally haematogenous spread, causing arthritis, septicaemia and meningitis.

Pathogenesis and epidemiology

Gonococcal infection has been reported only in humans. The infection is limited to the mucosa of the anterior urethra in men and the cervix of women. In the newborn, **gonococcal conjunctivitis** may occur due to cross-infection from the mother's birth canal.

Three virulence factors have been identified:

- an **endotoxin** which inhibits the ciliary activity of the fallopian tubes and retards the expulsion of the gonococcus
- an **enzyme** which destroys the protective immunoglobulins (secretory IgA) of the mucosa
- **β-lactamase** is produced by some strains — penicillinase-producing *N. gonorrhoeae* (PPNG).

Diagnosis

Gram smears show Gram-negative pairs of the typical kidney-shaped gonococci inside neutrophils (Fig. 27.2). **Swabs** from the urethra cultured on lysed blood or chocolate agar yield oxidase-positive, translucent colonies; and rapid carbohydrate utilization tests are also diagnostic (see Ch. 14).

Treatment

A choice of antibiotics is available: a large, single, curative oral dose of amoxicillin (with probenecid to delay renal excretion); ceftriaxone; spectinomycin (for β-lactamase-positive gonococci); or erythromycin (children or pregnant women).

177

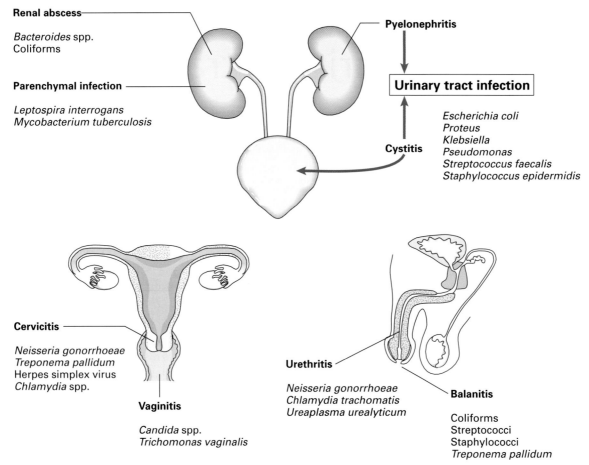

Fig 27.1 Major infectious agents of the genitourinary tract.

Non-specific urethritis

One of the most common sexually transmitted diseases, non-specific urethritis is seen more in men than in women. It is caused by more than one agent, but *Chlamydia trachomatis* is the most common cause. A mycoplasmal organism ('bacteria' without a cell wall), *Ureaplasma urealyticum*, may also cause significant morbidity.

Clinical features

Acute purulent urethral discharge resembles that of gonorrhoea; cervicitis occurs in women.

Diagnosis

Smears and swabs of urethral or cervical discharge are diagnostic. Culture is now rarely done. Smears are examined for

Table 27.1 Sexually transmitted diseases

Disease	Agent
Bacterial infections	
Gonorrhoea	*Neisseria gonorrhoeae* (the gonococcus)
Syphilis	*Treponema pallidum*
Vaginitis	*Gardnerella vaginalis*, anaerobes
Chancroid	*Haemophilus ducreyi*
Viral infections	
Genital herpes	Herpes simplex virus (type 2 mainly)
Genital warts	Papillomavirus
Hepatitis B[a]	Hepatitis B virus
AIDS[a]	Human immunodeficiency virus (HIV)
Others	
Lymphogranuloma venereum	*Chlamydia trachomatis* types L_1–L_3
Granuloma inguinale (donovanosis)	*Calymmatobacterium granulomatis* (a *Klebsiella*-like microorganism)
Pubic lice (crabs)	*Phthirus pubis*
Genital scabies	*Sarcoptes scabiei*
Non-specific urethritis	*Chlamydia trachomatis* types D to K
Trichomoniasis	*Trichomonas vaginalis*
Vaginal thrush	*Candida albicans*

[a] Not always sexually transmitted.

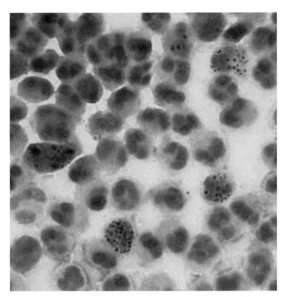

Fig. 27.2 Smear of a urethral pus exudate in gonorrhoea showing polymorphs and intracellular Gram-negative gonococci.

intracytoplasmic inclusions by immunofluorescence. Serology for chlamydial antigens by indirect immunofluorescence with monoclonal antibody or by enzyme-linked immunosorbent assay (ELISA).

Treatment

Tetracycline is given for up to 10 days; relapses are common owing to the diverse aetiology of the disease.

Syphilis

One of the classic diseases with **protean manifestations** (i.e. affecting virtually all organ systems of the body), syphilis is not uncommon, especially in some developing countries where commercial sex is practised widely. The disease, important due to its late and severe sequelae, is also associated with concomitant HIV infection.

Aetiology

The disease is caused by *Treponema pallidum*, the syphilis spirochaete.

Clinical features

Syphilis has an incubation period of 10–90 days (average 3 weeks) and is characterized by four main clinical stages: primary, secondary, tertiary, and late or quaternary (Fig. 27.3).

Primary syphilis. A painless red papule develops at the inoculation site of the spirochaete, some 3 weeks after the contact; this may be in the labia, vagina, cervix, penis or the oral mucosa. The papule then produces the **chancre** of primary syphilis: a flat, red, indurated, **highly infectious** ulcer with a serous exudate. Inguinal lymph nodes are enlarged. The chancre disappears spontaneously within 3–8 weeks.

Secondary syphilis. This stage is reached 6–8 weeks later and lasts for 1–3 months. A generalized mucocutaneous spread of the spirochaetes ensues at this stage and the lesions appear as papules on the skin and **oral ulcers** (see Ch. 35). The ulcers may coalesce to give the characteristic 'snail tracks' in about a third of those affected. **These lesions**, like the primary chancre, **are highly infectious**. Other manifestations are generalized lymphadenopathy and **condylomata** (warts) of the anus and vulva; rarely periostitis, arthritis and glomerulonephritis may be seen.

Tertiary syphilis. The most destructive phase of the disease occurs 3–10 years after primary syphilis. Lesions appear as characteristic **gummata** or granulomatous nodules of the skin, mucosa, bone and other internal organs. Gummata commonly break down to produce shallow, punched-out ulcers. In the oral cavity gumma may rarely break down to produce palatal perforations, leading to **oronasal fistulae**. **These lesions are not infective** as the tissue damage is due to a delayed type of hypersensitivity reaction.

Late or quaternary syphilis. Occurs 10–20 years after primary syphilis. The two main clinical forms of late syphilis

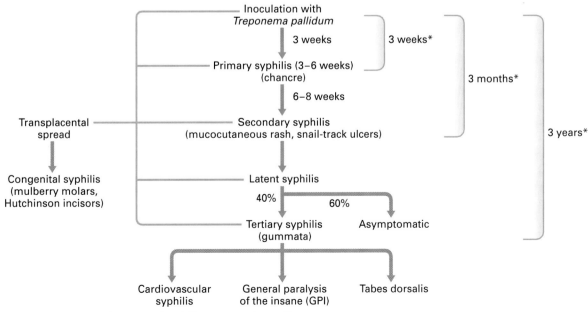

Fig. 27.3 Natural history of untreated syphilis. * Approximate figures.

are **cardiovascular syphilis** and **neurosyphilis**, with resultant pathology of the aorta and the nervous system, respectively.

Latent syphilis. This may be seen in some after many years without any symptoms. The disease lies dormant without any clinical signs (except for positive serology) and may manifest as cardiovascular or neurosyphilis.

Congenital syphilis. Treponema pallidum is one of the few microorganisms that has the ability to cross the placental barrier; thus the fetus may be infected during the second or third trimester from a syphilitic mother (either in the primary or secondary stage of syphilis). The disease will manifest in the infant as:

- **latent infection** — no symptoms but positive serology
- **early infection** — lesions such as skin rashes, saddle nose, bone lesions and meningitis appear up to the end of the second year of age
- **late infection** — after the second year of age: lesions include **Hutchinson's incisors** (notching of incisor teeth), **mulberry molar teeth** (due to infection of the enamel organ in the fetus), interstitial keratitis, bone sclerosis, arthritis, deafness.

Diagnosis

Direct microscopy. Spirochaetes in exudate from primary or secondary lesions are identified by dark-ground microscopy; now rarely done. Care should be taken to differentiate *T. pallidum* from oral spirochaetes when oral lesions are examined. *Note: T. pallidum* cannot be grown in laboratory media, but can be propagated in the testes of rabbits.

Serology. Antigens used for syphilis serology are of two types:

- **Cardiolipin or lipoidal antigen**: although not derived from the spirochaete it is sensitive for detecting antibody. The most popular test which uses this antibody is the **VDRL** (Venereal Diseases Reference Laboratory) test; it is simple and sensitive, but biological false-positive reactions are common. As the antibody disappears after treatment it can be used to monitor the efficacy of antimicrobial therapy (Table 27.2).
- **Specific treponemal antigen**: using *T. pallidum* as antigen gives fewer false-positive reactions and tests remain positive after treatment. The tests are *T. pallidum* haemagglutination test (**TPHA**), fluorescent treponemal antibody-absorption test (**FTA-Abs**), which detects both IgM and IgG antibody, and **ELISA**. The last is increasingly used as a screening test to detect IgG antibody, although some false positives may result.

The interpretation of syphilis serology is complex (because of the many medical conditions which yield false-positive reactions) and is not discussed here.

Treatment

Penicillin (large doses, for up to 3 weeks) is the drug of choice. Erythromycin or tetracycline can be used if the patient is hypersensitive.

Table 27.2 Serological tests for syphilis

Stage of disease	VDRL	TPHA	FTA-Abs
Primary	+ or −	−	+
Late primary	+	+ or −	+
Secondary and tertiary	+	+	+
Late (quaternary)	+	+	+
Latent	+ or −	+	+
Treated syphilis	−	+	+
Congenital syphilis	+	+	+

VDRL, Veneral Diseases Reference Laboratory; TPHA, *Treponema pallidum* haemagglutination; FTA-Abs, fluorescent treponemal antibody-absorpton.
Note: The efficacy of treatment can be monitored by the VDRL test.

Notes on some common sexually transmitted diseases

HIV infection

This is a pandemic infection commonly transmitted by sexual intercourse, and is also a disease of enormous importance for health-care personnel (see Ch. 30).

Trichomoniasis

A common protozoal infection in women is caused by *Trichomonas vaginalis*. It is transmitted mainly by sexual intercourse: in men the infection is often symptomless; in women it manifests as a chronic vaginal infection ranging from a yellow, offensive discharge with vaginitis to symptomless or low-grade infection.

- **diagnosis** is by culture of swabs in special media or examination of direct smear for motile, flagellated protozoa
- **treatment**: metronidazole.

Candidiasis

Candidiasis is a yeast infection commonly transmitted by sexual intercourse; it is frequently seen in women but rare in men. *Candida albicans* is the most frequent causative yeast; the disease is characterized by white false membranes in the vulva and the vagina, which may be accompanied by a watery discharge; many cases are symptomless.

Diagnosis and treatment are as described in Chapter 22.

Herpes genitalis

Mainly due to herpes simplex type 2 virus, but as a result of sexual promiscuity type 1 viruses (which are more or less confined to oral regions) are frequently implicated. The lesions are vesicular and painful, and seen in anogenital regions. The primary lesion, associated with fever and inguinal lymphadenopathy, is more protracted and painful than the secondary recurrences. Asymptomatic infection is common in both men and women, hence sexual spread of the disease is common.

Diagnosis and treatment are as described in Chapter 21.

Hepatitis B

See Chapter 29.

Control of sexually transmitted diseases

Although control is difficult, **tracing of sexual partners** of infected individuals is essential to prevent spread of disease in the community. Patients are requested to name consorts and the latter should submit themselves to examination and treatment. In the long term, prevention of sexually transmitted diseases, including HIV infection, is far more important in reducing health-care costs of the community.

URINARY TRACT INFECTIONS

Urinary tract infections are common, especially in women, despite the availability of a spectrum of antibiotics. They are defined as follows:

- **bacteriuria**: multiplication of bacteria in urine within the renal tract (more than 10^5 organisms per millilitre of urine is considered to be significant bacteriuria, i.e. evidence of urinary tract infection)
- **pyuria**: presence of pus cells (polymorphs) in urine
- **cystitis**: infection of the bladder
- **pyelonephritis**: infection of the pelvis and parenchyma of the kidney
- **urethritis**: infection of the urethra.

Cystitis, pyelonephritis or urethritis may occur either singly or in combination.

Important pathogens

Causative agents are many and varied (see Fig. 27.1) but *Escherichia coli* is the most common, accounting for 60–80% of infections. Some *E. coli* strains are more invasive than others, possibly as a result of the possession of capsular or K antigens which inhibit phagocytosis, and their superior ability to adhere to the uroepithelium with the aid of the pili on cell surfaces.

Other organisms that commonly cause infection include:

- *Staphylococcus saprophyticus*: commonly seen in sexually active women under 25 years of age
- *Proteus mirabilis*: causes about 10% of the infections
- *Klebsiella* spp.: resistant to a number of antibiotics (multiply antibiotic-resistant)
- *Staphylococcus aureus* and *Pseudomonas aeruginosa*: seen after instrumentation or catheterization.

Note: **acute** urinary tract infection is mostly **monomicrobial** in origin, while **polymicrobial** infection with more than one organism is common in **chronic** infections.

Clinical features

Urinary tract infection is mainly a disease of women, with a male to female ratio of 1:10. Clinical features of cystitis include dysuria, urgency, suprapubic pain, increased frequency and haematuria. Fever, loin pain and tenderness are signs of pyelonephritis.

Laboratory diagnosis

- **Microscopy**: wet films and Gram-stained films used for detection of red blood cells, polymorphs, bacteria and epithelial cells.
- **Culture**: usually on nutrient agar and MacConkey's agar. As the number of organisms in the sample indicates the degree of infection, this can be assessed semiquantitatively by appropriate plating out.

Treatment

An array of oral antibiotics excreted in urine in high concentrations is available, including trimethoprim, co-trimoxazole, ciprofloxacin and nitrofurantoin. Therapy depends on the aetiological agent and its antibiotic sensitivity pattern.

DENTISTRY AND GENITOURINARY INFECTIONS

It is important that the dentist is aware of sexually transmitted diseases as many of them manifest in the oral cavity as a result of deviant sexual habits and the escalating sex industry in both developed and developing countries. Indeed, some would consider the oral cavity as a sexual organ. Furthermore, organisms that may cause sexually transmitted diseases (e.g. herpes, HIV infection) may have the propensity to be transmitted in the dental clinic environment, from the patient to the dentist, by direct contact or indirectly via contaminated instruments if appropriate infection control measures are not implemented.

Urinary tract infections are of no direct relevance to dentistry except insofar as patients are taking antibiotics, which may either affect the oral flora or, rarely, interact with drugs prescribed by the dentist. Indeed, the potential of metronidazole to kill anaerobic bacteria was first detected by an astute dentist who noted the resolution of acute ulcerative gingivitis in a patient under his care who was undergoing treatment for vaginal trichomonal infection with this drug (at that time prescribed solely as an antiprotozoal agent).

KEY FACTS

- The **predominant vaginal flora** in adult women comprises lactobacilli; other microorganisms are diphtheroids, streptococci, anaerobes and coliforms
- The urine in the bladder is normally sterile, but the voided urine often becomes contaminated with flora on the distal portions of the urethra

- The **flushing action** of the urine is the most **important defence factor** of the urethra in both males and females
- A large group of infections are transmitted by sexual intercourse (both heterosexual and homosexual) and varying patterns of sexual behaviour can result in infections manifesting in the oral cavity, oropharynx and the rectum

KEY FACTS *(continued)*

- **Gonorrhoea**, caused by *Neisseria gonorrhoeae* (the gonococcus), causes acute urethritis with purulent discharge

- *Gonorrhoea may involve the rectum and oropharynx with resultant pharyngitis, sore throat, tonsillitis and gingivitis (especially from orogenital contact)*

- Virulence factors of *Neisseria gonorrhoeae* include an endotoxin, a protease that destroys secretory IgA, and β-lactamase production in some (PPNG)

- **Syphilis** caused by *Treponema pallidum* (syphilis spirochaete) is a classic disease with **protean manifestations** and is characterized by four main clinical stages

- *In primary syphilis, chancre (a flat, red, indurated, highly infectious ulcer with a serous exudate) seen both on the oral and vaginal mucosae is the hallmark feature*

- *Secondary syphilis is characterized by a generalized mucocutaneous spread of spirochaetes and lesions that appear as*

papules on the skin, and infectious oral ulcers (snail-track ulcers)

- *In tertiary syphilis non-infective lesions appear as characteristic gummata or granulomatous nodules of the skin, mucosa, bone and other internal organs. Intraorally, gummata may break down to produce palatal perforations, leading to oronasal fistulae*

- The two main clinical forms of **late or quaternary syphilis** are cardiovascular syphilis and neurosyphilis

- *Dental lesions in congenital syphilis include Hutchinson's incisors (notching of incisor teeth) and mulberry molar teeth (due to infection of the enamel organ in the fetus)*

- **Syphilis** is mainly **diagnosed by serology** with either the specific treponemal antigen or with cardiolipin or lipoidal antigens

- Causative agents of **urinary tract infection** are many but *Escherichia coli* **is the most** common, accounting for 60–80% of infections

FURTHER READING

Greenwood, D, Slack, R, and Peutherer, J (eds) (1997). *Medical microbiology* (14th edn). Churchill Livingstone, Edinburgh.

Mims, C, Playfair, J, Roitt, I, Wakelin, D, and Williams, R (1998). Urinary tract infections; Sexually transmitted diseases. In *Medical microbiology* (2nd edn), Chs 18, 19. Mosby, London.

Shanson, DC (1999). Infections of the urinary tract; sexually transmitted diseases. In *Microbiology in clinical practice* (3rd edn), Ch. 20. Butterworth-Heinemann, Oxford.

Siegel, MA (1996). Syphilis and gonorrhea. *Dental Clinics of North America* 40, 369–383.

28 Skin and wound infections

NORMAL FLORA

The skin has a thriving microbial community; there are about 10^3–10^4 organisms per square centimetre of skin. These bacteria may be:

- normal or resident flora — a stable population of organisms in terms of numbers and composition
- transient flora — essentially 'in transit' but may multiply for a short period; are eliminated quickly because of competition from the normal flora.

The main resident flora of the skin includes staphylococci — principally *Staphylococcus epidermidis* (asymptomatic carriage of *S. aureus* is common in specific niches such as the anterior nares and axillae, and in hospital personnel), propionibacteria, micrococci and diphtheroids. Most of them are located superficially in the stratum corneum but some are found in the hair follicles and act as a reservoir, replenishing the superficial flora after hand-washing. The composition of the normal flora in areas of the body such as the scalp, axillae and pubic area differs considerably because of ecological differences such as the pH, temperature and nutrients (e.g. sebum, fatty acids, urea).

Continuous desquamation of the stratum corneum and the impervious nature of the epithelium are major barriers for invading organisms. Other antimicrobial defences include **lysozyme** (in sweat, sebum and tears), **bacteriocins** produced by commensals, and **fatty acids** produced from hydrolysis of sebum triglycerides.

SKIN INFECTIONS

The major forms of skin infections and the agents involved are shown in Table 28.1.

Bacterial skin infections

Staphylococcal infections

Boils, styes, carbuncles, sycosis barbae and angular cheilitis are all caused by *staphylococci*. A **boil** is a common, circumscribed infection of the hair follicle with central suppuration; pus eventually discharges and the boil heals, leaving no scar. **Carbuncles**, now rare, are large abscesses, which occur at the back of the neck, especially in people with diabetes. They are associated with constitutional upset and malaise. **Sycosis barbae**

is a staphylococcal skin infection involving the shaving area of the face.

Streptococcal infections

In contrast to staphylococcal infections, which generally remain localized, streptococcal infections of the skin tend to spread subcutaneously, and may lead to the following conditions.

Cellulitis. *Streptococcus pyogenes* group A is the most common offender, although *Staphylococcus aureus* may be involved in some. Cellulitis is a serious disease as subcutaneous spread of infection may carry the pathogen to lymphatic and blood vessels, resulting in marked constitutional upset and septicaemia.

Erysipelas. A distinctive type of cellulitis caused by *Streptococcus pyogenes* is usually seen in the elderly. Lesions are typically on the face and limbs; the lesion distribution on the face is often butterfly-like with a characteristic 'orange-peel' texture of skin and induration; the patient may be acutely ill with high fever and toxaemia.

Impetigo. A disease of young children: vesicles appear on the skin around the mouth and later become purulent, with characteristic honey-coloured crusts; both *Streptococcus pyogenes* and *Staphylococcus aureus* are involved.

Necrotizing fasciitis

Necrotizing fasciitis is a rapidly progressing infection involving the full thickness of the skin down to the fascial planes, causing extensive necrosis and tissue loss. The skin looks initially normal, but the infection spreads surreptitiously along the fascial planes, destroying the blood supply to the skin, which discolours and becomes necrotic within hours (hence the tabloid term 'flesh-eating bacteria'). The patient is severely ill with toxaemia and shock, and may die within 24 hours. Formerly called 'streptococcal gangrene', it can be caused by a mixed flora comprising staphylococci, strict anaerobes and Enterobacteriaceae; the major offending organism is *Streptococcus pyogenes*. Management entails excision of skin, antibiotics and supportive therapy.

Angular cheilitis (syn. Angular stomatitis)

Inflammation of one or both angles of the mouth, especially in denture-wearing elderly people, may be related to 183

Table 28.1 Agents of some important skin infections[a]

Aetiological agent	Skin infection
Bacteria	
Staphylococcus aureus	Abscesses (boils), impetigo, pustules, carbuncles, toxic epidermal necrolysis (Ritter's disease), omphalitis, angular cheilitis, sycosis barbae
Beta-haemolytic streptococci	Cellulitis, impetigo, erysipelas
Propionibacterium acnes	Acne
Mycobacterium tuberculosis	Lupus vulgaris
Mycobacterium ulcerans	Swimming pool granuloma
Mycobacterium leprae	Leprosy
Actinomyces israelii	Actinomycosis (cervicofacial)
Treponema pallidum	Syphilis
Haemophilus ducreyi	Chancroid
Viruses	
Herpes simplex virus	Cold sore, herpetic whitlow
Varicella–zoster virus	Chickenpox, shingles
Papovaviruses	Papillomas, warts
Coxsackievirus A	Hand, foot and mouth disease
Fungi	
Candida spp.	Chronic mucocutaneous candidiasis
	Angular cheilitis
Various dermatophytes	Ringworm, etc.

[a] Infections caused by protozoa and insects are not given.

Staphylococcus aureus and/or *Candida* infection. However, many other predisposing factors are involved and the dentist should be aware of the management of this condition (see Ch. 35).

Acne

Caused by *Propionibacterium acnes*, acne is a common and disfiguring facial infection of adolescents. The disease is a disorder of the pilosebaceous system and is believed to occur as a result of the production of fatty acids and lipases by bacteria, which initiates an inflammatory response and blocks the ducts which drain the sebum from the gland to the skin surface. Hormonal imbalances also play a role. Long-term, low-dose antibiotic therapy may alleviate acne in chronic cases.

Leprosy

Caused by *Mycobacterium leprae*. The organism lives in human skin and nerves and is transmitted by prolonged contact to cause a chronic granulomatous disease. There are two types: the **lepromatous** and the **tuberculoid** forms (see Ch. 19).

Gram-negative infections

Gram-negative infections, less frequent than Gram-positive infections, are mostly associated with the moist areas of the skin such as the groin, axillae and perineum. Organisms involved include *Pseudomonas aeruginosa* and *Bacteroides* spp.

Diagnosis of bacterial skin infections

Swabs and smears of pus and exudate from the lesions are adequate; Gram-stained smears will generally indicate whether staphylococci or streptococci are involved. Swabs inoculated on blood agar (both aerobically and anaerobically) demonstrate the nature of haemolysis produced by streptococci (α-, β- or no haemolysis); subsequent confirmation of

the identity of isolates is by appropriate tests (e.g. coagulase test, API tests).

Viral skin infections

Herpes simplex viruses (human herpesviruses 1 and 2) cause recurrent **cold sores** and **genital lesions**; **herpetic whitlow** may be an occupational disease of dentists and nursing staff. Varicella–zoster virus (HHV-3) may cause **chickenpox** (primary lesion) and **shingles** of the skin (either in the facial dermatomes or others). Human herpesvirus 6 and human parvovirus B19 cause **exanthem subitum** and the 'slapped cheek' syndrome, respectively; both are innocuous self-limiting diseases which causes facial rash and redness, mainly in children (see Ch. 21). Papovaviruses cause the common **wart**, and coxsackievirus A16 infection may result in **hand, foot and mouth disease** (Table 28.1).

Note that many infectious diseases such as rubella, chickenpox, measles and glandular fever manifest as macules (spots) or papules (pimples) on the skin.

Diagnosis of viral skin infections

Diagnostic methods include serology for antibody studies; swab or vesicular fluid for tissue culture; and electron microscopy (see Ch. 6).

Fungal skin infections

Fungal skin infections are mainly caused by dermatophytes and the yeast *Candida*. As their name implies, dermatophytes (which include *Microsporum*, *Epidermophyton* and *Trichophyton*) live in keratinized tissues, especially hair, nails and the skin squames. *Candida* species are common opportunist pathogens which may cause both skin and mucosal infections (see Ch. 35).

WOUND INFECTIONS

Surgical wound infection

Surgical wound infection accounts for approximately a quarter of hospital-acquired (**nosocomial**) infections. It is a significant cause of morbidity, prolonging the hospital stay of surgical patients, and frequently results in death.

Aetiology

Staphylococcus aureus and *Escherichia coli* are the major pathogens, but other coliforms such as *Pseudomonas aeruginosa* and *Klebsiella* spp. may be involved. If the wound is contaminated (e.g. large bowel), anaerobes, *Clostridium* spp. and *Bacteroides* spp. may also be involved. Most wound infections are polymicrobial in nature.

Clinical features

Wound edges become reddened, with or without pus formation; sometimes a wound abscess may form unnoticed in the deeper layers and eventually discharge through the suture line. Patients may or may not be pyrexial, depending on the degree of infection. Surgical wound infection may result in:

- spread of infection either to adjacent tissues or into the blood, causing **septicaemia** (see below)
- **wound dehiscence** (breakdown of the wound), necessitating resuture.

Pathogenesis and epidemiology

The infection could be either **endogenous** or **exogenous**. The source of an exogenous infection could be an infected person in an adjoining bed, or a carrier, who might be a member of staff. Reservoirs of infection include human skin, environmental dust and inanimate objects (**fomites**) such as bed linen. The mode of cross-infection could be **direct** or **indirect contact**, or the **airborne** route. Many factors affect the incidence of wound infection; these include:

- type of wound — **clean** (i.e. no incision through respiratory, gastrointestinal or genitourinary tract); **contaminated** (e.g. following surgery in a site with a normal flora); or **infected** (e.g. drainage of an abscess)
- overcrowded wards
- length of stay in hospital (shorter hospital stay carries a lesser risk of infection)
- length of the operation (longer operation carries a greater infectious risk)
- presence of foreign bodies and drains
- general health of the patient.

Prevention

Infection may be avoided by:

- rigid observation of **aseptic** and **antiseptic techniques** during both patient preparation and the operation itself
- rigid observation and implementation of **infection control theatre protocols**
- appropriate theatre **clothing**, as transmission of infection from humans is the single most important cause of wound infection

- **positive-pressure ventilation** within the operating room to prevent ingress of contaminated air and dust from the external hospital environment
- **isolation** of patients with discharging wounds to prevent the dissemination of pathogens, i.e. **source isolation**, where the patient is the source of infection (compare **protective isolation** of susceptible patients, for instance a bone marrow transplant patient, from infectious agents)
- carefully chosen **preoperative antibiotic prophylaxis** in specific situations (e.g. colonic surgery).

Infections of burns

Major burns create large, moist, exposed surfaces that are ideal for bacterial growth because the protective skin cover has been lost.

Aetiology

Common organisms that infect burns are *Streptococcus pyogenes*, *Pseudomonas aeruginosa* and *Staphylococcus aureus*; infection is usually polymicrobial.

Pathogenesis and epidemiology

Bacteria colonize burn wounds within 24 hours if appropriate prophylaxis is not given, with eventual cellulitis of adjacent tissues and septicaemia. *Streptococcus pyogenes*, in particular, is a frequent cause of septicaemia; *P. aeruginosa* has a special ability for surviving in burnt tissue and in burns wards, but it is not as virulent as *S. pyogenes*.

Diagnosis of wound infections

Swabs of exudate, tissue or pus are cultured on conventional media (blood agar, MacConkey's agar, Robertson's medium); the smears of the tissue or exudate are Gram-stained and examined for organisms.

Clostridial wound infections

Wound infections described above, which are suppurative, differ clinically from those caused by clostridia (Gram-positive, anaerobic, spore-forming rods; Ch. 13). These infections are severe, but fortunately rare. The two major clostridial wound infections are **tetanus**, caused by *Clostridium tetani*, and **gas gangrene**, due to three different but related organisms: *C. perfringens*, *C. novyi* and *C. septicum*.

Tetanus

See Chapter 25.

Gas gangrene

Gas gangrene is caused by *Clostridium perfringens* (60–65%), *C. novyi* (20–40%) and *C. septicum* (10–20%).

Clinical features. Spreading gangrene of the muscles is accompanied by toxaemia and shock. The involved tissues are black and oedematous with a foul-smelling serous exudate; they exhibit the sign of **crepitus** (palpable crackling on pressure due to subcutaneous movement of gas bubbles) as a result of the production of gaseous metabolites by the multiplying clostridia.

Pathogenesis and epidemiology. A serious disease with a high mortality rate, very often requiring the excision or amputation of the affected area or limb, gas gangrene is a result of the toxins and enzymes produced by clostridia thriving on damaged and devitalized tissues, which provide ideal conditions for anaerobic growth. The organisms produce a variety of toxins, one of which is a **lecithinase** which damages cell membranes; other enzymes produce gaseous by-products within tissue compartments, helping further spread of infection.

Clostridia can be commonly isolated from faeces, and their spores are ubiquitous in nature.

Laboratory diagnosis (See Chapter 6).

Treatment. Gas gangrene is treated with:
- **surgical debridement**, including wide excision or even amputation of affected areas
- **antibiotics**: large doses of penicillin, with or without metronidazole
- **hyperbaric oxygen** may be given, if available, to reduce anaerobiosis of affected tissues.

Prevention. Debridement and amputation should be performed as appropriate. Prophylactic penicillin should be administered for surgical procedures in the area of the thigh, perineum and buttocks (as clostridia are commensals in these regions).

KEY FACTS

- The skin has a thriving microbial community of **resident** and **transient** flora; there are about 10^3–10^4 organisms per cm^2 of skin
- The principal resident flora of the skin are *Staphylococcus epidermidis*, propionibacteria, micrococci and diphtheroids
- **Asymptomatic carriage** of *Staphylococcus aureus* is common in sites such as the **anterior nares** and axillae, and in hospital personnel
- **Boils, styes, carbuncles, sycosis barbae** and **angular cheilitis** may be all due to staphylococcal infection
- Subcutaneous spread of infection or **cellulitis** is caused by *Streptococcus pyogenes* (group A), sometimes with *Staphylococcus aureus*
- **Necrotizing fasciitis** is the term given to rapidly progressing infection involving the full thickness of the skin including the fascial planes, causing **extensive necrosis, tissue loss, toxaemia and shock**
- *Angular cheilitis or stomatitis is mainly caused by* Staphylococcus aureus *and/or* Candida *infection; but other predisposing factors are involved*

- **Acne**, a common, disfiguring facial infection of adolescents is caused by *Propionibacterium acnes*
- *Mycobacterium leprae*, the agent of **leprosy**, lives in human skin and nerves and is transmitted by prolonged contact to cause two types of chronic granulomatous disease: **the lepromatous** and the **tuberculoid forms**
- *Surgical wound infections account for approximately a quarter of hospital-acquired (nosocomial) infections*
- *Staphylococcus aureus* and *Escherichia coli* are the major agents of surgical infection
- **Factors affecting** the incidence of **wound infection** include the type of wound (clean, contaminated or infected), overcrowded wards, length of stay in hospital, length of the operation, foreign bodies and drains, and the general health of the patient
- Common organisms that infect **burns** are *Streptococcus pyogenes*, *Pseudomonas aeruginosa* and *Staphylococcus aureus*; infection is usually **polymicrobial**
- The two major **clostridial wound infections** are tetanus, caused by *Clostridium tetani*, and **gas gangrene**, due to *C. perfringens*, *C. novyi* or *C. septicum*

FURTHER READING

Mims, C, Playfair, J, Roitt, I, Wakelin, D, and Williams, R (1998). Infections of the skin, muscle, joints, bone and hemopoietic system. In *Medical microbiology* (2nd edn), Ch. 23. Mosby, London.

Murray, PR, Rosenthal, KS, Kobayashi, GS, and Pfaller, MA (1998). Superficial, cutaneous and subcutaneous mycoses. In *Medical microbiology* (3rd edn), Ch. 69. Mosby Year Book, St Louis.

Shanson, DC (1999). Skin infections and infestations. In *Microbiology in clinical practice* (3rd edn), Ch. 17. Butterworth-Heinemann, Oxford.

29 Viral hepatitis

A clear understanding of viral hepatitis is essential for all dental practitioners, particularly in view of the serious sequelae of the disease and the potential of transmitting the infection in the dental clinic. Hepatitis can be due to a number of causes such as infections, alcohol abuse, trauma or drug-induced toxicity. However, in global terms viral infections are by far the single most important agent of hepatitis. These include infections with herpes simplex virus, cytomegalovirus and Epstein–Barr virus, but the vast majority of viral liver diseases are one of the following:

- hepatitis A (infectious hepatitis, short incubation hepatitis)
- hepatitis B (serum hepatitis)
- hepatitis C
- hepatitis D (delta hepatitis)
- hepatitis E (enterically transmitted hepatitis)
- hepatitis G.

These may be classified into two groups depending on the viral transmission route:

1. **Faecal–oral route**: hepatitis A and hepatitis E (highly unlikely to be transmitted in dentistry).
2. **Parenteral route**: hepatitis B, hepatitis C, hepatitis D and possibly hepatitis G (could be transmitted in dentistry).

Data from the World Health Organization (WHO) indicate that viral hepatitis B infection alone accounts for more than 1 million deaths worldwide. In terms of morbidity, there are around 350 million hepatitis B chronic carriers and another 100 million chronic carriers of hepatitis C.

The various types of viral hepatitis differ in severity of infection, morbidity, mortality rate, presence or absence of a carrier state, and frequency of long-term sequelae such as cirrhosis and cancer. The main differences between the hepatitides caused by these viruses are shown in Table 29.1.

SIGNS AND SYMPTOMS OF HEPATITIS

The common symptoms and signs of hepatitis include malaise, jaundice, dark urine and pale, fatty stools. These, together with results of serum and urine biochemistry and specific serology tests, facilitate the diagnosis of viral hepatitis. Investigation typically reveals abnormal liver function with raised levels of serum transaminases and bilirubin, and bilirubinuria. Specific serologic tests are now available to detect hepatitis A, B, C, D and E antibodies.

HEPATITIS A

The hepatitis A virus (HAV) is a small (27 nm) RNA virus belonging to the picornavirus group (which also includes poliovirus and coxsackieviruses). The virus is inactivated by ultraviolet light, exposure to water at 100°C for 5 minutes and by exposure to 2% glutaraldehyde for 15 minutes.

Epidemiology

Hepatitis A commonly occurs in developing parts of the world where sewage disposal measures and food hygiene are unsatisfactory. Only 10–13% of the population in developed countries have been exposed to the virus by the age of 20 years. It is usually contracted by the faecal–oral route from contaminated food and water. Children and young people are most often infected, and for this reason a history of hepatitis in childhood would, in most instances, be indicative of a hepatitis A infection.

Clinical features

The mean incubation period is 30 days (range 2–7 weeks). Patients are infectious before the onset of symptoms during the prodromal phase and just before the onset of clinical disease.

Jaundice is common in adults and rare in young children. There are no chronic sequelae. Some patients continue to excrete HAV in faeces during weeks 1 to 3 of the illness, and HAV may also be present in saliva (100 particles per mL) throughout this period.

Diagnosis

Diagnosis is by demonstration of HAV antigen in faeces. Serological tests demonstrate IgM class anti-HAV antibodies in serum during the acute or early convalescent phase (IgG class antibodies appear later in the disease and confer enduring protection against the disease).

Unlike hepatitis B, there is no carrier state associated with the disease. This, together with its faecal–oral transmission, implies that hepatitis A transmission in the dental clinic is highly unlikely.

Table 29.1   Epidemiological and clinical features of hepatitis viruses

	Hepatitis A	Hepatitis B	Hepatitis C	Hepatitis D	Hepatitis E	Hepatitis G
Synonym	Infectious hepatitis	Serum hepatitis	Hepatitis C	Delta hepatitis	Hepatitis E	Hepatitis G
Type of virus	ssRNA	dsDNA	ssRNA	ssRNA	ssRNA	RNA
Incubation period	2–7 weeks	1–6 months	2–26 weeks	2–12 weeks	6–8 weeks	?
Transmission	Faecal–oral	Predominantly parenteral	Parenteral and faecal–oral	Parenteral	Faecal–oral	Parenteral
Carrier state	No	Yes	Yes	Yes	No	?
Severity of hepatitis	±	++	+	+	±	±
Immunity:						
Passive immunization	Hyperimmune globulin	Hyperimmune globulin	None	Hyperimmune globulin	No	?
Active immunization	Vaccine (hepatitis A)	Vaccine (hepatitis B)	None	Vaccine (hepatitis B)	No	None

ds, double-stranded; ss, single-stranded.

Prophylaxis

Passive immunization by hyperimmune globulin is effective against clinical illness, particularly when administered in the early incubation period. However, the main use of short-term, pre-exposure prophylaxis is for travellers to hepatitis A endemic areas, such as some parts of the developing world. Several vaccines of inactivated HAV produced in human cell culture are available. Immunization (two doses, initial and a booster 6–12 months after) is safe and effective and recommended for professionals working with institutionalized patients. A combined vaccine for hepatitis A and B is now available.

Hepatitis A and dentistry

Hepatitis A virus is not a significant infection risk in dentistry as the route of transmission is faecal–oral. Close contact with saliva may transmit infection as saliva can contain some HAV. Rarely infection has been transmitted by needlestick injury, and there is a report of transmission from a surgeon to a patient. Universal infection control measures are adequate to prevent transmission in dental practice.

HEPATITIS B

The hepatitis B virus (HBV) is a DNA hepadnavirus (*hepa-*, liver + DNA) which is structurally and immunologically complex. Electron microscopy of HBV reveals three distinct particles (Fig. 29.1):

- Dane particle (42 nm) — the complete infective virus
- spherical forms (22 nm) — non-infective
- tubular forms (22 nm × 100 nm) — non-infective.

Being a **hepatotropic** virus, HBV will reside and multiply in hepatocytes after entering the body, and cause hepatic injury and inflammation (hepatitis) to varying degrees. When it multiplies in the hepatocytes, for some unknown reason the virus particles described above are produced in different proportions within the liver cell cytoplasm. As a result of overpro-

duction of these non-infective spheres and tubules, which are the surface proteins of the virus (hence called hepatitis B surface antigens or HBsAg), they circulate freely in the serum for prolonged periods after the acute hepatitis episode.

The central **core** of the HBV consists of a single-stranded DNA, an enzyme (DNA polymerase) and a core antigen (HBcAg). Although this antigen is rarely found in serum, a breakdown product of HBcAg, termed 'e' antigen (HBeAg), may be found in serum and is a marker of active infection.

Epidemiology

The prevalence of hepatitis B varies greatly in different parts of the world: it is higher in African and Asian countries than in the Americas, Australia and western Europe (Fig. 29.2); in urban than in rural areas; in men than in women. In developed countries the risk of exposure to hepatitis B is high in certain categories of people, as shown in Table 29.2. Several variants of HBV are now known, and when these involve re-arrangement of the surface antigens, existing vaccines may not be protective. This has come to light as a few individuals who

Table 29.2   Hepatitis B high-risk population groups

Selected patient groups
  Patients requiring frequent large-volume transfusions of *unscreened* blood/blood products (e.g. in haemophilia)
  Institutionalized patients with learning difficulties
  Patients with a recent history of jaundice
  Patients in renal dialysis units
  Immunosuppressed/immunodeficient patients

Population groups
  Injecting drug abusers
  Promiscuous homosexual men
  Female prostitutes
  Migrants from developing countries
  Health-care and laboratory personnel (especially surgeons)

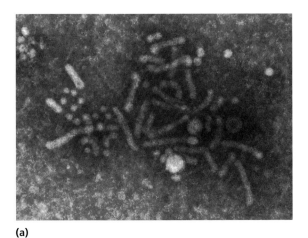

(a)

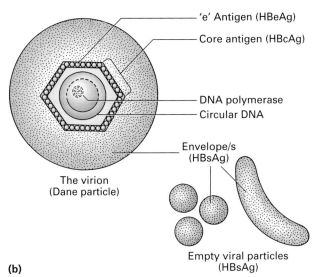

'e' Antigen (HBeAg)

Core antigen (HBcAg)

DNA polymerase

Circular DNA

Envelope/s
(HBsAg)

The virion
(Dane particle)

Empty viral particles
(b)   (HBsAg)

Fig. 29.1 Hepatitis B virus: (a) scanning electron micrograph; (b) hepatitis B virus and particles.

had been successfully immunized against HBV but who were at high risk of infection nevertheless contracted hepatitis B. A variant HBV, HBV-2, has been described in West Africa, the Middle East, Spain, France, Taiwan, New Zealand and the USA, and another has been reported from Italy, Greece and the UK. Both variants are able to infect persons immunized against the usual form of HBV.

Carrier state and identification of carriers

Most patients who contract hepatitis B recover within a few weeks without any sequelae (Fig. 29.3). However, serological markers of previous HBV infection are invariably present in these patients for prolonged periods. Such markers take the form of antibodies to various components of the HBV. A minority (2–5%) fail to clear HBV by 6–9 months and consequently develop a chronic carrier state. This state more frequently follows **anicteric** HBV infection (i.e. infection without jaundice). The converse of this is that a majority of infections that lead to jaundice resolve without a carrier state; hence a history of jaundice in a patient in most instances indicates little or no risk in terms of hepatitis B transmission.

The chronic carriers of hepatitis B infection fall into two main groups: those with **chronic persistent hepatitis** (the so-called 'healthy carrier' state) and those with **chronic active hepatitis** (Fig. 29.3). In chronic persistent hepatitis the patient does not develop liver damage and is generally in good health, although the liver cells persistently produce viral antigen (HBsAg) because of the integration of the viral genome into the DNA of the hepatocytes. The second group of chronic carriers are extremely infectious as they harbour the infective Dane particles in their blood. In addition, they are very susceptible to cirrhosis and hepatocellular carcinoma. Nonetheless, the chronic active hepatitis group represents a small minority of hepatitis B patients. In general, infection with HBV leads to complete recovery in most individuals, while only about 2–5% develop a carrier state. These two disease states elicit characteristic serological profiles in the affected individual during various phases of the disease, as shown in Figures 29.4 and 29.5.

Diagnosis and serological markers

Diagnosis of HBV is complicated by the variety of serological markers and the complex sequelae of the disease itself. Table 29.3 summarizes the significance of the serological markers described below.

1. Hepatitis B surface antigen (HBsAg) indicates that the person is a carrier and potentially infective. This state can

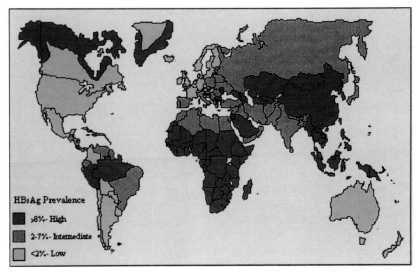

HBsAg Prevalence

■ ≥8% - High

■ 2-7% - Intermediate

□ <2% - Low

Fig. 29.2 Geographic distribution of chronic hepatitis B virus infection. (Courtesy of Centers for Disease Control and Prevention, USA.)

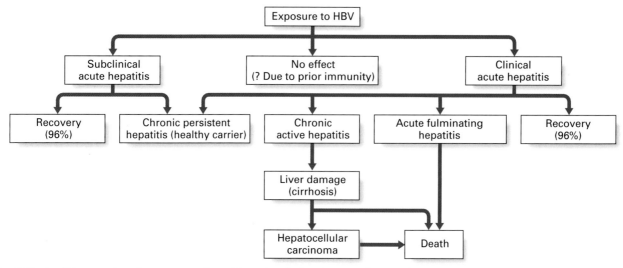

Fig. 29.3 Possible sequelae of exposure to hepatitis B virus (values in parentheses indicate percentage recovery).

persist for months until recovery, or for years in chronic carrier states.

2. Antibody to hepatitis B surface antigen (anti-HBs) appears in serum during the recovery phase and is long-lived; its presence indicates recovery and immunity to further HBV infection; also seen in high titre after successful vaccination for HBV, as the active ingredient of the hepatitis B vaccine is HBsAg.

3. Hepatitis B 'e' antigen (HBeAg) is indicative of active disease or high infectivity. Infectivity of this particle is so high that even 0.0001 mL serum containing the particle may transmit the disease; its prolonged persistence in serum indicates possibility of chronic liver damage.

4. Antibody to hepatitis B 'e' antigen (anti-HBe) appears in the serum soon after the appearance of HbeAg and indicates partial recovery from infection and a low level of

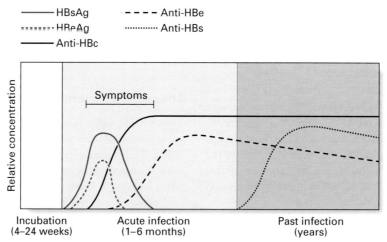

Fig. 29.4 Typical profile of hepatitis B serological markers after recovery from infection.

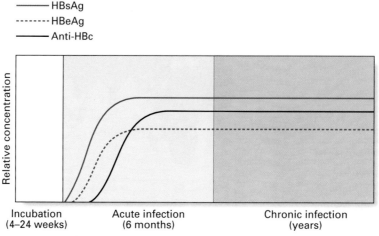

Fig. 29.5 Hepatitis B chronic carrier state: no seroconversion.

Table 29.3 Serological markers of hepatitis B infection and their interpretation

HBsAg	HBeAg	Anti-HBe	Anti-HBs	Risk status
+	Unknown	Unknown	–	High/low risk
+	+	–	–	High risk
+	–	+	–	Low risk
–	–	+	+	Immune due to previous infection
–	–	–	+	Immune due to vaccination

infectivity; its absence, in the presence of HBeAg, indicates high infectivity and possible chronic carrier state.

5. The core antigen (HBcAg) is present in the liver but not in the serum.
6. Antibody to hepatitis B core antigen (anti-HBc) in serum is indicative of active or very recent infection; it is a sensitive indicator of previous exposure to HBV infection as it outlasts all other antibodies.

Hepatitis B and dentistry

More than 380 health-care workers, including dental surgeons, have been infected with hepatitis B in clinical settings. Most were surgeons; in dentistry the risk of infection is greater among oral surgeons and periodontists than among general dental practitioners. Universal infection control procedures were often lacking when transmission occurred.

The number of health-care workers contracting infection reported since the introduction of the vaccine programme in 1987, especially in dentistry, has been small. However, there is an ever-present danger of hepatitis B transmission in dentistry if dental personnel are not vaccinated, or are vaccinated but with inadequate seroconversion (see below).

Although the usual mode of transmission of hepatitis B is from the patient to the dentist, there are at least eight recorded outbreaks where dentists have transmitted the disease to patients.

Intraorally, the greatest concentration of hepatitis B virus is at the gingival sulcus as a result of the continuous serum exudate, which is small in healthy people but greatly increased in diseased states e.g. periodontitis; the virus is present in mixed saliva but not in parotid or submandibular saliva (Table 29.4).

Special precautions are **not** necessary when treating carriers of hepatitis B (or any other disease), as universal infection control measures, routinely employed in dentistry irrespective of the clinical status of the patient (see Ch. 36), should prevent disease transmission.

Table 29.4 Concentration of hepatitis B in body fluids

High	Moderate	Low/undetectable
Blood	Mixed saliva	Urine
Wound exudates	Semen Vaginal fluid	Sweat, tears Breast milk Parotid/submandibular saliva

Prophylaxis

See Chapter 10.

Treatment

In chronic carriers of the virus **interferon therapy** may be successful in eliminating the carrier state.

HEPATITIS C

Some years ago the term 'non-A non-B hepatitis' (NANBH) was used to describe a disease complex with probable infective origin, that did not belong to either hepatitis A or hepatitis B. Subsequent research demonstrated that NANBH is due to infective agents transmitted by both the parenteral and the enteric route. One such parenterally transmitted agent was named 'hepatitis C virus' (HCV) and another, enterically transmitted, NANBH was termed 'hepatitis E virus'.

Aetiology

Hepatitis C is caused by an enveloped RNA virus related to the flaviviruses. The virus has yet to be grown in culture or visualized ultrastructurally. It may exist as one of at least six different genotypes. Some patients may be infected with more than one genotype. The viral RNA can remain intact for at least 7 days at room temperature. Thus, although the infectivity of HCV is still unclear, it is essential that adherence to universal infection control is observed at all times.

Epidemiology

Hepatitis C is globally prevalent. According to the World Health Organization, about 3% of the world population has been infected with hepatitis C and there are more than 170 million chronic carriers at risk of developing liver cirrhosis or cancer. There may, however, be considerable regional and ethnic group variation (Fig. 29.6).

Blood, blood products, intravenous immunoglobulins and donated organs have transmitted HCV, although newer methods of HCV detection have reduced but not entirely eradicated such risk. Injecting drug abusers, transfusion recipients and haemophiliac patients receiving blood products are other groups who are at risk. The disease occurs in 5–10% of transfusion recipients, leading to chronic hepatitis in about half of them.

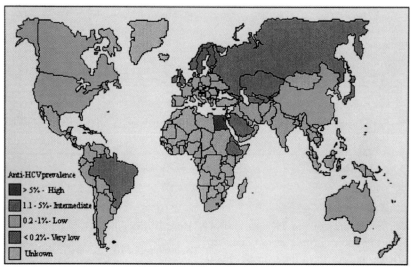

Fig. 29.6 Prevalence of hepatitis C virus infection among blood donors. (Courtesy of Centers for Disease Control and Prevention, USA.)

Diagnosis

The diagnosis of HCV infection is serological. Assays using the enzyme-linked immunosorbent assay (ELISA) technique can detect antibodies to HCV envelope or core proteins. Polymerase chain reaction (PCR) assays are also very sensitive and specific and can detect early infection. Most HCV-infected persons are HCV-seropositive within 6 months of infection. Because of this delay in antibody response donated blood may not be screened effectively.

Clinical features

- The incubation period varies from 2 weeks to 26 weeks (average 6–7 weeks).
- The initial infection is often asymptomatic, especially in children and young adults, while some 40% of adults may have acute symptoms. Hence many are unaware of their infection or the eventual outcome.
- A minority can have persistent viraemia without serologic or clinical evidence of hepatic disease. Infection with HCV rarely gives rise to fulminant hepatic failure.
- About 25% of infected patients develop jaundice and up to 60% can have histologic evidence of chronic liver disease. Cirrhosis may eventually develop in up to 80% of chronically HCV-infected persons.
- Interestingly, the link between HCV and hepatocellular carcinoma appears to be even stronger than that for HBV.
- Factors thought to influence the extent of liver disease include HCV genotype, gender, age at infection and the extent of immunodeficiency.

Sequelae of chronic HCV infection

Persistent chronic infection develops in approximately 80% of infected persons and the course of infection may run for 20 or more years. Approximately 70% of those with chronic HCV will develop chronic liver disease. The virus may also cause mixed cryoglobulinaemia, thyroid disorders, diabetes mellitus, thrombocytopenia and lichen planus.

Treatment

Infection can be managed with interferon alfa, aciclovir and tribavirin (ribavirin). These, in essence, attempt to clear the virus and the viraemia and reduce the risk or slow down the development of liver sequelae. Interferon is moderately effective, with reported success rates varying from 15% to 50%.

Prevention

At present there is no passive or active immunization programme for HCV infection. All immunization methods appear to be unsatisfactory as re-exposure of HCV-infected patients to different strains of HCV still results in reinfection. This reflects the possible different types of HCV and their rapid rate of mutation. By the same token, prophylaxis with immunoglobulins confers little, if any, immunity.

Hepatitis C and dentistry

- Possible oral manifestations of HCV infection include **lichen planus, oral malignancy** and **salivary gland disease**; the underlying pathogenic mechanisms of these HCV-related lesions are not clear but may reflect immunogenetic factors or the presence of anti-epithelial antibodies.
- There is no unequivocal evidence of transmission of HCV as a consequence of dental treatment.
- Saliva of up to 50% of patients with acute and chronic hepatitis C infection may contain HCV-RNA; other studies have failed to detect HCV in saliva.
- Needlestick injuries are the most common way in which HCV is transmitted in clinical settings, although healthcare workers are not at especial risk of infection. The risk of HCV infection after a needlestick injury with HCV-contaminated blood may be 3–10% (approximately 10 times greater than for HIV).
- Studies of dental staff in the UK and Taiwan have shown no raised incidence of HCV infection, but their counterparts in the USA (particularly oral surgeons) may be liable to HCV carriage.

- Immunoglobulin therapy or interferon therapy has been suggested as a possible management procedure for a needlestick injury involving blood from an HCV-infected patient. The efficacy of either approach remains to be determined.

HEPATITIS D (DELTA HEPATITIS)

Delta hepatitis is caused by a 'defective' RNA virus which coexists with HBV (Fig. 29.7). Hepatitis D virus (HDV) is the smallest animal virus known and contains a nucleoprotein, a delta antigen and an outer surface protein. The outer coat of the delta virus is 'borrowed' HBsAg and hence the virus cannot survive independently without the hepatitis B viral particles. Consequently, delta infection is only seen as a:
- co-infection in a hepatitis B patient
- superinfection in a hepatitis B carrier.

Both usually cause an episode of acute hepatitis. Co-infection usually resolves, while superinfection frequently causes chronic delta infection leading to chronic active hepatitis (Fig. 29.8).

Epidemiology

It has been estimated that about 15 million persons are infected with HDV worldwide, as about 5% of HBV carriers are HDV-positive. In non-endemic areas such as the USA and northern Europe, HDV is confined mainly to persons frequently exposed to blood and blood products, particularly drug addicts. Up to 4% of US blood donors have evidence of previous HDV infection. It is noteworthy that HDV infection is not common in most groups in South-East Asia. Geographic areas with a high incidence of delta hepatitis are the Amazon basin, parts of Africa, the Middle East and Arab countries, where 30–90% HBsAg carriers with liver disease are infected. Delta infection occurs rarely in the susceptible population of northern Europe and is virtually confined to parenteral drug abusers.

Routes of delta transmission appear to be similar to those of hepatitis B, the infection being most commonly seen among persons at high risk of acquiring hepatitis B infection (see Table 29.2). The transmission and epidemiology of HDV infection are much the same. In general, it is a parenterally transmitted infection which has become a major problem in injecting drug abusers. It is also transmitted by sexual or close contact with HDV-infected persons. However, sexual transmission of HDV appears to be less common than for HBV, and HDV infection is uncommon in homosexual men.

Clinical features and diagnosis

The incubation period of HDV infection ranges from 2 weeks to 12 weeks and most infections lead to jaundice. The virus produces acute hepatitis, which usually resolves but may precipitate fulminant liver disease. The latter is 10 times more frequent in HDV infection than in HBV infection alone. Chronic hepatitis is a common sequel of HDV infection, and 70% of those affected develop cirrhosis. The role, if any, of HDV in hepatic carcinogenesis is unclear.

Diagnosis is by detection of delta antigen (using ELISA) in serum and/or by the appearance of delta antibody. Delta infection does not respond well to interferon therapy.

Prophylaxis

As the delta virus is dependent on HBV for replication, successful immunization with the hepatitis B vaccine will prevent delta infection.

Hepatitis D and dentistry

The main route of HDV transmission is parenteral, in either blood or blood products. Sexual transmission may occur sometimes within households, and perinatally if mothers are positive for HDV and HBeAg. It is unclear whether saliva is a vehicle.

There is at least one report of HDV transmission in dentistry in the USA, where up to 700 cases were recorded. At least four dentists were infected; one oral surgeon became a HBV carrier, and was thought to have infected several patients.

HEPATITIS E

Hepatitis E virus (HEV) is a relatively newly described RNA virus that bears some similarities to the Caliciviridae. As it is transmitted by the faecal–oral route the main agent is contaminated drinking water. Hepatitis E outbreaks are common in Africa, Asia and Latin America, especially in countries with poor sewage disposal facilities. In these geographic regions different HEV viruses are responsible for the infection. Intrafamilial and parenteral spread is rare. In most instances the disease follows a benign pattern like that of hepatitis A, with a low mortality rate of 1–2%. The infection is infrequently associated with fulminant hepatitis. The disease can be diagnosed by Western blot, ELISA and a polymerase chain reaction assay.

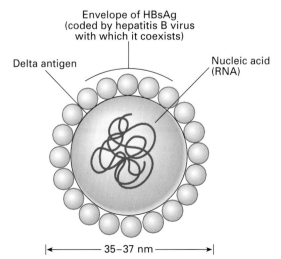

Envelope of HBsAg
(coded by hepatitis B virus
with which it coexists)

Delta antigen

Nucleic acid
(RNA)

35–37 nm

Fig. 29.7 Hepatitis D (delta) virus.

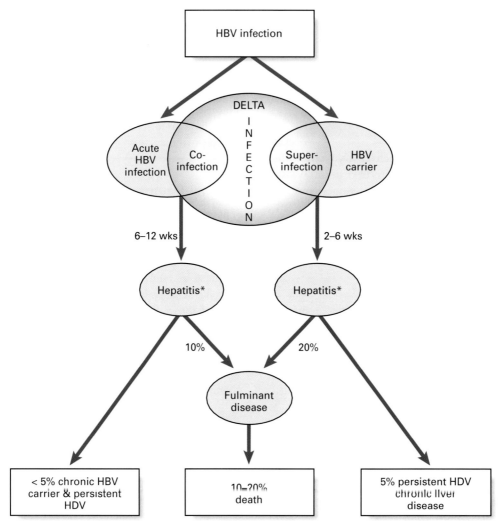

Fig. 29.8 Sequelae of hepatitis delta virus infection.

Due to its mode of transmission, the virus does not pose a major risk of cross-infection in dentistry.

HEPATITIS F?

In 1994 an investigator reported finding viral particles in the stool of post-transfusion, non-A, non-B, non-C, non-E hepatitis cases. Injection of these particles into Indian Rhesus monkeys presumably caused hepatitis, named 'hepatitis F'. However, no other investigator has been able to confirm these findings, and the original observation is now thought to be incidental.

Thus, there is no hepatitis F virus as yet. Unfortunately, though, this alphabetic position in the viral nomenclature has been occupied.

HEPATITIS G

It has become increasingly evident that there are patients with acute or chronic hepatitis who are not infected by the hepatitis viruses A to E described above (hence the designation non-A–E hepatitis). Another hepatitis agent isolated in 1967 from a surgeon (whose initials were G.B.) with acute hepatitis has been transmitted in tamarins. This particular virus, first termed the GB agent, was thought to be two novel RNA viruses of the Flaviviridae family, and were designated hepatitis GB virus A (GBV-A) and hepatitis GB virus B (GBV-B). To add to the confusion, other closely related viruses, hepatitis GBV-C and hepatitis G virus, have been found in humans with chronic hepatitis, and recovered from patients with non-A–E hepatitis. All these viruses appear to be identical and fall under the common term 'hepatitis G', at least for the time being.

Infections with these viruses appear more common among injecting drug abusers and people with haemophilia. Hepatitis G virus does not seem to elicit a strong immune response.

Hepatitis G and dentistry

Hepatitis G virus RNA is present in whole saliva of infected individuals, but transmission through this route has not been determined. No data is available on the transmission of hepatitis G or the rate of HGV carriage in dental staff.

No vaccine is available; implementation of universal infection control measures should be adequate to prevent transmission of this virus in dentistry.

TRANSFUSION TRANSMITTED VIRUS

Transfusion transmitted virus (TTV) causes post-transfusion hepatitis; it has not yet been given an alphabetic nomenclature. Described in 1997, it is a non-enveloped, single-stranded DNA virus possibly belonging to the Parvoviridae family. It has been isolated from persons in UK, Japan and Brazil, especially older blood donors. The most remarkable feature of TTV is the extraordinarily high prevalence of chronic viraemia in apparently healthy people, up to nearly 100% in some countries. It may be transmitted parenterally but this route has not been confirmed. No information on TTV salivary carriage or transmission in dental settings is available.

KEY FACTS

- Viruses are by far the most important agents of hepatitis, and include hepatitis A, B, C, D, E and G (the existence of hepatitis F has been queried)
- These **hepatotropic viruses** are classified into two groups depending on the transmission route — the **faecal–oral route**: hepatitis A and hepatitis E (highly unlikely to be transmitted in dentistry); and the **parenteral route**: hepatitis B, C and D and possibly hepatitis G (could be transmitted in dentistry)
- The various types of viral hepatitis differ in severity of infection, morbidity, mortality rate, presence or absence of a carrier state, and frequency of long-term sequelae such as cirrhosis and cancer
- *Hepatitis A virus: 27 nm, RNA virus, belongs to the picornavirus group; clinical disease mild; no chronic carrier state*
- *Hepatitis A vaccine is safe and effective and recommended for professionals working with institutionalized patients. A combined vaccine for hepatitis A and B is available*
- **Hepatitis B virus (HBV)** is a double-shelled DNA virus; on electron microscopy three distinct particles are seen: the infective Dane particle and the non-infective, spherical and tubular forms
- The central **core** of the HBV consists of single-stranded DNA, an enzyme (DNA polymerase) and a core antigen (HBcAg). Although this antigen is rarely found in serum, a breakdown product of HBcAg, termed 'e' antigen (HBeAg), may be found in serum and is a marker of active infection
- HBV is transmitted by **body fluids**: blood to blood contact, perinatal and sexual transmission are the major routes
- *The diagnosis of HBV is serological with initial screening for HBsAg*
- Appearance of anti-HBs heralds recovery and immunity to further HBV infection; high titres of anti-HBs are seen as successful vaccination for HBV (as the active ingredient of the hepatitis B vaccine is HBsAg)
- *HBV vaccine is safe, effective and relatively long-lasting, and also protects against hepatitis D infection*
- *The number of dental-care workers contracting hepatitis B since the introduction of the vaccine programme has been small, but there is an ever-present danger of HBV transmission if personnel are not vaccinated, or vaccinees do not seroconvert (up to 5%). Hence antibody levels should be ascertained after a vaccine course*
- *Intraorally, the greatest concentration of HBV is at the gingival sulcus as a result of the continuous serum exudate, which is small in health but greatly increased in diseased states*
- *Hepatitis C is due to an enveloped RNA virus that may have up to six different genotypes. Some patients may be infected with more than one genotype*
- *Persistent chronic HCV infection may develop in some 85% of those infected and the course of infection may run up to 20 years*
- *Possible oral manifestations of HCV infection include **lichen planus, oral malignancy** and **salivary gland disease***
- *Saliva of up to 50% of patients with acute and chronic hepatitis C infection may contain HCV-RNA; some studies have failed to detect HCV in saliva*
- *The risk of infection after a needlestick injury with HCV-contaminated blood may be 3-10% (compare 0.4% for HIV and 0.007% for HBV)*
- **Delta hepatitis** is caused by a 'defective' RNA virus (HDV) which coexists with HBV and hence is seen as a **co-infection** in a hepatitis B patient or a **superinfection** in a hepatitis B carrier
- The transmission and epidemiology of HDV infection are similar to HBV, and the virus is a major problem, especially in injecting drug abusers
- **Hepatitis E virus** is an RNA virus that resembles the Caliciviridae, transmitted via the faecal–oral route; the main agent is contaminated drinking water
- **Hepatitis G virus** is a flavivirus, present in whole saliva of infected individuals, common among injecting drug abusers and haemophiliac patients; disease associations have yet to be defined
- **Transfusion transmitted virus (TTV)** is a recently described, hepatotrophic, non-enveloped, single-stranded DNA virus; causes post-transfusion hepatitis; may be transmitted parenterally. No information on TTV salivary carriage or transmission in dental settings is available

FURTHER READING

Bendinelli, M, Pistello, M, Maggi, F, Fornai, C, Freer, G, Vatteroni, ML (2001). Molecular properties, biology, and clinical implications of TTvirus, a recently identified widespread infectious agent of humans, *Clinical Microbiology Reviews* 14, 98–104.

Karaylannis, P, and Thomas, H (1997). Hepatitis G virus: identification, prevalence and unanswered questions. *Gut* 40, 294–296.

Klein, RS, Freeman, K, Taylor, PE, et al (1999). Occupational risk of hepatitis C virus infection among New York City dentists. *Lancet* 338, 1539–1542.

Molinari, JA (1996). Hepatitis C virus infection. *Dental Clinics of North America* 40, 309–325.

Scully, C, and Samaranayake, LP (1992). *Clinical virology in oral medicine and dentistry.* Cambridge University Press, Cambridge.

Zuckerman, AJ, and Harrison, TJ (1994). Hepatitis viruses. In Zuckerman, AJ, Banatvala, JE, and Pattison JR (eds) *Principles and practice of clinical virology* (3rd edn), Ch. 2. John Wiley, Chichester.

Human immunodeficiency virus infection, AIDS, and infections in compromised patients

By the beginning of the year 2001 approximately 36 million people worldwide had become infected with human immunodeficiency virus (HIV) and some 22 million had died of acquired immune deficiency syndrome (AIDS). Although HIV infection is now a global pandemic, AIDS was described only in 1981, in young homosexual men in the USA. However, the disease appears to have originated in Africa, where cases have been revealed from as long ago as 1959. The virus causes depletion of CD4-positive T helper lymphocytes over many years, as a consequence of which patients succumb to opportunistic infections, particularly *Pneumocystis carinii* pneumonia and oral candidiasis, and neoplasms, especially Kaposi's sarcoma.

After infection with HIV there is a prolonged asymptomatic period that may last up to 10 years, but the risk of developing severe immunodeficiency and AIDS increases with time. Thus the clinical spectrum of HIV infection is broad, ranging from asymptomatic or mild infection to severe clinical illness and profound immunodeficiency. The variety of clinical manifestations seen in AIDS has spawned a number of definitions of the disease. However, the Centers for Disease Control and Prevention in the USA have rationalized and revised these to include all patients with CD4-positive cell counts of less than 200 per microlitre.

The battle to conquer HIV infection and AIDS is fought on many fronts, consuming millions of dollars, and thus far all efforts at producing a preventive vaccine have failed. However, the introduction of new antiviral regimens such as highly active antiretroviral therapy (HAART) has increased life expectancy in HIV infection and dramatically reduced complications, suppressing viral replication to undetectable levels.

The impact of HIV and AIDS on the practice of clinical dentistry has been enormous, first because of the regimentation in infection control it has spawned throughout the profession, and second because of the many oral manifestations and their management which the practising dentist has to be aware of.

Definitions

- **HIV infection**: infection with the human immunodeficiency virus — an RNA retrovirus.
- **HIV disease**: the resulting immunodeficiency and the appearance of attendant diseases (i.e. not all HIV-infected persons will have symptomatic disease).
- **Acquired immune deficiency syndrome**: a term given to a group of disorders characterized by a profound cell-mediated immunodeficiency consequential to irreversible suppression of T lymphocytes by the HIV. These disorders are called **AIDS-defining illnesses**, and include parameters such as CD4 lymphocyte count below $200 \times 10^6/L$, oropharyngeal candidiasis, hairy leukoplakia, etc. (Table 30.1).

Retroviridae

Human immunodeficiency virus is a lymphotrophic virus which belongs to the family Retroviridae. The latter RNA viruses comprise a single taxonomic group made up of three subfamilies:

- **lentiviruses** cause slowly progressive disease and are cytopathic in nature; they include HIV-1 and HIV-2
- **oncoviruses** include those that cause tumours: human T-cell leukaemia virus (HTLV-I) which causes adult T-cell leukaemia-lymphoma (ATLL); and HTLV-II, associated with hairy cell leukaemia
- **spumaviruses** are not recognized human pathogens.

The virus has a diameter of 100 nm, and its structure is described below. There are two types: **HIV-1** is the most prevalent; **HIV-2** is a variant that originated in West Africa and has spread to Central Africa, Europe and South America. Type 1 is classified into two major groups: M, containing 10 genetically distinct subtypes (A–J), and O, containing a heterogeneous collection of viruses. Type 2 HIV, except for its antigenic and nucleic acid profile, has similar biological properties to HIV-1.

The structure of HIV is shown in Figure 30.1. It consists of:

1. An envelope containing virus-specific 'coat' proteins (e.g. glycoproteins gp41 and gp120) which can act as antigens. Glycoprotein gp120 has a 'rugger ball' configuration and plays an important role in the initial events leading to infection. These coat proteins undergo almost continuous structural changes which hamper the development of effective vaccines.
2. Three **core proteins**, of which p24 is especially antigenic: antibodies to this form the basis of most serologic testing (the HIV test).

Table 30.1 Centers for Disease Control classification of HIV infection

Absolute CD4 cell count (×10⁶/L)	Clinical group		
	A	B	C
> 500	A1	B1	C1
200–499	A2	B2	C2
< 200	A3	B3	C3

Group A: acute HIV infection, asymptomatic phase or persistent generalized lymphadenopathy.
Group B: symptomatic but not AIDS-defining (see text).
Group C: conditions meeting CDC/World Health Organization AIDS defining criteria.

3. A **genome of RNA** comprising two identical molecules of single-stranded RNA.
4. Two molecules of an enzyme, **reverse transcriptase** (an RNA-dependent DNA polymerase), essential for transcribing the RNA code of the virus to a DNA code during viral multiplication (so that it may integrate into the host cell DNA).

Stability of HIV

The survival of HIV under varying conditions has been investigated.

- HIV is destroyed by heat (autoclave and hot-air oven); the virus is inactivated by a factor of 100-fold each hour at a temperature over 60°C
- the virus may survive up to 15 days at room temperature and at body temperature (37°C)
- disinfectants: 2% glutaraldehyde and hypochlorite (10 000 p.p.m. available chlorine, equivalent to 1:10 dilution of domestic bleach) kills 10⁵ units of virus in a few minutes. The virucidal activity of alcohol is relatively low compared to this.

Important: the above figures indicate the limits of survival at very high starting concentrations of HIV (up to 1000 times more than the levels found in the blood of patients) under experimental conditions. Also, the efficacy of the mentioned disinfectants is affected by a variety of factors such as the associated organic bioburden. Hence care and strict adherence to protocols are essential when dealing with HIV.

Viral replication

See Chapter 10.

Transmission of HIV

The virus is most commonly acquired by having sex with an infected partner. The virus can enter the body through the lining of the vagina, vulva, penis, rectum or mouth during sex. The infection can also be transmitted by exchange of infected blood, or other body fluids such as breast milk, and is not transmitted by social or casual, non-sexual contact. Currently, heterosexual sex is the major mode of transmission worldwide.

Other notable transmission modes include sharing of needles, vertical transmission in utero, breast-feeding, and transfusion of infected blood or blood products (factor VIII concentrate). Occasional cases of HIV infection result from needlestick injuries in health-care settings. The question of HIV transmission among health-care workers, including dentists, is addressed at the end of this chapter.

Saliva and HIV transmission

There is only a very slim possibility that HIV may be transmitted by saliva, for the following reasons.

1. Only a small minority of HIV-infected individuals harbour the virus in whole saliva (e.g. in one study HIV was detected in mixed saliva of 5% of infected individuals and in only one of 15 parotid saliva samples). In any case HIV virions cannot exist in cell-free state in saliva, and estimates are that there is less than

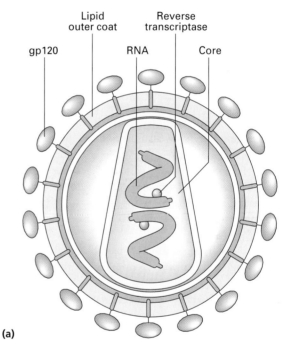

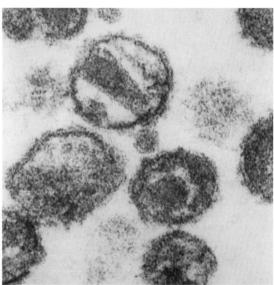

Fig. 30.1 Human immunodeficiency virus: (a) structure; (b) scanning electron micrograph of virions showing the pyramid-shaped central core.

one infectious particle of HIV per millilitre of mixed saliva.

2. Saliva contains IgA group antibodies to HIV proteins (p24, gp120, gp160) which may neutralize the infectivity of the virus and are the basis of salivary kits used for HIV testing in epidemiological studies.

3. Other HIV inhibitory factors in saliva include high-molecular-weight mucins thought to entrap the virus, proline-rich proteins, and a serine protease inhibitor termed **salivary leucocyte protease inhibitor** (SLPI). The latter possibly blocks cell surface receptors needed for entry of HIV into cells.

4. The virus loses its infectivity when exposed to mixed saliva for 30 minutes.

5. Animal studies have shown that it is not possible to transmit HIV by surface application of the virus on the oral mucosa, although it was transmitted in this manner through vaginal mucosa.

6. The dose of HIV required for infection is far higher than that for hepatitis B virus (the risk of acquiring hepatitis B infection from a contaminated needlestick injury is 6–30%, compared with a 0.4% risk of contracting HIV infection).

Epidemiology

The main groups of individuals affected are:

- **Promiscuous individuals**, both **homosexuals** and **heterosexuals**: 75% of all infection has been acquired through sexual intercourse; the current male to female ratio is 3.2 (infections in homosexuals were levelling off due to increased awareness of the disease and safe sex practices, but a recent increase has been reported)
- **injecting drug abusers**: some 10% of infection globally; 26% in the USA
- **persons receiving blood or blood products**: about 1% globally (mainly a problem of the developed world)
- **offspring of infected mothers**: varying transmission rates reported, 10–50%; most infection acquired at birth, with a few in utero and breast-feeding accounting for the rest.

The global pandemic

At the time of writing (December 2001) approximately 40 million persons worldwide have been infected with HIV and some 24 million have succumbed to severe disease (i.e. AIDS); 90% of the latter are living in developing countries, especially in Asia and Africa. The estimated annual increase worldwide is about 20%, but this varies widely in different geographic locales. For instance, the annual increase is about 11% in the Americas, 26% in Africa and 167% in Asia, indicating the staggering explosion of the disease in the latter region. This reflects to a great extent the close link between the disease and the economic, social and cultural issues and taboos in each region.

Currently HIV infection is the leading cause of death in US men aged 25–44 years. In some countries, such as the Ivory Coast, HIV/AIDS is the leading cause of death; and in Uganda, it causes 80% of deaths in adults aged 20–39 years.

ACQUIRED IMMUNE DEFICIENCY SYNDROME

Natural history of the disease

Acquired immune deficiency syndrome is an insidious disease, characterized by **opportunistic infections** (fungal, viral and mycobacterial), **malignancies** (especially Kaposi's sarcoma and lymphomas that may be virally induced) and **auto-immune disorders** (Fig. 30.2).

The average time to development of AIDS is 8–11 years in most adults in the developed world, and much less in the developing world due to aggravating cofactors such as malnutrition and intercurrent infection (e.g. malaria). A few individuals (some 2%) have not developed AIDS despite antibody positivity. Overall, almost half of those diagnosed with AIDS are dead. Untreated, the median survival is about 1 year from the time of diagnosis, and 95% are dead within 5 years.

A significant proportion of individuals (up to 60%) who are infected with HIV produce antibodies within a few weeks, at which time they develop an acute **seroconversion illness** similar to glandular fever. Symptoms of such seroconversion include fever, malaise, rash, oral ulceration and, occasionally, encephalitis and meningitis. In some the disease may then become quiescent and asymptomatic for several years (range 1–15 years or more) for reasons yet unknown. Some of them may have **persistent generalized lymphadenopathy** (PGL) where the enlarged lymph nodes are painless and asymmetrical in distribution and involve submandibular and neck nodes. In the HIV disease classification, patients with these symptoms are categorized as group A (Table 30.1).

Progressive disease leads to other features including fatigue, fever, weight loss, candidiasis, diarrhoea, hairy leukoplakia, herpes zoster and perianal herpes, and these illnesses are sometimes referred to as the **AIDS defining complex**. Patients with these symptoms and signs of progressive illness are categorized as group B.

Finally, a percentage of HIV-infected individuals develop **full-blown AIDS** (from 50% to 70% depending on drug therapy and other associated cofactors; median life expectancy is 18 months). These individuals are in group C. The AIDS-defining conditions are subdivided into opportunistic infections and secondary neoplasms, and include Kaposi's sarcoma,

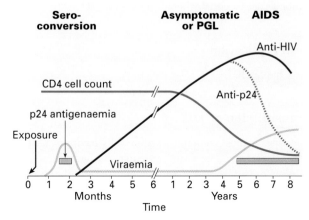

Fig. 30.2 Key events in HIV infection. PGL, persistent generalized lymphadenopathy.

Table 30.2 Opportunistic infections, neoplasms and miscellaneous complications of HIV disease

Opportunistic infections

Mucocutaneous	Human herpesviruses 1, 2, 3, 4, 5, 8
	Human papillomaviruses
	Molluscum contagiosum
	Non-tuberculous mycobacteria
	Candida albicans
	Staphylococcus aureus
	Histoplasmosis
Gastrointestinal	Cryptosporidiosis
	Microsporidiosis
	Isosporiasis
	Giardiasis
Respiratory	*Pneumocystis carinii*
	Aspergillosis
	Candidosis
	Cryptococcosis
	Histoplasmosis
	Zygomycosis (mucormycosis)
	Strongyloidosis
	Mycobacteria including TB
	Staphylococcus aureus
	Streptococcus pneumoniae
	Haemophilus influenzae
	Toxoplasmosis
	Cytomegalovirus (CMV)
Meningitis	Creutzfeldt–Jakob agent
Encephalitis	Papovaviruses
	Cryptococcus neoformans
	Toxoplasma gondii

Neoplasms
Kaposi's sarcoma
Lymphoma
Squamous cell carcinoma
Leukaemia

Miscellaneous
Encephalopathy
Thrombocytopenic purpura
Lupus erythematosus
Seborrhoeic dermatitis

Pneumocystis carinii pneumonia (PCP) and many other exotic infections (Table 30.2).

The CDC disease classification also incorporates **blood CD4 lymphocyte count**, as a decrease in the latter is associated with adverse prognosis (Table 30.1).

Opportunistic infections and neoplasms in AIDS

The opportunistic infections, neoplasms and other features of AIDS and its prodrome are listed in Table 30.2.

Pneumocystis carinii *pneumonia*

This pneumonia is caused by an extracellular protozoan, *Pneumocystis carinii*, which grows slowly in its trophozoite and cyst forms within the lung alveoli. Seen in 80% of patients, it is the immediate cause of death in 20% of those dying with AIDS. It is treated with aerosolized pentamidine.

Toxoplasmosis

Protozoal infection with *Toxoplasma gondii* is seen in 15% of AIDS patients, affecting especially the central nervous system.

Atypical mycobacteriosis

Atypical mycobacteriosis is present in about 40% of patients in the West; caused by *Mycobacterium avium* **complex** (MAC) infections due to mycobacteria such as *Mycobacterium avium* and *Mycobacterium intracellulare*. In some countries up to a quarter of HIV-positive people are infected with *Mycobacterium tuberculosis*, which may be increasingly drug-resistant (MDR-TB: see Ch. 19).

Candidiasis and herpesvirus infections

See below.

Orofacial manifestations of HIV infection

The earliest indicators of HIV infection may manifest in the oral cavity, and some 50 disease entities that may affect the orofacial region of HIV-infected patients have been described. The more common orofacial manifestations of HIV infection are (Table 30.3):

- **fungal infections** — oral candidiasis (erythematous and pseudomembranous variants mainly); linear gingival erythema and angular cheilitis (both are possibly due to mixed bacterial and fungal infections)
- **viral infections** — hairy leukoplakia, Kaposi's sarcoma, herpes infections, papillomas
- **bacterial infections** — gingivitis and periodontitis
- **cervical lymphadenopathy** and **lymphomas** such as non-Hodgkin's lymphomas (not discussed further).

Table 30.3 Oral manifestations of HIV disease

Strongly associated	Less common	Rare
Cervical lymphadenopathy Candidiasis: erythematous pseudomembranous	Herpesviruses: herpes simplex virus varicella–zoster virus cytomegalovirus	Mycobacterial, cryptococcal or histoplasmal ulcers Addisonian pigmentation Osteomyelitis
Hairy leukoplakia	Periodontitis and gingivitis	Cranial neuropathies
Kaposi's sarcoma	Human papillomavirus	Other infections
Recurrent ulcers	Non-Hodgkin's lymphoma Parotitis Xerostomia	

Oral candidiasis

Oral candidiasis (usually erythematous or pseudomembranous candidiasis) is very common in HIV infection, especially at the early stage of the disease; it is a reliable and ominous prognostic indicator of the disease progression to AIDS (the earlier the appearance of oral candidiasis, the worse the prognosis). Oesophageal candidiasis frequently accompanies oral candidiasis and is usually managed by azole drugs, commonly fluconazole. However, azole resistance is increasingly common.

Linear gingival erythema and angular cheilitis are possibly due to mixed fungal and bacterial infections (see Ch. 35).

Viral infections

Viral infections include herpetic stomatitis, herpes zoster, Kaposi's sarcoma and others such as hairy leukoplakia and papillomas of viral origin.

Herpetic stomatitis. A 10% prevalence of herpetic stomatitis in HIV-infected persons has been reported. Herpes simplex infections are mainly intraoral, sometimes extensive and persistent, but rarely disseminate. A minority suffer from herpes zoster and papillomavirus infections. The latter manifest as oral papillomas, warts or condylomata.

Kaposi's sarcoma. Caused by human herpesvirus 8, this is a multifocal systemic tumour due to proliferating microvascular and fibroblastic processes, seen mostly in sexually transmitted HIV infection.

Hairy leukoplakia. This classically appears as an asymptomatic, greyish-white to white, corrugated lesion on the tongue, either unilaterally or bilaterally (Fig. 30.3). The aetiological agent is the Epstein–Barr virus. (*Note*: it is also seen in patients belonging to other risk groups, and uncommonly in healthy individuals.) As more than three-quarters of HIV-infected patients with hairy leukoplakia develop AIDS within 3 years, it is considered to indicate a poor prognosis.

Necrotizing (ulcerative) gingivitis and necrotizing (ulcerative) periodontitis

An unusual type of recalcitrant, aggressive periodontal disease has been identified in those who are infected with HIV. The

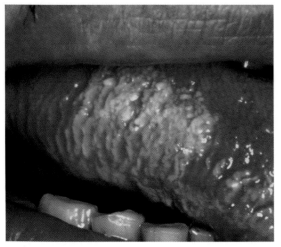

Fig. 30.3 Hairy leukoplakia of the lateral border of the tongue in a patient with AIDS.

disease begins as a form of gingivitis, which mimics acute ulcerative gingivitis. However, it differs from the latter as the disease progresses unceasingly despite routine management protocols such as metronidazole therapy, debridement and scrupulous oral hygiene. The anterior gingiva is most commonly affected. In some patients HIV gingivitis has a very destructive course, leading to periodontitis with loss of soft tissue and bone, sequestrum formation and, in extreme cases, tooth exfoliation.

DIAGNOSIS

History and clinical criteria are of the essence in the provisional diagnosis of HIV infection but laboratory investigations, **after appropriate professional counselling**, are required for confirmation of the disease.

The first step in serodiagnosis is the enzyme-linked immunosorbent assay (ELISA) or agglutination screening tests for serum antibodies. Up to about 2% of the ELISA tests are either false positive or false negative: hence a positive ELISA must be re-tested in duplicate samples. If two or more of the latter three ELISA results are positive, confirmatory testing has to be done by a **western blot assay**. Thus, the principles and ethics of diagnosis are:

1. Apply a minimum of two methodologically different assays.
2. Repeat the test 2–3 months later, as there is a 'window' period between acquisition of infection and the development of antibodies (Fig. 30.2)
3. Do not divulge positive results until confirmed using the strictest criteria. Maintain confidentiality of the results at all times.

MANAGEMENT

A number of antimicrobial agents are used in the management of HIV and its related infections. The two main groups of drugs used to suppress HIV proliferation are:

1. **Reverse transcriptase inhibitors**: these drugs inhibit the reverse transcriptase enzyme of HIV, and are subdivided into:
   - **nucleoside (analogue) reverse transcriptase inhibitors**, including zidovudine (azidothymidine, AZT), the first drug introduced in this category; didanosine (ddI); lamivudine (3TC); stavudine (d4T); and zalcitabine (ddC)
   - **non-nucleoside** reverse transcriptase inhibitors, e.g. nevirapine.
2. **Protease (proteinase) inhibitors**: saquinavir, ritonavir, indinavir and nelfinavir inhibit proteins essential for viral reproduction, such as reverse transcriptase and integrase.

Combination therapy with nucleoside analogues and protease inhibitors is far more effective than monotherapy with individual drugs. However, the side effects and the cost of treatment are both barriers to such 'cocktail' therapy.

A large number of antimicrobial drugs are also used prophylactically to prevent emergence of fungal, bacterial and viral infections, and as therapeutic supportive measures to prolong the quality of life in these patients.

PREVENTION OF HIV INFECTION

- Public education programmes aiming at changing sexual behaviour, especially the use of **barrier contraceptives**, will continue to be the mainstay of HIV prevention into the foreseeable future.
- Free distribution of **sterile needles** to injecting drug abusers has proved useful.
- Transmission in health-care settings can be prevented by appropriate **protective workwear** (see Ch. 37).
- The likelihood of a HIV vaccine becoming available within the next 5 years is low, owing to the rapid rate of virus mutation from one generation to another and also because the virus resides within lymphocytes and other cells, thus evading antibody responses. However, a number of candidate vaccines are undergoing trials and the approach to vaccine development is shown in Figure 30.4.

HIV transmission and dental health-care workers

The risk to dental professionals

A number of prospective surveillance studies indicate that there is no risk of HIV transmission by either saliva or blood in routine dental care. However, accidental injuries via contaminated needles are associated with a very low risk of infection (0.4%). In view of the thousands of infected patients treated since the advent of the AIDS pandemic, it is highly unlikely that the occupational hazard of dentists contracting HIV infection is greater than that for other health-care workers. Additionally, the susceptibility of HIV to many disinfectants, the hygienic environment in most dental surgeries and the use of disposable instruments reduce the risk still further.

The HIV-infected dental health-care worker

The disclosure of possible HIV transmission to five patients by an infected dentist (in Florida, USA) has raised important ethical, moral and legal issues pertaining to continued delivery of dental care by infected dental personnel. (However, the dental transmission route has been questioned and it is believed that the patients acquired the infection from high-risk activities.)

The consensus of professional opinion is that it is the ethical and moral responsibility of dentists who believe that they may be infected with HIV to obtain medical advice and, if found to be infected, to act upon the medical advice, if necessary by modifying the practice of dentistry in some way or by ceasing practice altogether.

INFECTIONS IN COMPROMISED PATIENTS

A **compromised patient** is a person whose **normal defence mechanisms are impaired**, making the individual more susceptible to infection (e.g. individuals with damaged heart valves, diabetes and immunodeficiency states, including AIDS).

Although the majority of compromised patients are hospitalized, a significant proportion are ambulant community-dwellers and likely to seek routine dental care. It is important to note that the drugs and dental treatment provided may interfere with the compromised state and the medications prescribed.

Mechanisms leading to immunocompromised states

Immunodeficiency disease can be either **primary** (developmental or genetically determined), which is rare, or **secondary**, due to procedures such as irradiation and cytotoxic drug therapy.

Primary immunodeficiency

Rarely children are born with congenital deficiency of the immune system. These include deficiencies in B cells, with

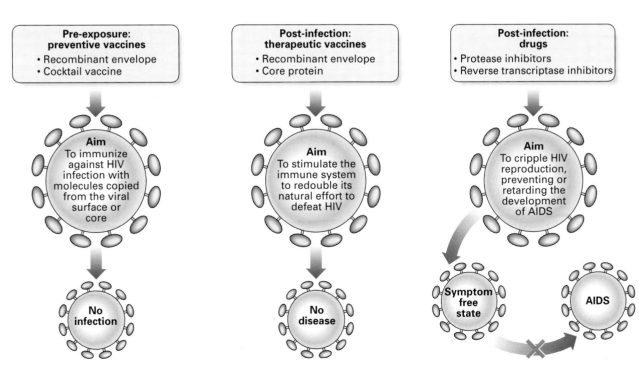

Fig. 30.4 Current approaches to HIV vaccine production and post-infection drug therapy.

Table 30.4   Main causes of secondary immunodeficiency

Drugs
    Methotrexate
    Cytarabine

Malignant disease
    Acute leukaemia
    Hodgkin's disease

Infections
    AIDS
    Severe viral infections

Deficiency states
    Iron deficiency

Autoimmune disease
    Rheumatoid arthritis

Others
    Diabetes mellitus
    Irradiation

depressed immunoglobulin production, T-cell deficiency (e.g. thymic aplasia), combined B-cell and T-cell deficiency, and neutrophil dysfunction.

Secondary immunodeficiency

Secondary immunodeficiency can be due to disease or therapy (Table 30.4).

Disease. Diseases include neoplasms of the **lymphoid system** leading to lymphomas (Hodgkin's disease), leukaemia and multiple myeloma, and — of special interest — **AIDS** due to HIV infection (see above). Other diseases such as **diabetes, renal failure, rheumatoid arthritis** and **autoimmune disease** (e.g. systemic lupus erythematosus) diminish immunity by often complex and incompletely understood mechanisms.

Therapy. Modern medical treatment, especially drugs, radiotherapy and surgical removal of the spleen, may diminish or abolish immune function.

- **drugs**: immunosuppressives, cytotoxic drugs and steroid therapy
- **radiotherapy** is widely used in cancer treatment and is a popular regimen for therapy of head and neck cancer; in addition to the general depressive effect of radiotherapy on immune cells, it has localized effects on salivary glands and oral mucosa leading to **xerostomia** and **mucositis** of the oral mucosa, respectively — the latter results in secondary oral infections
- **splenectomy** results in increased susceptibility to infection with encapsulated bacteria such as *Streptococcus pneumoniae*.

Types of infection

Infection may be caused by **endogenous commensal flora** of low pathogenicity (e.g. oral candidiasis) or **exogenous organisms** acquired from the environment (e.g. drug-resistant hospital staphylococci, MRSAs). Both virulent organisms and even the most harmless commensals may cause life-threatening disease. Some examples are given in Table 30.5.

Oral infections in immunocompromised patients

Important cofactors for oral infection

Cofactors important in oral infection include:
- the duration and depth of immunosuppression
- previous or current antimicrobial treatment (e.g. broad-spectrum antibiotics promote fungal infection)
- the degree of oral hygiene and quality of oral care provided
- the nature of the cytotoxic or immunosuppressive drug used (e.g. methotrexate in particular causes oral ulceration, which may become secondarily infected).

Clinical presentation

The presentation of oral infections varies widely, depending on the cofactors mentioned above. Some conditions are more commonly associated with a particular category of compromised patient than others. For instance, in acute leukaemia the response to dental plaque is exaggerated, leading to gross gingival swelling, but periodontal disease is not a significant

Table 30.5   Examples of organisms that cause infection in compromised patients

Agent	Infection
Bacteria	
Enterobacteriaceae	Urinary tract infection, pneumonia, septicaemia, meningitis
Mycobacterium tuberculosis and other mycobacteria	Tuberculosis, disseminated disease
Staphylococcus aureus	Septicaemia, pneumonia
Streptococcus pneumoniae	Septicaemia
Fungi	
Candida spp.	Thrush, systemic candidiasis, chronic mucocutaneous disease
Cryptococcus neoformans	Meningoencephalitis
Aspergillus and *Mucor* spp.	Disseminated disease
Viruses	
Herpes simplex virus	Severe cold sores
Cytomegalovirus	Pneumonia
Protozoa	
Pneumocystis carinii	Interstitial pneumonia (in AIDS)
Toxoplasma gondii	Severe toxoplasmosis

Table 30.6 Diseases of infective origin seen in different compromised patient populations

Condition	Cytotoxic therapy	Radiotherapy	AIDS	Acute leukaemia
Mucositis	+	+	−	+
Ulceration	+	+	+	+
Xerostomia	+	+	+	−
Sialadenitis	−	+	±	−
Osteomyelitis	+	+	−	−
Candidiasis	+	+	+	+
Herpes infection	+	−	+	+
Periodontal diseases	−	+	+	+
Dental caries	−	+	−	−

problem during cytotoxic therapy. Oral problems encountered in immunocompromised patients are listed in Table 30.6.

Prevention of infection

General guidelines

Surveillance. Careful monitoring of the susceptible individual for signs of infection, is required; if these occur treatment should be instituted without delay.

Antibiotics. Avoid the abuse of antibiotics (particularly broad-spectrum antimicrobials) to minimize emergence of resistant flora.

Isolation. Severely ill patients (e.g. those with neutropenia) should be either isolated in a single room with only nursing staff admitted, or completely isolated (in a laminar air-flow bed or room) and provided with sterilized food.

Specific guidelines

Pretreatment management. Pretreatment management includes:
- a careful assessment of the patient's dental health before radiotherapy or immunosuppressive drugs are used
- appropriate restorative or surgical treatment (e.g. extraction of non-restorable teeth before radiotherapy to prevent osteomyelitis of the mandible)
- oral hygiene instruction and dietary advice (e.g. low-sugar diet, regular fluoride applications).

Management during treatment
- diagnosis and management should be carried out with the assistance of laboratory tests and reports.
- oral management of the patients must be closely linked with the medical treatment and it is essential that the dentist is regarded as part of the medical team.

XEROSTOMIA AND INFECTION

Xerostomia or dry mouth may be the result of:
- ageing
- drugs (e.g. cytotoxic therapy)
- radiotherapy
- Sjögren's syndrome (primary and secondary).

The resulting chronic dryness of the mucosa and the inadequate salivary cleansing mechanism increase the susceptibility of oral tissues to increased incidence of:
- caries
- periodontal diseases
- oral candidiasis
- ascending (bacterial) sialadenitis.

Other non-infective sequelae are difficulty in eating and swallowing dry food, and in wearing complete dentures; burning sensation of the oral mucosa; and changes in the sense of taste (**dysgeusia**).

A reduction or absence of salivary secretion has a profound effect on the composition of the normal oral flora. Reduced moisture levels tend to favour growth of bacteria resistant to drying, such as *Staphylococcus aureus*, and inhibit oral commensals adapted to high moisture levels. In addition, the pH of salivary secretions in these patients is low and the oxygen tension (E_h) is high, which may be unfavourable to the growth of bacteria such as *Veillonella*, commensal *Neisseria* and *Micrococcus* spp. Moreover, this environment favours the growth of *Candida* spp.

Sequelae of chronic xerostomia

Extensive dental caries

Dental caries may occur especially in the cervical and incisal surfaces of teeth and at the margins of dental restorations, sometimes subgingivally.

Prevention. Daily fluoride mouth rinsing, discontinuation of between-meals high-sucrose snacks, careful removal of dental plaque by proper, frequent brushing, and regular dental supervision. Severe caries may be controlled by fluoride application.

Periodontal disease

Periodontal disease, especially gingivitis, is common because of the lack of moisture.

Prevention. Mouthwashes containing 2% chlorhexidine will help control gingivitis and other oral infections.

Candidal infections

Candida-associated denture stomatitis, angular cheilitis and papillary atrophy of the tongue are frequent.

Prevention. See Chapter 35.

Ascending parotitis

Ascending parotitis is the result of the absence or reduced natural flushing action of the salivary flow in Stensen's duct.

Prevention. Treat with antibiotics: empirical therapy with penicillinase-resistant penicillins. Pus should be sent for culture and antibiotic sensitivities. Stimulate salivary secretion with sialagogues; if adequate amounts of saliva cannot be stimulated, use a proprietary saliva substitute.

KEY FACTS

- The **human immunodeficiency virus** (HIV), an enveloped, RNA retrovirus containing the enzyme reverse transcriptase, is the agent of **HIV disease**
- *Not all HIV-infected persons have symptomatic disease; some live a healthy symptom-free life for years*
- *Acquired immune deficiency syndrome (AIDS) is a group of disorders characterized by a profound cell-mediated immunodeficiency consequential to irreversible suppression of T lymphocytes by the HIV and associated with opportunistic infection, malignancies and autoimmune disorders*
- *AIDS-defining illnesses are characterized by a CD4 lymphocyte count below 200 mm², oropharyngeal candidiasis, hairy leukoplakia, etc.*
- Two major subtypes of HIV are known: **HIV-1** is more prevalent than **HIV-2**; both subtypes have similar biological properties
- The structure of HIV is characterized by an envelope containing virus-specific 'coat' proteins (e.g. glycoproteins, gp120); three **core proteins** (e.g. p24); a **genome of RNA**; and two molecules of an enzyme, **reverse transcriptase**
- *HIV is destroyed by heat (autoclave and hot-air oven) and disinfectants (2% glutaraldehyde and hypochlorite)*
- *HIV is transmitted by **blood-to-blood contact, sexual contact** and **perinatally***
- *HIV is unlikely to be transmitted by saliva as it is infrequently present in very low titres in saliva, and salivary IgA and serine protease inhibitors (SLPI) neutralize the virus*

- *Noteworthy opportunistic infections and neoplasms in AIDS include **Pneumocystis carinii pneumonia (PCP)**, toxoplasmosis, atypical mycobacteriosis, candidiasis, herpesvirus infections and Kaposi's sarcoma*
- *The earliest indicators of HIV infection may manifest in the oral cavity, and the more common of these are **oral candidiasis, hairy leukoplakia, Kaposi's sarcoma, recurrent ulcers and cervical lymphadenopathy***
- *Diagnosis of HIV is performed by screening with **ELISA tests** (agglutination test for serum antibodies) and subsequent confirmation by **Western blot assay***
- *The two main groups of drugs used to suppress HIV proliferation are the reverse transcriptase inhibitors (nucleoside and non-nucleoside) and protease inhibitors*
- **Barrier contraceptives** are the mainstay of HIV prevention for the foreseeable future
- A **compromised host** is a person whose normal defence mechanisms are impaired, making the individual more susceptible to infection
- **Immunodeficiency** disease can be either **primary** (developmental or genetically determined), which is rare, or **secondary**, due to procedures such as irradiation and cytotoxic drug therapy
- *The chronic dryness of the mucosa in **xerostomia** leads to caries, periodontal diseases, candidiasis and ascending (bacterial) sialadenitis*

FURTHER READING

BHIVA Guidelines Co-ordinating Committee (1997). British HIV Association guidelines for antiretroviral treatment of HIV seropositive individuals. *Lancet* 349, 1086–1092.

Dalgleish, AG, and Weiss, RA (1994). Human retroviruses. In Zuckerman, AJ, Banatvala, JE, and Pattison, JR (eds) *Principles and practice of clinical virology* (3rd edn), Ch. 24. John Wiley, Chichester.

EC Clearinghouse on Oral Problems Related to HIV Infection and WHO Collaborating Centre on Oral Manifestations of Immunodeficiency Virus (1993). Classification and diagnostic criteria for oral lesions in HIV infection. *Journal of Oral Pathology and Medicine* 22, 289–291.

Friedman-Kien, AE, and Cockerell, CJ (1996). *Color atlas of AIDS* (2nd edn). WB Saunders, Philadelphia.

Kemeny, L, Gyulai, R, Kiss, M, Nagy, F, and Dobozy, A (1997). Kaposi's sarcoma-associated herpesvirus/human herpesvirus-8: a new virus in human pathology. *Journal of the American Academy of Dermatology* 37, 107–113.

Lucht, E, and Nord, CE (1996). Opportunistic oral infections in patients infected with HIV-1. *Reviews in Medical Microbiology* 7, 151–163.

Norwak, MA, and McMichael, AJ (1995). How HIV defeats the immune system. *Scientific American* August, 42–49.

Samaranayake, LP (1991). When the dentist has HIV infection. *Dental Update* 18, 11–13.

Samaranayake, LP (1992). Oral mycoses in human immunodeficiency virus infection: a review. *Oral Surgery, Oral Medicine, Oral Pathology* 73, 171–180.

Samaranayake, LP, and Pindborg, JJ (1989). Hairy leucoplakia. *British Medical Journal* 298, 270–271.

Samaranayake, LP, and Scully, C (1989). Oral candidosis in HIV infection. *Lancet* ii, 1491–1492.

Oral microbiology

Oral and medical microbiology are closely interwoven subjects although the former is usually learnt in the final years of the dental curriculum (in conjunction with dental subjects such as oral medicine). The purpose of this section is to present concisely the many links between these two disciplines in order to give the student a broad, comprehensive view of oral microbiology at an early stage. Most importantly, perhaps, this section will demonstrate to the student the relevance of microbiology to the practice of dentistry.

- Normal oral flora, the oral ecosystem and dental plaque
- Microbiology of dental caries
- Microbiology of periodontal disease
- Dentoalveolar infections
- Oral mucosal and salivary gland infections

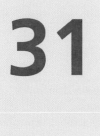

31 Normal oral flora, the oral ecosystem and dental plaque

NORMAL ORAL FLORA

Oral flora comprises a diverse group of organisms and includes bacteria, fungi, mycoplasmas, protozoa and possibly a viral flora which may persist from time to time. Bacteria are by far the predominant group of organisms and there are probably some 350 different cultivable species and a further proportion of unculturable flora, which are currently being identified using molecular techniques. This, together with the fact that the oral cavity has a wide range of sites (habitats) with different environmental conditions, makes the study of oral microbiology complex and difficult. Interestingly, despite the enormous diversity and complexity of the oral flora, many organisms commonly isolated from neighbouring ecosystems such as the gut and skin are not found in the mouth, indicating the unique and selective properties of the oral cavity with regard to microbial colonization.

The main bacterial genera found in the oral cavity are well characterized. Oral bacteria can be classified primarily as Gram-positive and Gram-negative organisms, and secondarily as either anaerobic or facultatively anaerobic according to their oxygen requirements. Some oral microbes are more closely associated with disease than others, while a proportion of the organisms are uncultivable. The following is a synopsis of the major bacterial genera isolated from the oral cavity. The student should refer to the appropriate chapters in Part 3 for detailed information on these organisms.

FLORA OF THE ORAL CAVITY

Gram-positive cocci

Genus Streptococcus

Gram-positive cocci in chains, non-motile, usually possessing surface fibrils, occcasionally capsulate; facultative anaerobes; variable haemolysis but α-haemolysis most common; selective medium: mitis salivarius agar (MSA).

mutans *group*
- **Main species**: *Streptococcus mutans* serotypes *c*, *e*, *f*; *S. sobrinus* serotypes *d*, *g*; *S. cricetus* serotype *a*; *S. rattus* serotype *b*; *S. ferus*; *S. macacae*; *S. downei* serotype *h*.
- **Cultural characteristics**: high, convex, opaque colonies; produce profuse extracellular polysaccharide in sucrose-containing media (Fig. 11.3); selective medium MSA + bacitracin agar.

- **Main intraoral sites and infections**: tooth surface, dental caries.

salivarius *group*
- **Main species**: *Streptococcus salivarius*; *S. vestibularis*.
- **Cultural characteristics**: large, mucoid colonies on MSA due to the production of extracellular fructans (polymer of fructose with a levan structure). *S. vestibularis* do not produce extracellular polysaccharide from sucrose; they produce urease and hydrogen peroxide, which lowers the pH and contributes to the salivary peroxidase system, respectively.
- **Main intraoral sites and infections**: dorsum of tongue and saliva; *S. vestibularis* mainly reside in the vestibular mucosa (hence the name); not a major oral pathogen.

anginosus *group*
- **Main species**: *Streptococcus constellatus*; *S. intermedius*; *S. anginosus.*
- **Cultural characteristics**: CO_2-dependent; form small, non-adherent colonies on MSA.
- **Main intraoral sites and infections**: gingival crevice; dentoalveolar and endodontic infections.

mitis *group*
- **Main species**: *Streptococcus mitis*; *S. sanguis*; *S. gordonii*; *S. oralis*; *S. crista.*
- **Cultural characteristics**: small, rubbery (*S. sanguis*) or non-adherent (*S. oralis* and *S. mitis*) colonies on MSA.
- **Main intraoral sites and infections**: mainly dental plaque; tongue and cheek; dental caries (?); infective endocarditis (except *S. mitis*).

Anaerobic streptococci (genus Peptostreptococcus*)*
- **Main species**: *Peptostreptococcus anaerobius*; *P. micros*; *P. magnus.*
- **Cultural characteristics**: strict anaerobes, slow-growing, usually non-haemolytic.
- **Main intraoral sites and infections**: teeth, especially carious dentine, periodontal and dentoalveolar abscesses in mixed culture.

Genus Stomatococcus
- **Main species**: *Stomatococcus* (formerly *Micrococcus*) *mucilagenosus.*

- **Cultural characteristics**: coagulase-negative; forms large colonies adherent to blood agar surface, facultative anaerobes.
- **Main intraoral sites and infections**: tongue mainly, gingival crevice; not a major opportunist pathogen.

Genera Staphylococcus *and* Micrococcus

See Chapter 11.

Gram-positive rods and filaments

These organisms are common isolates from dental plaque and include actinomycetes, lactobacilli, eubacteria and propionibacteria.

Genus Actinomyces

Short, Gram-positive pleomorphic rods
- **Main species**: *Actinomyces israelii*; *A. gerencseriae*; *A. odontolyticus*; *A. naeslundii* (genospecies 1 and 2); *A. myeri*; *A. georgiae*. The most important human pathogen is *A. israelii*.
- **Cultural characteristics**: ferments glucose to give characteristic patterns of short-chain carboxylic acids useful for speciating; strict or facultative anaerobes.
- **Main intraoral sites and infections**: *Actinomyces odontolyticus*, earliest stages of enamel demineralization, and the progression of small caries lesions appear related; *A. naeslundii* implicated in root surface caries and gingivitis; *A. israelii* is an opportunist pathogen causing cervicofacial and ileocaecal actinomycosis (Ch. 13). *Actinomyces gerencseriae* and *A. georgiae* are minor components of healthy gingival flora.

Genus Lactobacillus

Gram-positive bacilli
- **Main species**: *Lactobacillus casei*; *L. fermentum*; *L. acidophilus* (others include *L. salivarius*, *L. rhamnosus*).
- **Cultural characteristics**: catalase-negative, microaerophilic; complex nutritional requirements; aciduric, optimal pH 5.5–5.8. Selective medium, Rogosa agar.
- **Main intraoral sites and infections**: Common oral inhabitants, but comprise less than 1% of the oral flora. Dental plaque, usually in small numbers; advancing front of dental caries. As levels of salivary lactobacilli correlate well with intake of dietary carbohydrates, they are used to detect the cariogenic potential of the diet.

Genus Eubacterium

Pleomorphic, Gram-variable rods or filaments.
- **Main species**: *Eubacterium brachy*; *E. timidum*; *E. nodatum*; *E. saphenum*.
- **Cultural characteristics**: obligatory anaerobes, characterization ill-defined.
- **Main intraoral sites and infections**: dental plaque and calculus; implicated in caries and periodontal disease; comprise over 50% of the anaerobes of periodontal pockets; *E. yurii* is involved in 'corn-cob' formation in dental plaque (see Fig. 31.2).

Genus Propionibacterium

Gram-positive bacilli.
- **Main species**: *Propionibacterium acnes* (includes *P. propionicus*, formerly *Arachnia propionica*).
- **Cultural characteristics**: strict anaerobe; morphologically indistinguishable from *Actinomyces israelii* but produces propionic acid from glucose, unlike the latter.
- **Main intraoral sites and infections**: root surface caries, dental plaque. Possible involvement in dentoalveolar infections.

Other notable Gram-positive organisms

Rothia dentocariosa, a Gram-positive branching filament, is a strict aerobe, found in plaque and occasionally isolated from infective endocarditis.

Bifidobacterium dentium is a Gram-positive strict anaerobe regularly isolated from plaque; its role in disease is unclear.

Gram-negative cocci

Genus Neisseria

Gram-negative diplococci.
- **Main species**: *Neisseria subflava*; *N. mucosa*; *N. sicca*.
- **Cultural characteristics**: asaccharolytic and non-polysaccharide producing, facultative anaerobes.
- **Main intraoral sites and infections**: isolated in low numbers from tongue, saliva, oral mucosa and early plaque; may consume oxygen in early stages of plaque formation and provide conditions conducive for the growth of anaerobes; rarely associated with disease.

Genus Veillonella

Small, Gram-negative cocci.
- **Main species**: *Veillonella parvula*; *V. dispar*; *V. atypica*.
- **Cultural characteristics**: strict anaerobes; selective medium Rogosa vancomycin agar. Lack glucokinase and fructokinase and hence unable to metabolize carbohydrates; they therefore use lactate produced by other bacteria and raise the pH of plaque, and are thus considered to be beneficial in relation to dental caries.
- **Main intraoral sites and infections**: isolated from most surfaces including the tongue, saliva and dental plaque. No association with disease.

Gram-negative rods — facultative anaerobic and capnophilic genera

Genus Haemophilus

Gram-negative coccobacilli.
- **Main species**: *Haemophilus parainfluenzae*; *H. segnis*; *H. aphrophilus*; *H. haemolyticus*; *H. parahaemolyticus*.
- **Cultural characteristics**: all isolates are facultative anaerobes; growth is enhanced on heated blood agar (chocolate), requires haemin (X factor) and nicotinamide adenine dinucleotide (V factor) for growth.
- **Main intraoral sites and infections**: dental plaque, saliva and mucosae; dentoalveolar infections, acute sialadenitis, infective endocarditis.

Genus Actinobacillus

Gram-negative coccobacilli, microaerophilic or capnophilic (carbon dioxide-dependent).

- **Main species**: *Actinobacillus actinomycetemcomitans* (serotypes a–e).
- **Cultural characteristics**: freshly isolated strains contain fimbriae that are lost on subculture. Produces many virulence factors: leucotoxin, collagenase, protease that cleaves IgG.
- **Main intraoral sites and infections**: periodontal pockets; implicated in aggressive forms of periodontal disease (e.g. localised and generalised aggressive periodontitis).

Genus Eikenella

Gram-negative coccobacilli.

- **Main species**: *Eikenella corrodens*.
- **Cultural characteristics**: factor X-dependent and microaerophilic; produces corroding colonies on blood agar.
- **Main intraoral sites and infections**: dental plaque; dentoalveolar abscesses, infective endocarditis; possibly implicated in some forms of chronic periodontitis.

Genus Capnocytophaga

Carbon dioxide-dependent, Gram-negative fusiform rods with 'gliding' motility.

- **Main species**: *Capnocytophaga gingivalis*; *C. sputigena*; *C. ochracea*; *C. granulosa*; *C. haemolytica*.
- **Cultural characteristics**: capnophilic, medium-sized colonies with an irregular spreading edge.
- **Main intraoral sites and infections**: Plaque, mucosal surfaces, saliva; infections in immunocompromised, destructive periodontal disease? Some strains produce IgA1 protease.

Gram-negative rods — obligate anaerobic genera

These comprise a large proportion of the dental plaque. The classification of this group of organisms is fraught with difficulties, but the advent of new tests such as lipid analysis and molecular approaches have eased the problem to some extent. Most of the oral anaerobes were previously classified under the genus *Bacteroides*. However, advances in taxonomic methods have shown that they belong to two major genera, now termed *Porphyromonas* and *Prevotella*, which differ in their ability to metabolize sugar. Some of these organisms produce characteristic brown-black pigments on blood agar and are referred to collectively as '**black-pigmented anaerobes**'.

Genus Porphyromonas

Gram-negative pleomorphic rods, non-motile; six serotypes based on capsular polysaccharides (K antigen); asaccharolytic.

- **Main species**: *Porphyromonas gingivalis*; *P. endodontalis*; *P. catoniae*.
- **Cultural characteristics**: strict anaerobes, require vitamin K and haemin for growth.
- **Main intraoral sites and infections**: gingival crevice and subgingival plaque in small numbers. Associated with chronic periodontitis and dentoalveolar abscess; *P. gingi-*

valis is highly virulent in experimental infections, producing proteases, a haemolysin, collagen-degrading enzymes and cytotoxic metabolites; its capsule is an important virulent attribute; fimbriae helps adhesion. *Porphyromonas endodontalis* is mainly recovered from infected root canals.

Genus Prevotella

Gram-negative pleomorphic rods, non-motile; moderately asaccharolytic, producing acetic, succinic and other acids from glucose.

- **Main species**: pigmented species include *Prevotella intermedia*; *P. nigrescens*; *P. loeschii*; *P. corporis*; *P. melaninogenica*; Non-pigmented species include *P. buccae*; *P. oralis*; *P. oris*; *P. oulora*; *P. veroralis*; *P. dentalis* (*Bacteroides capillosus* and *B. forsythus* are other non-pigmented species that do not fall within the revised definition of the genus *Bacteroides* and are awaiting classification).
- **Cultural characteristics**: Strict anaerobes, usually require vitamin K and haemin for growth.
- **Main intraoral sites and infections**: periodontal pockets, dental plaque; chronic periodontitis and dentoalveolar abscess.

Genus Fusobacterium

Slender, cigar-shaped Gram-negative rods with rounded ends (see Fig. 18.1).

- **Main species**: *Fusobacterium nucleatum*; *F. alocis*; *F. sulci*; *F. periodonticum*.
- **Cultural characteristics**: require rich media for growth and are often asaccharolytic, strict anaerobes, usually non-haemolytic; *F. nucleatum* can produce ammonia and hydrogen sulphide from cysteine and methionine and is implicated as an odorigenic organism in halitosis.
- **Main intraoral sites and infections**: most common isolate is *F. nucleatum*; normal gingival crevice, tonsils (*F. alocis* and *F. sulci*) or periodontal infections (*F. periodonticum*); acute ulcerative gingivitis, dentoalveolar abscess.

Genus Leptotrichia

Gram-negative filaments with at least one pointed end.

- **Main species**: *Leptotrichia buccalis*.
- **Cultural characteristics**: strict anaerobes, with colonies resembling fusobacteria.
- **Main intraoral sites and infections**: dental plaque. No known disease association.

Genus Wolinella

Gram-negative curved bacilli, motile by polar flagella.

- **Main species**: *Wolinella succinogenes* (*W. recta* and *W. curva* are now assigned to the *Campylobacter* genus).
- **Cultural characteristics**: strict anaerobe.
- **Main intraoral sites and infections**: gingival crevice. Possible involvement in destructive periodontal disease.

Genus Selenomonas

Gram-negative curved cells with tufts of flagella.

- **Main species**: *Selenomonas sputigena*; *S. noxia*; *S. flueggei*; *S. inflexi*; *S. diane*.
- **Cultural characteristics**: strict anaerobe.

- **Main intraoral sites and infections**: gingival crevice. No known disease association.

Genus Treponema

Motile Gram-negative helical cells, in three main sizes (large, medium and small).
- **Main species**: *Treponema denticola*; *T. macrodentium*; *T. skoliodontium*; *T. socranskii*; *T. maltophilum*; *T. amylovarum*; *T. vincentii*.
- **Cultural characteristics**: all treponemes are strict anaerobes, and difficult to culture. Require enriched media with serum. Characterization poor; *T. denticola* is asaccharolytic; *T. socranskii* ferments carbohydrates to acetic, lactic and succinic acids.
- **Main intraoral sites and infections**: *T. denticola* is more proteolytic than others, and possesses proline aminopeptidase and and arginine-specific protease; it also degrades collagen and gelatin. Found in the gingival crevice; closely associated with acute ulcerative gingivitis, destructive periodontal disease.

Oral protozoa

Genus Entamoeba

Large, motile amoebae about 12 μm in diameter.
- **Main species**: *Entamoeba gingivalis*.
- **Cultural characteristics**: strict anaerobe; complex medium; cannot be easily cultured.
- **Main intraoral sites and infections**: periodontal tissues, especially in patients who have received radiotherapy and are on metronidazole. Its role, if any, in periodontal disease is unclear.

Genus Trichomonas

Flagellated protozoa, about 7.5 μm in diameter.
- **Main species**: *Trichomonas tenax*.
- **Cultural characteristics**: strict anaerobe; complex medium; difficult to grow in pure culture.
- **Main intraoral sites and infections**: gingival crevice; its role in disease is unclear.

For mycoplasmal and fungal infections of the oral cavity, please see Chapters 20 and 22, respectively.

THE ORAL ECOSYSTEM

Ecology is the study of the relationships between living organisms and their environment. An understanding of oral ecology is essential to comprehend the pathogenesis of diseases, such as caries and periodontal disease, caused by oral bacteria.

The oral environment

The human mouth is lined by stratified squamous epithelium. This is modified in areas according to function (e.g. the tongue) and interrupted by other structures such as teeth and salivary ducts. The gingival tissues form a cuff around each tooth and there is a continuous exudate of crevicular fluid from the gingival crevice. A thin layer of saliva bathes the surface of the oral mucosa.

The mouth, being an extension of an external body site, has a natural microflora. This **commensal** (or indigenous, or resident) flora exists in harmony with the host, but disease conditions supervene when this relationship is broken. The predominant dental diseases in humans (caries and periodontal disease) are caused in this manner. In addition to the commensal flora there are others (such as coliforms) which survive in the mouth only for short periods (**transient flora**).

The oral ecosystem comprises the oral flora, the different sites of the oral cavity where they grow (i.e. habitats) and the associated surroundings.

Oral habitats

The major oral habitats are:
- buccal mucosa
- dorsum of tongue
- tooth surfaces (both supragingival and subgingival)
- crevicular epithelium
- prosthodontic and orthodontic appliances, if present.

Buccal mucosa and dorsum of tongue. Special features and niches of the oral mucosa contribute to the diversity of the flora; for instance, the cheek mucosa is relatively sparsely colonized, whereas the papillary surface of the tongue is highly colonized because of the safe refuge provided by the papillae. The papillary surface of the tongue has a low redox potential, promoting the growth of anaerobic flora, and thus may serve as a reservoir for some of the Gram-negative anaerobes implicated in periodontal disease. Further, the keratinized and non keratinised mucosae may offer refuge to variants of oral flora.

Teeth. The surfaces of the teeth are the only non-shedding area of the body that harbours a microbial population. Large masses of bacteria and their products accumulate on tooth surfaces to produce dental plaque, present both in health and disease. Plaque is a classic example of a **natural biofilm** and is the major agent initiating caries and periodontal disease. In the latter situations there is a shift in the composition of the plaque flora away from the species that predominate in health (see Chs 32 and 33).

A range of habitats are associated with the tooth surface (Fig. 31.1). The nature of the bacterial community varies depending on the tooth concerned and the degree of exposure to the environment: smooth surfaces are colonized by a

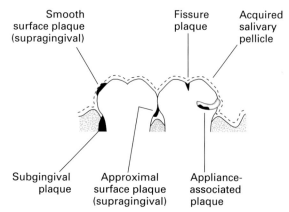

Fig. 31.1 Habitats associated with tooth surfaces and the nomenclature of plaque derived from these habitats.

Table 31.1 Specific and non-specific host defence factors of the mouth

Defence factors	Main function
Non-specific	
Epithelial desquamation	Physical removal of microbes
Saliva flow	Physical removal of microbes
Mucin/agglutinins	Physical removal of microbes
Lysozyme	Cell lysis (bactericidal, fungicidal)
Lactoferrin	Iron sequestration (bactericidal, fungicidal)
Apolactoferrin	Iron sequestration (bactericidal, fungicidal)
Sialoperoxidase system	Hypothiocyanite production (neutral pH); hypocyanous acid production (low pH)
Histidine-rich peptides	Antibacterial and antifungal activity
Salivary leucocyte protease inhibitor	Blocks cell surface receptors needed for entry of HIV
Specific	
Intraepithelial lymphocytes and Langerhans cells	Cellular barrier to penetrating bacteria and/or antigens
Secretory IgA	Prevents microbial adhesion and metabolism
IgG, IgA, IgM	Prevent microbial adhesion; opsonins; complement activators
Complement	Activates neutrophils
Neutrophils/macrophages	Phagocytosis

smaller number of species than pits and fissures; subgingival surfaces are more anaerobic than supragingival surfaces.

Crevicular epithelium and gingival crevice. Although this habitat is only a minor region of the oral environment, bacteria that colonize the crevicular area play a critical role in the initiation and development of gingival and periodontal disease. A vast literature on this subject is available.

Prosthodontic and orthodontic appliances. If present and not kept scrupulously clean, dental appliances may act as inanimate reservoirs of bacteria and yeasts. Yeasts on the fitting surface of full dentures can initiate *Candida*-associated denture stomatitis due to poor denture hygiene.

Factors modulating microbial growth

Different microenvironments in the mouth support their own microflora which differ both qualitatively and quantitatively. The reasons for such variations are complex and include anatomical, salivary, crevicular fluid and microbial factors, among others.

Anatomical factors

Bacterial stagnation areas are created as a result of:
- the shape of the teeth
- the topography of the teeth (e.g. occlusal fissures)
- malalignment of teeth
- poor quality of restorations (e.g. fillings and bridges)
- non-keratinized sulcular epithelium.

These areas are difficult to clean, either by the natural flushing action of saliva or by toothbrushing.

Saliva

Whole (mixed) saliva bathing oral surfaces is derived from the major (parotid, submandibular and sublingual) and minor (labial, lingual, buccal and palatal) salivary glands. It is a complex mixture of inorganic ions including sodium, potas-

sium, calcium, chloride, bicarbonate and phosphate; the concentrations of these ions varies diurnally and in stimulated and resting saliva. The major organic constituents of saliva are proteins and glycoproteins (such as mucin), which modulate bacterial growth (Table 31.1) in the following ways:
- adsorption on the tooth surfaces forms a salivary pellicle, a conditioning film that facilitates bacterial adhesion
- acting as a readily available, primary source of food (carbohydrates and proteins)
- aggregation of bacteria, thereby facilitating their clearance from the mouth, or deposition on surfaces, contributing to plaque formation
- inhibition of the growth of exogenous organisms by non-specific defence factors (e.g. lysozyme, lactoferrin and histatins which are bactericidal and fungicidal) and specific defence factors (e.g. immunoglobulins, mainly IgA)
- maintenance of pH with its excellent buffering capacity (acidic salivas promote growth of cariogenic bacteria).

Gingival crevicular fluid

There is a continuous but slow flow of gingival crevicular fluid in health, and this increases during inflammation (e.g. gingivitis). The composition of crevicular fluid is similar to that of serum and thus the crevice is protected by these 'surrogate' specific and non-specific defence factors of serum. Crevicular fluid can influence the ecology of the crevice by:
- flushing microbes out of the crevice
- acting as a primary source of nutrients: proteolytic and saccharolytic bacteria in the crevice can utilise the crevicular fluid to provide peptides, amino acids and carbohydrates for growth; essential cofactors (e.g. haemin) can be obtained by degrading haem-containing molecules such as haemoglobin
- maintaining pH conditions
- providing specific and non-specific defence factors: IgG predominates (IgM and IgA are both present to a lesser extent)
- phagocytosis: 95% of leucocytes in the crevicular fluid are neutrophils.

Microbial factors

Microbes in the oral environment can interact with each other both in promoting and suppressing the neighbouring bacteria. Mechanisms that accomplish this include:

- competition for receptors for adhesion by prior occupation of colonizing sites and prevention of attachment of 'latecomers'
- production of toxins, such as bacteriocins, that kill cells of the same or other bacterial species; e.g. *Streptococcus salivarius* produces an inhibitor (enocin) that inhibits *S. pyogenes*
- production of metabolic end-products such as short-chain carboxylic acids which lower the pH and also act as noxious, antagonistic agents
- use of metabolic end-products of other bacteria for nutritional purposes (e.g. *Veillonella* spp. use acids produced by *Streptococcus mutans*)
- coaggregation with same species (homotypic) or different species (heterotypic) bacteria, e.g. corn-cob formation (Fig. 31.2).

These mechanisms, which enable the commensal oral flora to suppress or inhibit the growth of exogenous, non-oral organisms and thereby exclude them from their habitat are called **colonization resistance**.

Miscellaneous factors

Local environmental pH. Many microbes require a neutral pH for growth. The acidity of most oral surfaces is regulated by saliva (mean pH 6.7) Depending on the frequency of intake of dietary carbohydrates the pH of plaque can fall to as low as 5.0 as a result of bacterial metabolism. Under these conditions acidophilic bacteria can grow well (e.g. lactobacilli) while others are eliminated by competitive inhibition.

Oxidation–reduction potential. The oxidation–reduction potential of the environment (redox potential or E_h) varies in different locations of the mouth. For instance, redox potential falls during plaque development from an initial E_h of over +200 mV (highly oxidized) to −141 mV (highly reduced) after 7 days. Such fluctuations favour the growth of different groups of bacteria.

Antimicrobial therapy. Systemic or topical antibiotics and antiseptics affect the oral flora; for instance, broad-spectrum antibiotics such as tetracycline can wipe out most of the endogenous flora and favour the emergence of yeast species.

Diet. Fermentable carbohydrates are the main class of compounds that alter the oral ecology. They act as a major source of nutrients, promoting the growth of acidogenic flora. The production of extracellular polysaccharides facilitates adherence of organisms to surfaces, while the intracellular polysaccharides serve as a food resource.

Iatrogenic factors. Procedures such as dental scaling can radically alter the composition of the periodontal pocket flora of diseased sites and shift the balance in favour of colonization of such sites by flora that are associated with health.

Nutrition of oral bacteria

Oral bacteria obtain their food from a number of sources. These include **host resources**:

- remnants of the host diet always present in the oral cavity (e.g. sucrose, starch)
- salivary constituents (e.g. glycoproteins, minerals, vitamins)
- crevicular exudate (e.g. proteins)
- gaseous environment (although most require only a very low level of oxygen)

and **microbial resources**:

- extracellular microbial products of the neighbouring bacteria, especially in dense communities such as plaque
- intracellular food storage (glycogen) granules.

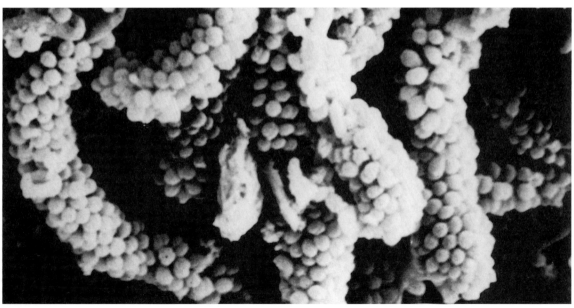

Fig. 31.2 Scanning electron micrograph of supragingival plaque showing corn-cob formation: cocci aggregated around an axial filamentous organism (×5000).

Acquisition of the normal oral flora

1. The infant mouth is sterile at birth, except perhaps for a few organisms acquired from the mother's birth canal.
2. A few hours later the organisms from the mother's (or the nurse's) mouth and possibly a few from the environment are established in the mouth.
3. These **pioneer species** are usually streptococci, which bind to mucosal epithelium (e.g. *Streptococcus salivarius*).
4. The metabolic activity of the pioneer community then alters the oral environment to facilitate colonization by other bacterial genera and species. For instance, *S. salivarius* produces extracellular polymers from sucrose, to which other bacteria such as *Actinomyces* spp. can attach.
5. When the composition of this complex ecosystem (comprising several genera and species in varying numbers) reaches equilibrium, a **climax community** is said to exist. (*Note*: this is a highly dynamic system.)
6. Oral flora on the child's first birthday usually consist of streptococci, staphylococci, neisseriae and lactobacilli, together with some anaerobes such as *Veillonella* and fusobacteria. Less frequently isolated are *Lactobacillus*, *Actinomyces*, *Prevotella* and *Fusobacterium* species.
7. The next evolutionary change in this community occurs during and after tooth eruption when two further niches are provided for bacterial colonization: the hard tissue surface of enamel and the gingival crevice. Organisms that prefer hard-tissue colonization, such as *Streptococcus mutans*, *S. sanguis* and *Actinomyces* spp., then selectively colonize enamel surfaces, and those preferring anaerobic environments, such as *Prevotella* spp., *Porphyromonas* spp. and spirochaetes, colonize the crevicular tissues. However, the anaerobes do not appear in significant numbers until adolescence. For instance, only 18–40% of 5-year-olds have spirochaetes and black-pigmented anaerobes compared with 90% of 13–16-year-olds.
8. A second childhood (in terms of oral bacterial colonization) is reached if all teeth are lost as a result of senility. Bacteria that colonize the mouth at this stage are very similar to those in a child before tooth eruption.
9. Introduction of a prosthetic appliance at this stage changes the microbial composition once again. Growth of *Candida* species is particularly increased after the introduction of acrylic dentures, while it is now recognized that the prevalence of *Staphylococcus aureus* and lactobacilli is high in those aged 70 years or over. The denture plaque is somewhat similar to enamel plaque; it may also harbour significant quantities of yeast.

DENTAL PLAQUE

Dental plaque is a tenacious microbial deposit which forms on the hard-tissue surfaces of the mouth, comprising living, dead and dying bacteria and their products, together with host compounds mainly derived from saliva.

Composition

The organisms in dental plaque are surrounded by an organic matrix which comprises about 30% of the total plaque volume. The matrix is derived from the products of both the host and plaque constituents. In the gingival area, proteins from the crevicular exudate become incorporated into the plaque. This matrix acts as a food reserve and as a cement, binding organisms both to each other and to various surfaces.

The microbial composition of dental plaque can vary widely between individuals; some people are rapid plaque-formers, others slow. Further, there are large variations in plaque composition within an individual, for example:

- at different sites on the same tooth
- at the same site on different teeth
- at different times on the same tooth site.

Distribution

Plaque is found on most dental surfaces in the absence of oral hygiene. In general it is found in anatomical areas protected from the host defences, e.g. occlusal fissures, interproximally or around the gingival crevice. Plaque samples are described in relation to their site of origin and are categorized as **Supragingival**:

- fissure plaque — mainly in molar fissures
- approximal plaque — at contact points of teeth
- smooth surface — e.g. buccal and palatal surfaces,

subgingival, or **appliance-associated**:

- full and partial dentures (denture plaque)
- orthodontic appliance-related plaque.

Microbial adherence and plaque formation

Adherence of a microbe to an oral surface is a prerequisite for colonization and it is the initial step in the path leading to subsequent infection or invasion of tissues. The complex interaction of the factors that prevent microbial colonization on oral surfaces are shown in Figure 31.3.

Dental plaque formation

Plaque formation is a complex process comprising a number of different stages.

1. **Pellicle formation**. Adsorption of host and bacterial molecules to the tooth surface forms the acquired salivary

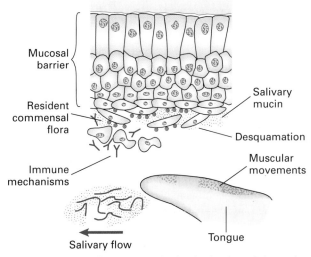

Fig. 31.3 Factors affecting microbial colonization of the oral mucosa.

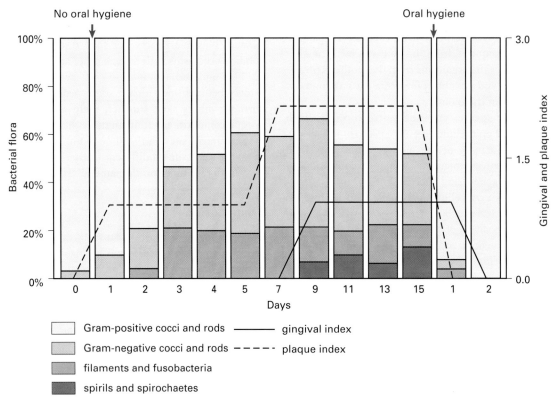

Fig. 31.4 Results from an experimental study showing the predominant groups of organisms comprising the pioneer and the climax community of plaque. Note the relationship between the plaque index and the gingival index.

pellicle. A thin layer of salivary glycoproteins is deposited on the surface of a tooth within minutes of exposure to the oral environment. Oral bacteria initially attach to the pellicle and not directly to enamel (i.e. hydroxyapatite).

2. **Transport.** Bacteria approach the vicinity of the tooth surface prior to attachment, by means of natural salivary flow, Brownian motion or chemotaxis.

3. **Long-range interactions** involve physicochemical interactions between the microbial cell surface and the pellicle-coated tooth. Interplay of van der Waals' forces and electrostatic repulsion produces a reversible phase of net adhesion.

4. **Short-range interactions** consist of stereochemical reactions between adhesins on the microbial cell surface and receptors on the acquired pellicle. This is an irreversible phase in which polymer bridging between organisms and the surface helps to anchor the organism, after which the organisms multiply on the virgin surface. Doubling times of plaque bacteria can vary considerably (from minutes to hours), both between different bacterial species and between members of the same species, depending on the environmental conditions.

5. **Coaggregation or coadhesion**: fresh bacteria now attach on to the already attached first generation of cells; these may be bacteria of the same genus or different but compatible genera.

6. **Biofilm formation**: the above process continues with a resultant confluent growth and the formation of a biofilm, which matures in complexity as time progresses. This is a complex, competitive, sequential and dynamic colonization process by different categories of oral bacteria. Broadly speaking, the **pioneer group** of organisms that selectively colonize the salivary pellicle are Gram-

positive cocci and rods. These are followed by Gram-negative cocci and rods, and finally by filaments, fusobacteria, spirils and spirochaetes. Such an example of a natural succession of plaque flora has been elegantly demonstrated in 'experimental gingivitis' studies where groups of individuals, initially subjected to meticulous oral hygiene, were then followed-up during a phase of no oral hygiene, and the freshly developing plaque flora were monitored closely. Results of such a study are shown in Figure 31.4.

One major component of a biofilm is the extracellular matrix. This comprises microbial polysaccharides and additional layers of salivary glycoprotein (or crevicular fluid components, depending on the site). The metabolic products of the early plaque colonizers can radically alter the immediate environment (e.g. create a low redox potential suitable for anaerobes), leading to new colonizers inhabiting the plaque, with a resultant gradual increase in microbial complexity, biomass and thickness. As a result of this dynamic process the plaque mass reaches a critical size at which a balance between the deposition and loss of plaque bacteria is established; this community is termed the **climax community** (Fig. 31.5).

7. **Detachment**: the bacteria that colonize this climax community may detach and enter the **planktonic** phase (i.e. suspended in saliva) and be transported to new colonization sites, thus restarting the whole cycle.

Calculus formation

Calcium and phosphate ions derived from saliva may become deposited within deeper layers of dental plaque (as saliva is supersaturated with respect to these ions). If the plaque is allowed to grow undisturbed then the degenerating bacteria in a climax community may act as seeding agents of mineralization. The process is accelerated by bacterial phosphatases and proteases that degrade some of the calcification inhibitors in saliva (statherin and proline-rich proteins). These processes lead to the formation of insoluble calcium phosphate crystals which coalesce to form a calcified mass of plaque, termed **calculus**.

Many toothpastes now contain pyrophosphate compounds which adsorb excess calcium ions, thus reducing intraplaque mineral deposition. In general, mature calculus is composed of 80% (dry weight) mineralized material, mostly hydroxyapatite and the remainder (20%) organic compounds.

Structure

The structure of calculus is shown in Figure 31.5. Predominant flora are cocci, bacilli and filaments (especially in the outer layers), and occasionally spiral organisms. The bacteria near the enamel surface tend to have a reduced cytoplasm to cell-wall ratio, suggesting that they are metabolically inactive. Supragingival calculus contains more Gram-positive organisms, while subgingival calculus tends to contain more Gram-negative species.

In some areas (especially the outer surface) cocci attach and grow on the surface of filamentous microorganisms giving a 'corn-cob' arrangement. The filamentous bacteria tend to orient themselves at right angles to the enamel surface, producing a palisade effect (like books on a shelf).

The cytoplasm of some bacteria (mainly cocci) contains glycogen-like food storage granules, available as a ready source of nutrition during periods of adversity.

Calculus has a rough surface and is porous, thus serving as an ideal reservoir for bacterial toxins that are harmful to the periodontium (e.g. lipopolysaccharides). Hence removal of calculus is essential to maintain good periodontal health.

The role of dental plaque in caries and periodontal disease is discussed in Chapters 32 and 33, respectively.

The role of oral flora in systemic infection

Recently it has been recognized that plaque-related oral diseases, especially periodontitis, may alter the course and pathogenesis of a number of systemic diseases. These include:

- Cardiovascular disease:
  - infective endocarditis
  - coronary heart disease: atherosclerosis and myocardial infection
  - stroke
- Bacterial pneumonia
- Diabetes mellitus
- Low birth weight babies.

This is a resurgence of a common belief called '*focal infection theory*' that was popular in the late 19th and early 20th century.

Three mechanisms linking oral infections to secondary systemic disease have been proposed:

- **Metastatic infection**: *microbes gaining entry* into the circulatory system through breaches in the oral vascular barrier as in the case of bacteraemias produced during tooth extractions (see Ch. 24), and resultant disease such as infective endocarditis.
- **Metastatic injury**: *products of bacteria* such as cytolytic enzymes, exotoxins and endotoxins gaining access to the cardiovascular system, in individuals suffering from periodontitis.
- **Metastatic inflammation**: caused by *immunological injury* due to oral organisms. Thus soluble antigens may enter the bloodstream from the oral route, react with circulating specific antibodies and form macromolecular complexes leading to immune mediated disease such as Beçhet's syndrome.

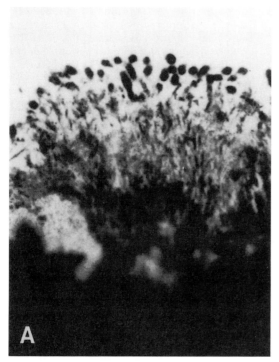
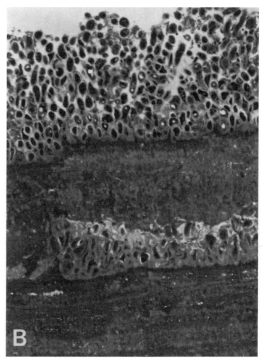

Fig. 31.5 Micrographs of (A) smooth surface plaque showing the many relationships between different bacterial forms, including palisading and corn-cob formation and (B) mature plaque with compact bacteria and calcification at the base (approx. ×5000).

Of these the mechanisms linking oral infection and periodontal disease have been studied the most and the following are now known:

1. Factors that place individuals at high risk for periodontitis may also place them at high risk for systemic disease such as cardiovascular disease. These include tobacco smoking, stress, ageing, race or ethnicity and male gender.
2. Subgingival biofilms: these enormous reservoirs of especially Gram-negative bacteria comprise a continuous source of lipopolysaccharide (LPS, i.e. endotoxins) which induces major vascular responses. Further, LPS upregulates endothelial cell adhesion molecules, and secretion of OL-1 and TNF-∝ etc.
3. Periodontium is a reservoir of cytokines: the pro-inflammatory cytokines TNF-∝ and IL-1β, gamma interferon and prostaglandin E_2 reach high concentrations in periodontitis. Spill over of these mediators into the circulation may induce or aggravate systemic effects.

Apart from the well established link between endocarditis and dental bacteraemias there is no firm evidence to indicate that the other postulated diseases above are either initiated or perpetuated by oral flora and their byproducts. The evidence available is circumstantial at best with a multitude of confounding factors. Therefore further research is necessary to confirm or refute these observations. Nonetheless, it is safe to state that good oral health is important not only to prevent oral disease but also to maintain good general health.

KEY FACTS

- The oral flora comprise a diverse group of organisms and includes bacteria, fungi, mycoplasmas, protozoa and possibly viruses
- There are probably some 350 different **cultivable species** and a further proportion of **unculturable flora**, currently identified using molecular techniques
- Streptococci are the predominant supra-gingival bacteria; they belong to four main **species groups**: *mutans*, *salivarius*, *anginosus* and *mitis*
- The predominant cultivable species in subgingival plaque are *Actinomyces*, *Prevotella*, *Porphyromonas*, *Fusobacterium* and *Veillonella* spp.
- The oral ecosystem comprises the oral flora, the different **sites** of the oral cavity where they grow (i.e. habitats) and the associated **surroundings**
- The major oral habitats are the keratinized and unkeratinized buccal mucosa including the dorsum of the tongue, tooth surfaces, crevicular epithelium, and prosthodontic and orthodontic appliances, if present
- **Adherence** of a microbe to an oral surface is a prerequisite for colonization and is the initial step in the path leading to subsequent infection or invasion of tissues
- Saliva modulates bacterial growth by (a) providing a **pellicle** for bacterial adhesion, (b) acting as a **nutrient source**, (c) **coaggregating** bacteria, (d) providing non-specific (e.g. lysozyme, lactoferrin and histatins) and specific (e.g. mainly IgA) **defence factors**, and (e) maintaining **pH**

- Microbes interact with each other by **competing** for receptors for adhesion, production of **bacteriocins** plus **antagonistic metabolic end-products**, and by **coaggregation**
- Large masses of bacteria and their products accumulate on tooth surfaces to produce dental plaque, present both in health and disease; plaque is an example of a natural **biofilm**
- Stages in the plaque formation are **transport, adhesion/coadhesion** of bacteria leading to **irreversible attachment**, and **colonization**
- *Dental plaque can be defined as a tenacious, complex microbial community, found on tooth surfaces, comprising living, dead and dying bacteria and their products, embedded in a matrix of polymers mainly derived from saliva*
- Recently it has been recognized that plaque-related oral diseases, especially periodontitis, may alter the course and pathogenesis of a number of systemic diseases. These include cardiovascular disease, infective endocarditis, bacterial pneumonia, diabetes mellitus and low birth weight babies. This is known as '**focal infection theory**'
- However, apart from the well-established link between endocarditis and dental bacteraemias there is no firm evidence to indicate that the other postulated diseases above are either initiated or perpetuated by oral flora and their byproducts

FURTHER READING

Bowden, GHW, and Hamilton, IR (1998). Survival of oral bacteria. *Critical Reviews in Oral Biology and Medicine* 9, 54–58.

Edgar, WM, and O'Mullane, DM (eds) (1996). *Saliva and oral health* (2nd edn). British Dental Association, London.

Lang, NP, Mombelli, A, and Attstrom, R (1997). Dental plaque and calculus. In Lindhe, J, Karring, T, and Lang, NP (eds) Clinical periodontology and implant dentistry (3rd edn), Ch. 3. Munksgaard, Copenhagen.

Li, X, Kolltveit, KM, Tronstad, L, Olsen, I (2000). Systemic disease caused by oral infection. *Clinical Microbiology Reviews* 13, 547–558.

Listgarten, MA (1994) The structure of dental plaque. *Periodontology 2000* 5, 52–65.

Marsh, PD, and Martin, MV (1999). *Oral microbiology* (4th edn). Butterworth-Heinemann, London.

Lehner, T (1992). *Immunology of oral diseases* (3rd edn). Blackwell, Oxford.

Samaranayake, LP, and Ellepola, ANB (2000). Studying *Candida albicans* adhesion. In An, Y, and Friedman, RJ (eds) *Handbook of bacterial adhesion: Principles, methods and applications*, pp. 527–540. Humana Press, New York.

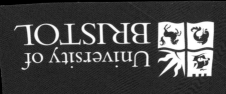
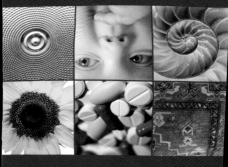

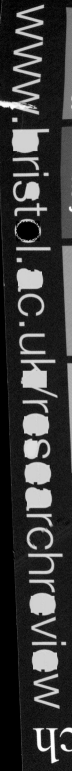

www.bristol.ac.uk/research review

Technology

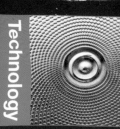

Society

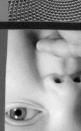

Science

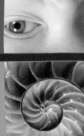

Nature

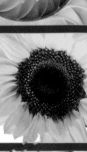

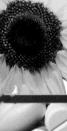

Health

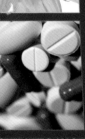

Arts

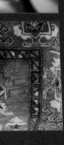

re:search

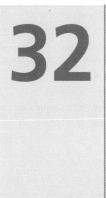

32 Microbiology of dental caries

Dental caries is a chronic endogenous infection caused by the normal oral commensal flora. The carious lesion is the result of demineralization of enamel — and later of dentine — by acids produced by plaque microorganisms as they metabolize dietary carbohydrates. However, the initial process of enamel **demineralization** is usually followed by **remineralization**, and cavitation occurs when the former process overtakes the latter. Once the surface layer of enamel has been lost, the infection invariably progresses to dentine, with the pulp becoming firstly inflamed and then necrotic.

Caries is defined as **localized destruction of the tissues of the tooth by bacterial fermentation of dietary carbohydrates**.

EPIDEMIOLOGY

Dental caries (with periodontal disease) is one of the most common human diseases and affects the vast majority of individuals. Although caries was not uncommon in the developing world, the recent affluence in these regions has resulted in a remarkable upsurge in caries due to the ready and cheap availability of fermentable carbohydrates. In contrast, caries prevalence is falling overall in the developed world due to the increasing awareness of cariogenic food sources and the general improvement in oral hygiene and the dental care delivery systems. Caries of enamel surfaces is particularly common up to the age of 20 years, after which it tends to stabilize. However, in later life, root surface caries becomes increasingly prevalent, due to gingival recession exposing the vulnerable cementum to cariogenic bacteria.

CLASSIFICATION

Dental caries can be classified with respect to the site of the lesion (Fig. 32.1):
- pit or fissure caries (seen in molars, premolars and the lingual surface of maxillary incisors)
- smooth surface caries (seen mainly on approximal tooth surfaces just below the contact point)
- root surface caries (seen on cementum or dentine when the root is exposed to the oral environment)
- recurrent caries (associated with an existing restoration).

CLINICAL PRESENTATION

The primary lesion of caries is a well-demarcated, chalky-white lesion (Fig. 32.2) in which the surface continuity of enamel has not been breached. This 'white spot' lesion can heal or remineralize and this stage of the disease is therefore reversible. However, as the lesion develops, the surface becomes roughened and cavitation occurs. If the lesion is not treated the cavitation spreads into dentine and eventually may destroy the dental pulp, finally leading to the development of a periapical abscess and purulent infection (see Ch. 34).

DIAGNOSIS

Diagnosis is usually by a combination of:
1. **Direct observation**.
2. **Probing**. Some do not advocate probing as this may create an incipient breach of the enamel and spread the infection from one tooth surface to another.
3. **Radiographs**. Early white-spot lesions may easily be missed because they cannot be detected by eye or by radiography. Similarly, it is possible for large carious lesions to develop in pits and fissures with very little clinical evidence of disease.
4. **Experimental methods**. Methods of potential practical value include laser fluorescence for diagnosis of buccal and lingual caries, and electrical impedance (resistance) to detect occlusal caries.
5. **Microbiological tests** may be helpful in the assessment of caries (see below).

AETIOLOGY

The major factors involved in the aetiology of caries (Fig. 32.3) are:
- host factors (tooth, saliva)
- diet (mainly the intake of fermentable carbohydrates)
- plaque microorganisms (i.e. supragingival plaque).

Host factors

Tooth structure

The structure of enamel, and of dentine in root caries, is important: some areas of the same tooth are much more 217

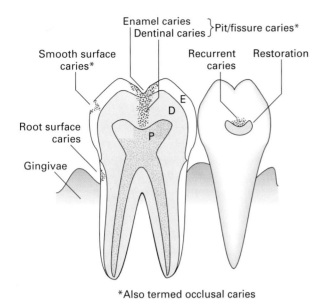

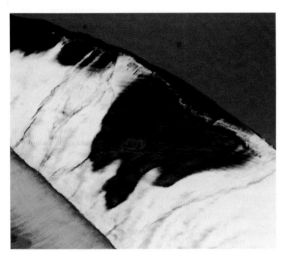

Fig. 32.1 Nomenclature of dental caries. D, dentine; E, enamel; P, pulp.

Fig. 32.2 Polarized light microscopic appearance of early enamel caries (ground section). The cone shaped body of demineralization is evident.

susceptible to carious attack than others, possibly because of differences in mineral content (especially fluoride).

Flow rate and composition of saliva

The **mechanical washing action** of saliva is a very effective mechanism in the removal of food debris and unattached oral microorganisms. It has a high **buffering capacity** which tends to neutralize acids produced by plaque bacteria on tooth surfaces, and it is supersaturated with **calcium** and **phosphorus ions**, which are important in the remineralization of white-spot lesions. Saliva also acts as a delivery vehicle for fluoride.

Diet

There is a direct relationship between dental caries and the intake of carbohydrates. The most cariogenic sugar is sucrose, and the evidence for its central role in the initiation of dental caries includes:

- increases in the caries prevalence of isolated populations with the introduction of sucrose-rich diets
- clinical association studies
- short-term experiments in human volunteers using sucrose rinses
- experimental animal studies.

Sucrose is highly soluble and diffuses easily into dental plaque, acting as a substrate for the production of extracellular polysaccharides and acids. Cariogenic streptococci produce water-insoluble **glucan** from sucrose, which in additon to facilitating **initial adhesion** of the organisms to the tooth surface serve as a **nutritional source** and a **matrix** for further plaque development. The relationship between sucrose and dental caries is complex and cannot be simply explained by the total amount of sugar consumed. The frequency of sugar intake rather than the total amount of sugar consumed appears to be of decisive importance. Also relevant are the **stickiness** and **concentration** of the sucrose consumed, both factors influencing the period for which sugar is retained in close contact with the enamel surface.

Carbohydrates other than sucrose, e.g. glucose and fructose, are also cariogenic, but less so than sucrose. Polyol carbohydrates, 'sugar alcohols' (e.g. xylitol), with low cariogenicity have been produced and are sought after as sugar substitutes in products such as chewing-gum and baby foods.

Microbiology

Microorganisms in the form of dental plaque are a prerequisite for development of dental caries. The different types of plaque and the factors involved in their development are described in Chapter 31.

Specific and non-specific plaque hypothesis

Although *mutans* streptococci have been recognized as the major group of organisms involved in caries, there is some controversy as to whether one or more specific groups of bac-

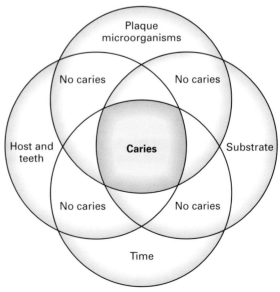

Fig. 32.3 Interplay of major aetiologic factors in dental caries (all four factors must act simultaneously for caries to occur).

teria are principally involved in caries — the **specific plaque hypothesis** — or the disease is caused by a heterogeneous mixture of non-specific bacteria — the **non-specific plaque hypothesis**.

There is conflicting opinion for and against the specific plaque hypothesis:

- *mutans* streptococci are involved in the initiation of almost all carious lesions in enamel
- *mutans* streptococci are important, but not essential
- the association of *mutans* streptococci and caries is weak and no greater than for other bacteria.

Given the extreme variation in the composition of supragingival plaque from the same site in the same mouth at different times, it is unlikely that the initiation and progression of all carious lesions are associated with specific organisms such as *Streptococcus mutans*. Further, other plaque bacteria also possess some of the biochemical characteristics thought to be important in cariogenicity. Therefore it seems likely that combinations of bacteria other than *mutans* streptococci and lactobacilli may be able to initiate carious lesions, and the plaque flora may be non-specific in nature. The current evidence implies that some bacteria (*mutans* streptococci, *Lactobacillus* spp. and *Actinomyces* spp.) may be more important than others in the initial as well as subsequent events leading to both enamel and root surface caries.

The role of mutans *streptococci*

There is a vast literature on the role of the *mutans* streptococci in caries. '*Streptococcus mutans*' is a loosely applied group name for a collection of seven different species (*S. mutans*, *S. sobrinus*, *S. cricetus*, *S. ferus*, *S. rattus*, *S. macacae* and *S. downei*) and eight serotypes (a–h). *Streptococcus mutans* serotypes c, e, f and *S. sobrinus* serotypes d, g are the species most commonly found in humans, with serotype c strains being most prevalent, followed by d and e. The others are rarely encountered. The evidence for the aetiological role of *mutans* streptococci in dental caries includes the following:

- correlations of *mutans* streptococci counts in saliva and plaque with the prevalence and incidence of caries
- *mutans* streptococci can often be isolated from the tooth surface immediately before development of caries
- positive correlation between the progression of carious lesions and '*S. mutans*' counts
- production of extracellular polysaccharides from sucrose (which help to cement the plaque organisms together and to the tooth surface)
- most effective streptococcus in caries studies in animals (rodents and non-human primates)
- ability to initiate and maintain microbial growth and to continue acid production at low pH values
- rapid metabolism of sugars to lactic and other organic acids
- ability to attain the critical pH for enamel demineralization more rapidly than other common plaque bacteria
- ability to produce intracellular polysaccharides (IPS) as glycogen, which may act as a food store for use when dietary carbohydrates are low
- immunization of animals with specific *S. mutans* serotypes significantly reduces the incidence of caries.

Note: not all strains of *mutans* streptococci possess all of the above properties, thus some strains are more cariogenic than

others. Caries may therefore be an infectious disease in a minority, with a highly pathogenic strain being transmitted from one individual to another. Despite this apparently strong relationship between *S. mutans* and caries, a number of longitudinal studies in children have failed to find such a strong correlation.

The role of lactobacilli

Lactobacilli were previously believed to be the causative agents of dental caries. They were considered to be candidate organisms for caries because of:

- their high numbers in most carious lesions affecting enamel (many studies have now shown its high prevalence in root surface caries too)
- the positive correlation between their numbers in plaque and saliva and caries activity
- their ability to grow in low pH environments (below pH 5) and to produce lactic acid
- their ability to synthesize both extracellular and intracellular polysaccharides from sucrose
- the ability of some strains to produce caries in gnotobiotic (germ-free) rats
- the fact that their numbers in dental plaque derived from healthy sites are usually low.

On the negative side, however, lactobacilli are rarely isolated from plaque before the development of caries and they are often absent from incipient lesions.

Although the role of lactobacilli in the carious process is not well defined, it is believed that:

- they are involved more in the progression of the deep enamel lesion (rather than the initiation)
- they are the pioneer organisms in the advancing front of the carious process, especially in dentine.

The role of Actinomyces *spp.*

Actinomyces spp. are associated with the development of root surface caries (root lesions differ from enamel caries in that the calcified tissues are softened without obvious cavitation). The evidence for the involvement of *A. viscosus* in root surface caries is based on:

- association studies in vivo
- in vitro experimental work with pure cultures
- experimental work in gnotobiotic rodents.

Despite the fact that *Actinomyces* spp. (especially *A. viscosus*) predominate in the majority of plaque samples taken from root surface lesions, some studies have reported both *mutans* streptococci and *Lactobacillus* spp. in these lesions. Furthermore, the sites from which these organisms were isolated appeared to have a higher risk of developing root surface caries than other sites. The role of *Actinomyces* spp. in caries is therefore not clear.

The role of Veillonella

Veillonella is a Gram-negative anaerobic coccus which is present in significant numbers in most supragingival plaque samples. As *Veillonella* spp. require lactate for growth, but are unable to metabolize normal dietary carbohydrates, they use lactate produced by other microorganisms and convert it into a range of weaker and probably less cariogenic organic acids, e.g. propionic acid. Hence this organism may have a **beneficial effect** on dental caries. This protective effect has been demonstrated in vitro and in animal experiments, but not in humans.

Plaque metabolism and dental caries

Plaque metabolism is a complex subject and the following is a very simplified account.

The main source of nutrition for oral bacteria is saliva. Although the carbohydrate content of saliva is generally low, increased levels (up to 1000-fold) are seen after a meal. To make use of these transient increases in food levels, oral bacteria have developed a number of regulatory mechanisms which act at three levels:

- transport of sugar into the organisms
- the glycolytic pathway
- conversion of pyruvate into metabolic end-products.

The bacterial metabolism of carbohydrate is critical in the aetiology of caries as the acidic end-products are responsible for enamel demineralization. The process begins when dietary sucrose is broken down by bacterial extracellular enzymes such as glucosyl and fructosyl transferases, with the release of glucose and fructose, respectively. These monosaccharides are then converted into polysaccharides that are either water-soluble or water-insoluble — glucans and fructans, respectively. Glucans are mostly used as a major bacterial food source; the insoluble fructans contribute to the plaque matrix while facilitating the adhesion and aggregation of plaque bacteria and serving as a ready, extracellular food source. Some of the sucrose is transported directly into bacteria as the disaccharide or disaccharide phosphate, which is metabolized intracellularly by invertase or sucrose phosphate hydrolase into glucose and fructose. During glycolysis, glucose is degraded immediately by bacteria via the Embden–Meyerhof pathway, with the production of two pyruvate molecules from each molecule of glucose. The pyruvate can be degraded further:

1. Under low sugar conditions pyruvate is converted into ethanol, acetate and formate (mainly by *mutans* streptococci).
2. In sugar excess, pyruvate is converted into lactate molecules.

Different species produce acids at different rates and vary in their ability to survive under such conditions. *Mutans* group streptococci, being the most acidogenic, and aciduric, are the worst offenders, and reduce the plaque pH to low levels, creating hostile conditions for other plaque bacteria. The resultant overall fall in pH to levels below 5.5 initiates the process of enamel demineralization. This characteristic fall in plaque pH, followed by a slow return to the original value in about an hour, produces a curve that is termed the 'Stephan curve'.

Ecological plaque hypothesis

A key feature of a number of caries studies is the absence of *mutans* streptococci at caries sites, suggesting that bacteria other than the latter can contribute to the disease process. Conversely, in some studies where *mutans* streptococci were found in high numbers, there was apparently no demineralization of the underlying enamel. This may be due to the presence of lactate-consuming species such as *Veillonella*, or to the production of alkali at low pH by organisms such as *Streptococcus salivarius* and *S. sanguis*. These and other related findings have led to the development of the 'ecological plaque hypothesis' of caries (Fig. 32.4). According to this proposal, cariogenic flora found in natural plaque are weakly competitive and comprise only a minority of the total community. With a conventional diet, levels of such potential cariogenic bacteria are clinically insignificant, and the processes of remineralization and demineralization are in equilibrium. If, however, the frequency of intake of fermentable carbohydrates increases, then the plaque pH level falls and remains low for prolonged periods, promoting the growth of acid-tolerant (aciduric) bacteria while gradually eliminating the communal bacteria that are acid-labile. Prolonged low pH conditions also initiate demineralization. This process would turn the balance in the plaque community in favour of *mutans* streptococci and lactobacilli. The hypothesis also explains to some extent the dynamic relationship between the bacteria and the host, so that alterations in major host factors such as salivary flow on plaque development can be taken into account.

MANAGEMENT OF DENTAL CARIES

The conventional approach to the treatment of dental caries was to remove and replace diseased tissue with an inert restoration. This approach made no attempt to cure the disease and the patient often returned some months later requiring further fillings due to new or recurrent caries. In contrast, the modern philosophy in caries management highlights:

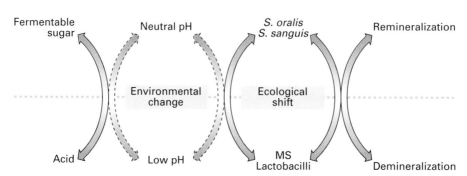

Fig. 32.4 Ecological plaque hypothesis. MS, *mutans* streptococci.

- early detection
- the importance of accurate diagnosis
- minimal cavity preparation techniques
- active prevention.

The result of such measures should be less, rather than more, demand for restorative treatment by individual patients.

Patient evaluation

In patients with a low incidence of caries, a case history and clinical and radiographical examination are probably adequate for treatment planning. However, for patients with rampant or recurrent caries, or where expensive crown and bridge work is planned, additional investigations are necessary. These include:
- assessment of dietary habits
- determination of salivary flow rate and buffering capacity
- microbiological analysis (discussed below).

Microbiological tests in caries assessment

Saliva samples can be used to establish the numbers of *Streptococcus mutans* and *Lactobacillus* spp. in the oral cavity, as follows.
1. A paraffin wax-stimulated sample of mixed saliva is collected.
2. In the laboratory the saliva is appropriately diluted and cultured on selective media (mitis salivarius bacitracin agar for *S. mutans*; Rogosa SL agar for *Lactobacillus* spp.).
3. The number of typical colonies (colony forming units or CFU) are then quantified and extrapolated to obtain the count per millilitre of saliva:
   - high caries activity: $> 10^6$/mL *S. mutans* and/or $> 100\,000$/mL *Lactobacillus* spp.
   - low caries activity: $< 100\,000$/mL *S. mutans* and $< 10\,000$/mL *Lactobacillus* spp.

Simplified detection kits for estimation of both lactobacilli and *S. mutans* in saliva are available. The results correlate well with laboratory plate counts, and the tests can be performed in the dental clinic without special facilities (Fig. 32.5).

The presence of high salivary levels of *S. mutans* or lactobacilli does not necessarily mean that the patient has an increased risk of developing dental caries, as it is a disease of multifactorial aetiology. Other factors, such as diet, buffering capacity, fluoride content of enamel and degree of oral hygiene, should also be considered. Further, the presence of large numbers of cariogenic organisms in saliva does not imply that all teeth are caries-prone, as the salivary organisms may have originated from a few foci with high caries activity. Therefore these tests at best give a generalized approximation of the caries risk. It should be noted that the microbiological tests used in caries assessment differ from conventional tests used in medical microbiology, where the presence of a pathogen indicates a positive diagnosis (e.g. syphilis). The main uses of microbiology tests in caries assessment are:
- to identify patients who have unusually high numbers of potential pathogens, so that these data can be taken into account when integrating all the factors that may contribute to the carious process in an individual patient
- to monitor the efficacy of caries prevention techniques, such as dietary and oral hygiene advice and the use of antimicrobial agents such as chlorhexidine.

Microbiology of root surface caries

Approximately 60% of individuals in the West aged 60 years or older now have root caries. This has arisen mainly because of the reduction in enamel caries and the consequential retention of teeth later into life, accompanied by gingival recession. The soft cemental surfaces thus exposed are highly susceptible to microbial colonization by virtue of their irregular and rough surfaces.

Early studies showed a high prevalence of *Actinomyces naeslundii*, *A. odontolyticus* and *Rothia dentocariosa* from human root surface caries. However, more recent data suggest a stronger association between lactobacilli, *mutans* streptococci and root caries. Indeed, the presence of lactobacilli is considered to be predictive of subsequent development of such lesions. The latter organisms, together with pleomorphic Gram-positive rods, are also frequent in the deeper dentinal parts of the lesion. The current information available suggests:
- a polymicrobial aetiology for caries initiation on root surfaces
- bacterial succession during the progression of the lesion.

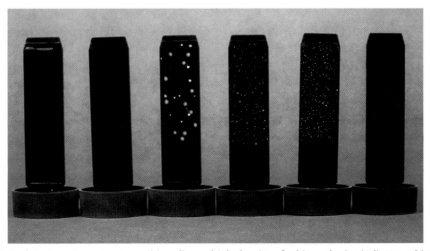

Fig. 32.5 Dip slide test to detect *mutans* streptococci in saliva: a high density of white colonies indicates a higher caries risk.

Prevention of dental caries

The major approaches to prevention of caries are:
- stopping or reducing between-meal consumption of carbohydrates, or substituting non-cariogenic artificial sweeteners (**sugar substitutes**), e.g. sorbitol, xylitol or lycasin
- making the tooth structure less soluble to acid attack by using **fluorides**
- using **sealants** to protect susceptible areas of the tooth (e.g. pits and fissures) that cannot easily be kept plaque-free by routine oral hygiene measures
- **reducing cariogenic flora** so that even in the presence of sucrose, acid production will be minimal (e.g. oral hygiene aids, antimicrobial agents and possibly immunization)
- **replacement** of cariogenic bacteria by organisms with low or no cariogenic potential.

The rationale for these procedures is outlined below.

Sugar substitutes

Artificial sweeteners or sugar substitutes cannot be absorbed and metabolized to produce acids by the vast majority of plaque bacteria. Two types of sugar substitutes are available:
- **nutritive sweeteners** with a calorific value, e.g. the sugar alcohols, sorbitol and xylitol, and lycasin (prepared from cornstarch syrup)
- **non-nutritive sweeteners**, e.g. saccharin and aspartame.

Fluoridation

Fluoride can be delivered to the tooth tissue in many ways. When administered systemically during childhood it is incorporated during amelogenesis. The best delivery vehicle is the domestic water supply (at a concentration of 1 part per million); failing this, tablets, topical applications of fluoridated gel or fluoridated toothpaste may be used.

Fluoride ions exert their anticariogenic effect by:
1. **Substitution** of the hydroxyl groups in hydroxyapatite and formation of fluoroapatite, which is less soluble in acid during amelogenesis.
2. Promotion of **remineralization** of early carious lesions in enamel and dentine.
3. Modulation of plaque metabolism by:
   - interference with bacterial membrane permeability
   - reduced glycolysis
   - inactivation of key metabolic enzymes by acidifying the cell interior
   - inhibition of the synthesis of intracellular polysaccharides, especially glycogen.

Fissure sealants

Sealants prevent caries in pits and fissures by eliminating stagnation areas and blocking potential routes of infection. Early lesions that are well sealed can be effectively arrested by this technique, whereas more extensive lesions may extend into pulp, as the trapped cariogenic bacteria are able to use the carious dentinal matrix as a source of nutrition.

Control of cariogenic plaque flora

Control may be achieved by mechanical cleansing, antimicrobial therapy, immunization and replacement therapy.

Mechanical cleansing techniques. Conventional toothbrushing with a fluoridated toothpaste is not very successful in reducing the caries incidence as it is entirely dependent on the motivation and skill of the patient. Further, it is unlikely that mechanical cleansing even with flossing, interdental brushes and wood sticks will affect pit and fissure caries.

Antimicrobial agents. Chlorhexidine as a 0.2% mouthwash is by far the most effective antimicrobial in plaque control.
1. Chlorhexidine disrupts the cell membrane and the cell wall permeability of many Gram-positive and Gram-negative bacteria.
2. It is able to bind tenaciously to oral surfaces and is slowly released into saliva.
3. It interferes with the adherence of plaque-forming bacteria, thus reducing the rate of plaque accumulation.
4. Compared with other bacteria involved in plaque formation, *mutans* streptococci are exquisitely sensitive to chlorhexidine, and are therefore preferentially destroyed.

Unfortunately, because of the problems of tooth staining and unpleasant taste, chlorhexidine is normally used only for short-term therapy.

Active immunization against dental caries. Using either **cell wall-associated antigens** (antigen I/II) or **glucosyltransferases** (extracellular enzymes) from *mutans* streptococci is effective in reducing experimental dental caries in rats and monkeys. The vaccine may produce its protective effect by:
- inhibition of the microbial colonization of enamel by secretory IgA
- interference with bacterial metabolism
- enhancement of phagocytic activity in the gingival crevice area due to the opsonization of *mutans* streptococci with IgA or IgG antibodies.

However, convincing proof that any of these mechanisms prevent the development of dental caries in vivo is lacking. Vaccination trials on humans have been unsuccessful because of fears of possible side effects, which would be unacceptable as caries is not a life-threatening disease. (The antibodies that develop after immunization with most antigens of *S. mutans* tend to cross-react with heart tissue, and the possibility that heart damage could result has made human vaccine trials very difficult.) Furthermore, the incidence of dental caries is falling in the West and the disease can be adequately controlled using other techniques.

A caries vaccine could, however, be useful for developing countries with limited dental services and increasing prevalence of caries, and also for prevention of disease in high-risk groups, for instance children with mental or physical disabilities.

Passive immunization. Experimental studies indicate that when the natural levels of oral *mutans* streptococci are suppressed by chlorhexidine, topical application of monoclonal antibodies against antigen I/II of *mutans* streptococci prevents recolonization by the organisms. Transgenic plants could be used to produce dimeric antibodies with specificity to antigen I/II of streptococci that are stable in the mouth and persist for longer periods than the monomeric antibody. These new developments have heightened the hopes of an alternative caries preventive strategy for the future.

Replacement therapy

Experimental studies indicate that genetically engineered, low-virulence mutants of *mutans* streptococci that are deficient in glucosyl transferase or deficient in lactate dehydrogenase activity can be 'seeded' into the oral environment. These organisms can replace their more virulent counterparts and prevent their re-emergence. It is feasible that replacement therapy of this nature may be exploited to control cariogenic flora in the future. However, assurances of the safety of these replacement strains are needed both by the public and the authorities before these methods are realized.

KEY FACTS

- **Caries** is defined as localized destruction of the tissues of the tooth by bacterial fermentation of dietary carbohydrates

- *Dental caries is a multifactorial, plaque-related chronic infection of the enamel, cementum or dentine*

- **Key factors** in the development of tooth caries are the **host** (susceptible tooth surface and saliva), plaque **bacteria**, and **diet** (mainly fermentable carbohydrates)

- The **initial caries lesion** is the **'white spot'** created by the demineralization of enamel; this is reversible and can be remineralized; cavitation represents irreversible disease

- The **specific plaque hypothesis** postulates that *mutans* streptococci are important in caries initiation, while heterogeneous groups of bacteria are implicated in the **non-specific plaque hypothesis**

- *Lactobacilli are implicated in the progression of caries, especially in the advancing front of the carious lesions (dentinal interface)*

- The properties of cariogenic flora that correlate with their pathogenicity are the ability to rapidly metabolize sugars to acids (**acidogenicity**), survive and grow under low pH conditions (**aciduricity**), ability to synthesize extracellular and intracellular polysaccharides

- *Strategies to control or prevent caries include: sugar substitutes, fluoridation (to increase enamel hardness mainly), fissure sealants and control of cariogenic flora (by antimicrobials, vaccination or passive immunization, or replacement therapy)*

- **Microbiologic tests** should be undertaken to identify **caries risk** factors in patients with extensive or recurrent caries, prior to delivering dental care (e.g extensive crown and bridge treatment)

- High **salivary or plaque counts** of *mutans* streptococci ($> 10^6$/mL) and lactobacilli ($> 10\,000$/mL) indicate high risk of disease

FURTHER READING

Bowden, GHW (1990). Microbiology of root surface caries. *Journal of Dental Research* 69, 1205–1210.

Bowen, WH, and Tabak, LA (eds) (1993). *Cariology for the nineties.* University of Rochester Press, New York.

Fejerskov, O, Ekstrand, J, and Burt, BA (eds) (1996). *Fluoride in dentistry* (2nd edn). Munksgaard, Copenhagen.

Kidd, EAM, and Joyston-Bechal, S (1996). *Essentials of dental caries* (2nd edn). Oxford University Press, Oxford.

Marsh, PD, and Marin, MV (1999). *Oral microbiology* (4th edn). Butterworth-Heinemann, London.

Russell, RRB (1994). The application of molecular genetics to the microbiology of dental caries. *Caries Research* 28, 69–82.

Tanzer, JM (1992). Microbiology of dental caries. In Slots, J, and Taubman, MA (eds) *Contemporary oral microbiology and immunology*, Ch. 22. Mosby Year Book, St Louis.

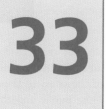

33 Microbiology of periodontal disease

Periodontal diseases can be defined as disorders of supporting structures of the teeth, including the gingivae, periodontal ligament and supporting alveolar bone. Everyone suffers from periodontal disease at some point, and it is one of the major diseases afflicting humankind. However, in most people the common chronic inflammatory diseases involving the periodontal tissues can be controlled, using mechanical cleansing techniques and good oral hygiene. A minority experience rapid progressive disease which requires assessment and management by **periodontologists**.

CLASSIFICATION OF PERIODONTAL DISEASE

Periodontal disease can be broadly categorized into **gingivitis** and **periodontitis**. These are yet again subdivided into numerous categories; a recent classification of periodontal diseases is given in Table 33.1. It should be noted that there is no universally acknowledged classification of periodontal disease and the clinical descriptors used relate to:

- the rate of disease progress (e.g. chronic, aggressive)
- lesion distribution (e.g. localized, generalized)
- age group of the person (e.g. prepubertal, juvenile, adult)
- association with systemic or developmental disorders.

Periodontitis usually develops from a pre-existing gingivitis; however, not *every* case of gingivitis develops into periodontitis.

ECOLOGY OF THE GINGIVAL CREVICE AND THE PERIODONTAL POCKET

The healthy gingival crevice is a unique environment. It is more anaerobic than most locales of the mouth and is constantly bathed by the gingival crevicular fluid (GCF) and its humoral and cellular defence factors including polymorphs. Dramatic changes ensue during the transition of the crevice into a periodontal pocket. The E_h falls further and becomes highly anaerobic and the flow of GCF increases. The mostly proteolytic bacteria living in the periodontal pocket raise the pH to alkaline levels (pH 7.4–7.8; compared to neutral values in health) which in turn promotes the growth of bacteria such as *Porphyromonas gingivalis*.

The exposed cemental surface of the tooth is first colonized mainly by streptococci and *Actinomyces* spp. Secondary colonizers such as *Prevotella* and *Porphyromonas* spp. can adhere to this layer of cells by coaggregation. Others such as *Peptococcus micros* can adhere to the crevicular epithelium. Thus the inhabitants and the ecology of a deep periodontal pocket are markedly different to that of the gingival crevice.

AETIOLOGICAL FACTORS

The main aetiological factors of periodontal diseases are:

- the host tissues
- specific and non-specific host defence mechanisms
- microorganisms in subgingival plaque.

Host tissues

The periodontium comprises the gingivae, periodontal ligament, cementum and alveolar bone (Fig. 33.1). Although the dentogingival junction is perhaps the most vulnerable site for microbial attack, it is not breached as long as oral hygiene is satisfactory. However, when plaque accumulates close to the gingival margin, the host defences are overcome and gingival inflammation (gingivitis) and subsequent periodontal inflammation with loss of attachment ensues (periodontitis).

Host defence factors

Both the specific and non-specific immune responses of the host to subgingival plaque are considered to play critical roles in the initiation, progression and recovery from periodontal diseases. One of the most important components of the host response is the gingival crevicular fluid, which contains both specific and non-specific defence factors (Table 33.2).

Polymorphonuclear leucocytes

Clinically healthy gingiva contain small numbers of polymorphonuclear leucocytes (PMNLs). Their numbers increase markedly during the onset of gingivitis and periodontitis. The PMNLs migrate from venules and enter the gingival sulcus through the junctional epithelial cells. When PMNLs encounter bacteria, phagocytosis ensues, and the ingested organisms are then killed with a combination of proteolytic and hydrolytic enzymes, and other cell-derived killing agents such as hydrogen peroxide and lactic acid. Although phagocytosis can occur in the absence of antibody, the presence of

Table 33.1 Classification of periodontal diseases

Gingival diseases
A. *Dental plaque-induced gingival diseases*
   1. Gingivitis associated with dental plaque only
   2. Gingival disease modified by systemic factors (e.g. puberty-associated gingivitis, pregnancy-associated gingivitis)
   3. Gingival disease modified by medications
   4. Gingival disease modified by malnutrition
B. *Non-plaque-induced gingival lesions*
   1. Specific bacterial origin (e.g. gonorrhoea)
   2. Viral origin (e.g. herpes)
   3. Fungal origin (e.g. linear gingival erythema)
   4. Genetic origin (e.g. hereditary gingival fibromatosis)
   5. Gingival manifestations of systemic conditions (e.g. allergic reactions)
   6. Traumatic lesions (factitious, iatrogenic, accidental) (e.g. chemical injury)

Periodontal diseases
A. *Chronic periodontitis*
   1. Localized
   2. Generalized
B. *Aggressive periodontitis*
   1. Localized
   2. Generalized
C. *Periodontitis as a manifestation of systemic disease*
   1. Associated with hematological disorders
      (i) Acquired neutropenia
      (ii) Leukaemias
      (iii) Others
   2. Associated with genetic disorders
      (i) Familial and cyclic neutropenia
      (ii) Down's syndrome
      (iii) Many other rare conditions
D. *Necrotizing periodontal diseases*
   1. Necrotizing ulcerative gingivitis (NUG)
   2. Necrotizing ulcerative periodontitis (NUP)
E. *Abscesses of the periodontium*
   1. Gingival abscess
   2. Periodontal abscess
   3. Pericoronal abscess
F. *Periodontitis associated with endodontic lesions*
   Combined periodontic-endodontic lesions
G. *Developmental or acquired deformities and conditions*

Table 33.2 Specific and non-specific defence factors in gingival crevicular fluid

Specific	Non-specific
B and T lymphocytes	Polymorphs Macrophages
Antibodies: IgG, IgA, IgM	Complement system Proteases Lysozyme Lactoferrin

immunoglobulins and complement enhance the process. The interaction between PMNLs and plaque bacteria may result in:

- death of the microorganism
- death of the leucocytes
- neutrophil autolysis and release of lysosomal enzymes (e.g. hyaluronidase, collagenase, elastase, acid hydrolase).

Thus, PMNLs may have both a protective and a damaging effect on host tissues. Phagocytosis, which may occur within the host tissues and possibly at the interface with subgingival plaque, is important in preventing the microbial ingress into the tissues.

Antibody

Locally derived specific antibodies (IgM, IgG and IgA) to subgingival plaque organisms are found in the GCF. An elevated titre of specific antibody to a periodontopathogen may be:

- protective
- involved in damaging hypersensitivity reactions to the host tissues
- non-specific and unrelated (i.e. an epiphenomenon).

The presence of antibody implies that the T-cell (helper and suppressor) and B-cell interactions occur in periodontal tissues. Cells required for a wide range of immune reactions, present in gingival tissues of periodontitis patients, possess antigen specificity for plaque bacteria. When stimulated, either antibodies (from B lymphocytes) or lymphokines (from T lymphocytes) are produced.

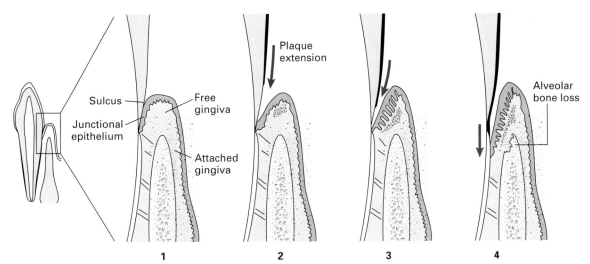

Fig. 33.1 The progression of a marginal periodontium from health to disease. (1) A healthy gingival sulcus with minimal supragingival plaque. (2) Established chronic gingivitis with minor inflammatory enlargement. (3) Long-standing chronic gingivitis with subgingival plaque extension into the pocket. (4) Chronic periodontitis with destruction of the periodontal membrane, alveolar bone loss and apical migration of the epithelial attachment.

Antibodies and complement present in the periodontal tissues interact to produce hypersensitivity reactions which may damage host tissues and also contribute to periodontal disease. There is evidence that all four types of hypersensitivity may be involved in the pathogenesis of periodontal disease.

Microorganisms in subgingival plaque

That dental plaque is essential in the aetiology of the common forms of chronic gingivitis and periodontitis is shown by the following.

1. Epidemiological data indicate a strong positive association between plaque levels and the prevalence and severity of periodontal diseases.
2. Clinical studies in healthy subjects have shown that discontinuation of oral hygiene results in plaque accumulation and subsequent onset of gingivitis (see Fig. 31.4). If plaque is then removed and oral hygiene recommended the tissues are restored to health.
3. The topical application of certain antimicrobial compounds (e.g. chlorhexidine gluconate) both inhibits plaque formation and prevents the development of gingivitis.
4. Periodontal disease can be initiated in gnotobiotic animals by specific periodontopathic bacteria isolated from human dental plaque (e.g. *Fusobacterium nucleatum*, *Porphyromonas gingivalis*) and the disease arrested by administering antibiotic active against that particular organism.

Microbiological studies of periodontal plaque flora

As most of the periodontal plaque flora is anaerobic, special care must be taken to preserve the viability of these organisms during sampling, dispersion and cultivation of plaque samples. Ideally, the sample should be taken from the advancing front of the lesion at the base of the pocket, although in practice this is difficult because of contaminants from the superficial plaque at the top of the pocket. The techniques involved in microbiological sampling of pocket flora include:

- **dark-field microscopy** to estimate the different morphological bacterial types (morphotypes) present, especially spirochaetes, which are not easily cultivable
- **cultural studies** using screening methods for the presence of a few, selected periodontopathic microorganisms, or in-depth studies using conventional culture techniques to isolate, identify and enumerate all cultivable flora
- conventional enzyme-linked immunosorbent assay (ELISA) and fluorescent antibody techniques
- **molecular biology** techniques using specific DNA probes, and determination of 16S RNA sequences by polymerase chain reaction to identify unculturable bacteria as well as the conventional pathogens; these techniques have revealed the presence of hitherto undescribed bacteria in periodontal pockets.

Specific and non-specific plaque hypotheses

Although bacteria are definitive agents of periodontal diseases there are conflicting views as to whether a single or a limited number of species are involved in the disease process — the **specific plaque hypothesis** — or disease is caused by any combination of a wider range of non-specific bacteria — the **non-specific plaque hypothesis**.

The specific plaque hypothesis

In certain disease states such as necrotizing ulcerative gingivitis the key aetiologic agents are fusobacteria and spirochaetes. Furthermore, this disease can be resolved by appropriate antibiotics active against anaerobes (e.g. metronidazole). Other studies have convincingly shown the direct involvement of *Actinobacillus actinomycetemcomitans* in aggressive (juvenile) periodontitis, and disease resolution after therapy with tetracycline, which is active against this organism. These observations led to the theory of specific plaque hypothesis.

The non-specific plaque hypothesis

This hypothesis proposes that collective groups of different bacteria have the total complement of virulence factors required for periodontal tissue destruction and that some bacteria can substitute for others absent from the **pathogenic consortium**. This hypothesis implies that plaque will cause disease irrespective of its composition, and it is supported by the clinical findings of numerous bacterial species in diseased periodontal pockets.

It is likely that the two theories represent the extremes of a complex series of host–parasite interactions.

The ecological plaque hypothesis

The ecological plaque hypothesis has also been proposed for the aetiology of periodontal disease. This postulates the following causative process:

1. The reaction of the host to natural **plaque accumulation** in the crevice is an **inflammatory response**.
2. The ensuing **increased GCF flow** provides complex host molecules that can be catabolized by the proteolytic Gram-negative anaerobes that already exist in small numbers in normal plaque flora.
3. The latter organisms **suppress the growth of species** common in the healthy crevice (i.e. facultative anaerobic Gram-positive bacteria mostly) and a **population shift** occurs in the resident flora.
4. These **periodontopathic flora** then produce virulence factors which overwhelm host defences for a time, resulting in **episodic tissue destruction** and disease activity.

This simple yet elegant hypothesis implies that periodontal disease is an endogenous or an opportunistic infection, caused by an imbalance in the composition of the resident microflora at a site, owing to an alteration in the ecology of the local habitat (Fig. 33.2).

Clinical implications

The non-specific plaque hypothesis and the ecology hypothesis imply that periodontal disease may be treated by reducing the plaque to an acceptable level and the maintenance of a healthy plaque, or by achievement of total plaque control. In contrast, the specific plaque hypothesis implies that therapy

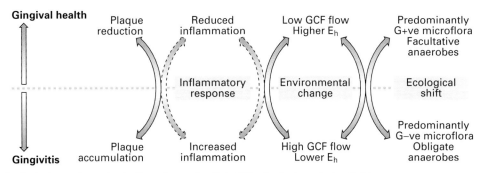

Fig. 33.2 The ecological plaque hypothesis. E_h, redox potential; GCF, gingival crevicular fluid.

should be directed at elimination of specific pathogens, for instance by appropriate antibiotic therapy.

Periodontal health and disease

Healthy gingival sulcus has a scant flora dominated by almost equal proportions of **Gram-positive** and **facultative anaerobic** organisms; spirochaetes and motile rods make up less than 5% of the organisms (Table 33.3). With increasing severity of disease the proportions of **strict anaerobic**, **Gram-negative**, and **motile** organisms increase significantly (Fig. 33.3).

A wide range of microbial products which are potentially toxic to host tissues have been identified in plaque bacteria; these virulence determinants are shown in Table 33.4. If these toxic products are released into the periodontal tissues, then rapid destructive inflammatory disease could be expected.

However, tissue destruction is usually slow, sporadic and episodic, suggesting the existence of powerful host defence mechanisms, of which little is known.

RELATIONSHIP BETWEEN CHRONIC MARGINAL GINGIVITIS AND PERIODONTITIS

Both chronic marginal gingivitis and periodontitis are destructive inflammatory diseases: the lesions of the former are confined to the gingivae; the latter involves both the connective tissue attachment of the tooth and the alveolar bone. Gingivitis is common both in adults and children, although early periodontitis is rarely seen before late adolescence. It is considered that chronic periodontitis is preceded by chronic gingivitis; however, in some cases gingivitis may exist for prolonged periods without progressing to periodontitis. The

Table 33.3 Microorganisms associated with various types of periodontal disease

Condition	Predominant microorganisms	Comments
Health	*Streptococcus sanguis* *Streptococcus oralis* *Actinomyces naeslundii* *Actinomyces viscosus* *Veillonella* spp.	Mainly Gram-positive cocci with few spirochaetes or motile rods
Chronic marginal gingivitis	*Streptococcus sanguis* *Streptococcus milleri* *Actinomyces israelii* *Actinomyces naeslundii* *Prevotella intermedia* *Capnocytophaga* spp. *Fusobacterium nucleatum* *Veillonella* spp.	About 55% of cells are Gram-positive with occasional spirochaetes and motile rods
Chronic periodontitis	*Porphyromonas gingivalis* *Prevotella intermedia* *Fusobacterium nucleatum* *Bacteroides forsythus* *Actinobacillus* *actinomycetemcomitans* *Selenomonas* spp. *Capnocytophaga* spp. Spirochaetes	About 75% of cells are Gram-negative (90% being strict anaerobes). Motile rods and spirochaetes are prominent
Aggressive periodontitis	*Actinobacillus actinomycetemcomitans* *Capnocytophaga* spp. *Porphyromonas gingivalis* *Prevotella intermedia*	About 65–75% of bacteria are Gram-negative bacilli. Few spirochaetes or motile rods present. These diseases may be associated with cellular immune or genetic defects

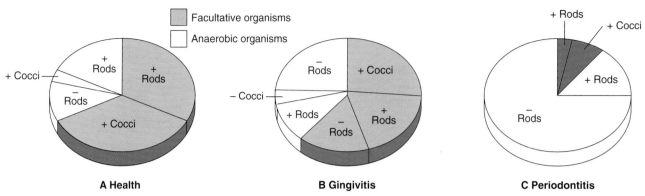

Fig. 33.3 Predominant plaque bacterial morphotypes in (A) health, (B) gingivitis and (C) periodontitis. +, Gram-positive; –, Gram-negative; shaded areas, facultative flora; white areas, anaerobic flora.

main stages in the development of chronic gingivitis and periodontitis are shown in Figure 33.1.

Chronic marginal gingivitis

Clinical presentation

The gingivae are red and swollen, with rounded edges; bleeding gums and halitosis are common. However, pain, discomfort and unpleasant taste is uncommon.

Pathogenesis

Plaque-associated gingivitis is divided into three separate but contiguous phases:
- the initial lesion — developing within 4 days of plaque accumulation
- the early lesion — seen after 7 days
- established lesion — for a variable period afterwards.

The initial lesion. Early histological examination shows an acute inflammatory reaction associated with vasculitis, perivascular collagen destruction, increase in crevicular fluid, and polymorphonuclear leucocytosis in the junctional epithelium and crevice. At this stage no clinical change is evident.

Table 33.4 Some microbial virulence determinants in periodontal disease

Adhesion and colonization
  Fimbriae
  Capsules
  Microbial antagonism and synergism
  'Corn-cob' formation

Tissue destruction
  Hyaluronidase
  Collagenase
  Acid phosphatase
  Epithelial cell toxin

Evasion of host immunity
  Leucocidins
  Proteases
  Cytotoxins
  Siderophores

The early lesion. After about 7 days clinically recognizable chronic gingivitis with gingival inflammation is seen. A dense infiltration of lymphocytes (75%) with macrophages and plasma cells can be observed, especially at the periphery of the lesion. The lymphocytic infiltrate occupies approximately 15% of the marginal connective tissue with areas of local collagen destruction. Polymorph infiltration of the gingival sulcus peaks 7–12 days following the onset of clinically detectable gingivitis.

The established lesion. This develops after a variable period of time when the above-mentioned changes in the gingival crevice support the growth of predominantly anaerobic flora. Histologically, a predominance of plasma cells and B lymphocytes are seen, together with a heavy neutrophil infiltrate in the junctional and the newly developed pocket epithelium. It is during this stage that periodontal pocket formation begins.

If oral hygiene is improved at this juncture without the removal of subgingival plaque then the lesion may persist for years without extending into the deeper periodontal tissues.

Microbiology

Gingivitis is related to the prolonged exposure of host tissues to a non-specific mixture of gingival plaque organisms. The microbiological features of the gingival pocket necessarily change during the transition from the initial lesion to the established lesion. In the initial stage, Gram-positive and facultative organisms predominate, including streptococci (see Table 33.3). In the early lesion, *Actinomyces* spp. increase together with proportions of capnophilic species such as *Capnocytophaga* spp. and obligately anaerobic Gram-negative bacteria. For example in one study, in the initial stage (of non-bleeding gingivitis) proportions of *Actinomyces israelii* and *A. naeslundii* almost doubled. When the disease progresses to the established lesion, where bleeding is seen, the flora further changes and levels of black-pigmented anaerobes such as *Porphyromonas gingivalis* and *Prevotella intermedia* increase quantitatively (e.g. 0.1–0.2% of total plaque flora), together with spirochaetes.

Treatment

Treatment is by thorough removal of plaque and calculus deposits, and the introduction of good oral hygiene.

The transition from gingivitis to periodontitis

Chronic marginal gingivitis may be present for up to 10 years in some individuals before progressing to periodontitis. This transition may be due to one or a combination of the following:

- selective overgrowth of one or more plaque species due to impairment of the host defences
- infection and proliferation of a newly arrived pathogen in the gingival area
- activation of tissue-destructive immune processes.

Chronic periodontitis (formerly adult periodontitis)

Periodontitis can be classified into various groups (Table 33.1), but chronic periodontitis is by far the most prevalent disease globally.

Morbidity

About 70–80% of all adults suffer from this universal disease, and chronic periodontitis comprises 95% of all periodontal diseases. Prevalence and severity increase with age.

Initiation and course

The juvenile form of aggressive periodontitis manifests around 13 years, with the onset of puberty; rather rapid progress with active and quiescent periods. The disease may manifest in adulthood, at any age. In both age groups the disease may either be localized or generalized.

Clinical presentation

All the features of the established lesion are present in addition to the following:

- gross gingival inflammation, fibrosis and some shrinkage (Fig. 33.4)
- bleeding pockets of more than 3 mm
- tooth mobility and migration
- irregular alveolar bone loss around the teeth
- gingival recession
- halitosis and offensive taste
- usually little or no pain
- no systemic disease.

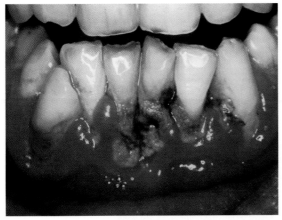

Fig. 33.4 Gross periodontal disease. Note the highly inflamed gingivae and calculus deposits.

Pathogenesis

The main processes that produce loss of attachment and pocket formation are:

1. The apical spread of subgingival plaque causes the junctional epithelium to separate from the tooth surface (i.e. **a new 'pocket' epithelium** is created).
2. Inflammatory tissue reactions below the pocket epithelium result in **destruction of the gingival connective tissue, periodontal membrane** and **alveolar bone**.
3. Apical proliferation of the junctional epithelium results in **migration of the epithelial attachment**.
4. The rate of tissue destruction is not constant but episodic, with periods of quiescence alternating with bouts of bone resorption. A number of patterns of disease activity can occur, ranging from **slowly progressive destruction** to **brief bursts of episodic activity** which may vary in intensity and duration in different sites in the same mouth. This makes microbiological sampling for disease activity extremely difficult.
5. While the entire dentition may be equally affected, more often the disease distribution is localized, with more severe destruction in molar areas and in anterior segments.

Microbiology

Microorganisms implicated in chronic periodontitis are listed in Table 33.3. The depth of the periodontal pocket creates a highly anaerobic locale with a shift from neutral to basic pH (7.4 to 7.8). The protein-rich fluid in the pocket encourages the growth of anaerobes, which possess many proteolytic enzymes. The subgingival plaque has two distinct zones: a zone of Gram-positive cocci and bacilli close to the tooth surface, and a zone of Gram-negative organisms next to the gingival crevice. In active pockets *Porphyromonas gingivalis*, *Actinobacillus actinomycetemcomitans*, *Prevotella intermedia* and *Fusobacterium nucleatum* may be present. Specific microbes are discussed below.

Spirochaetes. Significantly lower numbers of spirochaetes (Ch. 18) are present in healthy periodontal tissue, compared with diseased sites. Thus it was thought that a high percentage of spirochaetes in a subgingival sample strongly suggested a site undergoing — or about to experience — active, destructive disease. However, it is now clear that the number of spirochaetes cannot predict active periodontitis, and therefore the evidence for 'spirochaete specificity' is conflicting and confused. It is possible that one or more *Treponema* spp. are involved in the disease process.

Porphyromonas, Prevotella *and* Bacteroides *spp.* Although now divided into three species (Ch. 17), these organisms formerly belonged to a single group of organisms called 'black-pigmented *Bacteroides* species'. These bacteria are often isolated from periodontal pockets in large numbers and are believed to be intimately associated with all forms of periodontitis.

The evidence for the specificity of *Porphyromonas* and *Prevotella* species depends mainly on the following:

- clinical association studies
- the production of a wide range of factors in vitro which can impair the host defences and damage components of

the periodontium; these include proteases, collagenases, hyaluronidases and cytotoxins (Table 33.4)

- infections in experimental animals which have produced both soft tissue destruction and bone resorption.

Capnocytophaga and corroding bacteria. *Capnocytophaga* spp. (Ch. 14) are members of the commensal oral flora and were implicated as prime pathogens in periodontal infections at one time, especially in localized aggressive periodontitis (formerly localized juvenile periodontitis). Various corroding bacteria such as *Wolinella* spp. and *Eikenella corrodens* have been associated with a number of forms of periodontal disease. However, their precise role is uncertain.

Aggressive periodontitis

Periodontal diseases previously classified as juvenile periodontitis (localized and generalized), rapidly progressive periodontitis and prepubertal periodontitis are now categorized under this common heading.

Localized and generalized aggressive periodontitis (formerly localized/generalized juvenile periodontitis)

Morbidity. The condition is relatively rare, 0.1% in young whites, but is more common in West Africans and Asians. It appears around puberty, relatively common in girls; case clusters are usually seen in families.

Initiation and course. Approximately around 13 years, with onset of puberty; rather rapid progress with active and quiescent periods.

Clinical features. In the localized variant the incisors and/or first permanent molars in both jaws are affected for unknown reasons. Later, other teeth may be involved, producing the appearance of generalized alveolar bone loss (Fig. 33.5).

Alternatively, in the generalized variant of the disease many areas may be involved in a similar manner. The disease is insidious in nature and lesions are discovered incidentally on radiographs. In some generalized cases about 50% of the supporting alveolar bone is affected and teeth may be lost. The condition seldom manifests with gingivitis and patients present with adequate oral hygiene. In contrast to chronic periodontitis, little plaque or calculus is present in periodontal pockets. The disease may be inherited (autosomal recessive).

Microbiology and immunology. A majority of patients with aggressive periodontitis have peripheral blood lymphocytes with impaired ability to react to chemotactic stimuli. This deficiency may be associated with, or is a direct cause of, the presence of large numbers of *Actinobacillus actinomycetemcomitans*, a Gram-negative coccobacillus. Other organisms such as *Capnocytophaga* spp. and *Porphyromonas gingivalis* may be synergistically associated with the disease. The evidence for the specific involvement of *A. actinomycetemcomitans* in aggressive periodontitis includes:

1. A high incidence of the organism in subgingival plaque obtained from lesional sites.
2. High levels of antibody to *A. actinomycetemcomitans* which tend to fall after successful treatment.
3. The possession of a wide range of potentially pathogenic products, such as leucotoxins, ideally suited to a periodontopathic organism. However, all strains are not equally leucotoxic (compare *Escherichia coli* strains which are toxigenic and non-toxigenic).
4. Successful therapy with tetracycline is associated with disease regression and elimination of the organism from diseased sites.

Actinobacillus actinomycetemcomitans is a rare but recognized pathogen in medical microbiology, and has been implicated in

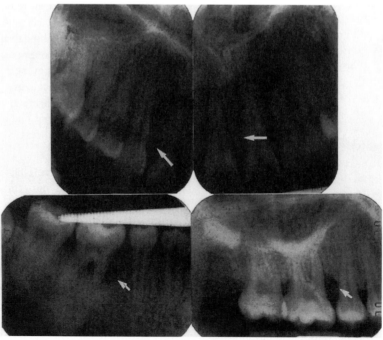

Fig. 33.5 Radiographic appearance of a patient with aggressive periodontitis showing localized periodontal bone loss (arrows).

actinomycosis (Ch. 13), abdominal and brain abscesses, septi-caemia and infective endocarditis.

Management. Mechanical therapy is the mainstay of treatment. In many, adjunct therapy with tetracycline (250 mg three times a day for 4 weeks) produces resolution, and may reduce the risk of reactivation.

NECROTIZING ULCERATIVE GINGIVITIS

Necrotizing ulcerative gingivitis, also known as acute necrotizing ulcerative gingivitis (ANUG), is rare in the West but may be seen in developing countries; it is commonly associated with poor and neglected oral hygiene, malnutrition and possibly systemic diseases.

Clinical features

The condition is characterized by acutely inflamed, red, shiny and bleeding gingivae with irregularly shaped ulcers which initially appear on the tips of the interdental papillae. If untreated, the ulcers enlarge and spread to involve the marginal, and rarely, the attached gingivae (Fig. 33.6). The lesions are extremely painful and are covered by a pseudomembrane (or slough) which can be wiped from the surface. The slough consists of leucocytes, erythrocytes, fibrin, necrotic tissue debris and microorganisms. Characteristically the patient's breath is malodorous. The patient may complain of an unpleasant metallic taste. There is little or no systemic upset, and mild submandibular lymphadenitis; involvement of the cervical lymph nodes occurs only in severe cases. Generalized fever or malaise is very uncommon.

If the disease is inadequately treated, tissue destruction slows down and the disease may enter a chronic phase with pronounced loss of supporting tissues (noma).

Aetiology

The main predisposing factors of ANUG are:
- poor oral hygiene
- severe malnutrition
- heavy smoking
- emotional stress
- primary herpetic gingivostomatitis

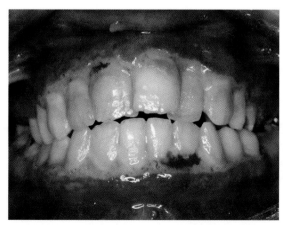

Fig. 33.6 Acute necrotizing ulcerative gingivitis. Note the loss of papillae, spontaneous bleeding and gross plaque accumulation.

- acquired immunosuppression such as recent measles infection
- infection with human immunodeficiency virus (see Ch. 30).

Microbiology

The disease is a specific, anaerobic, polymicrobial infection mainly due to the combined activity of fusobacteria (*Fusobacterium nucleatum*) and oral spirochaetes (*Treponema* spp.) — the so-called **fusospirochaetal complex**. The main evidence for the microbial specificity of ANUG is:
- microscopical association studies
- the ability of the complex to cause tissue destruction in other body sites, such as the tonsils (Vincent's angina, Ch. 23)
- animal studies
- rapid resolution of the disease and elimination of the fusospirochaetal complex after treatment with metronidazole
- invasion of the gingival soft tissues by both spirochaetes and fusiform bacilli.

Cultural studies indicate that medium-sized spirochaetes account for a third, and fusobacteria less than 5%, of the total flora. The remaining organisms comprise *Prevotella intermedia*, *Veillonella* and streptococci.

Diagnosis

The clinical appearance together with the offensive smell is pathognomonic. Confirmatory evidence is obtained by microscopy of a Gram-stained, deep gingival smear of the ulcerated lesion. A predominance of **three** components — **fusobacteria, spirochaetes** and **leucocytes** — is essential for a confident diagnosis (see Fig. 18.2); some, **but not all three**, of these components may be observed in primary herpetic stomatitis, gonococcal gingivitis, benign mucous membrane pemphigoid, desquamative gingivitis and some forms of leukaemia.

Management

1. Initial local debridement (with ultrasonic scaling, if possible) is essential.
2. Oral hygiene advice should be given and mouthwashes, e.g. chlorhexidine, prescribed.
3. Metronidazole (200 mg three times daily for 4 days) is the drug of choice.

Noma or cancrum oris

In some developing countries (e.g. sub-Saharan Africa), an extremely severe form of ANUG called **noma** or **cancrum oris** is seen in children. Typically, the child is less than 10 years old, malnourished (especially with regard to protein) and has a recent history of viral infection, e.g. measles. As a result the specific immune system of the child may be compromised, and the initial necrotic lesion may spread locally from the gingivae into the cheek and sometimes to the face, causing extensive tissue loss and severe disfigurement. Noma is extremely rare in developed countries.

CLINICAL IMPLICATIONS OF MICROBIOLOGICAL TESTS IN PERIODONTAL DISEASE

Microbiological tests are useful in the management of periodontal disease to **identify** sites of active tissue destruction, and **monitor** the effects of treatment and decide when recall is necessary. The presence of a specific putative pathogen associated with any of the periodontal diseases mentioned above could be detected by:

- direct microscopy of one or more smears of samples obtained from the affected site
- cultural studies of the predominant cultivable pathogens, using media that select the specific pathogen (e.g. tryptic soy-serum bacitracin vancomycin (TSBV) medium to select *A. actinomycetemcomitans*)
- enzymatic studies using commercially available test kits

that use synthetic substrates (e.g. BANA: benzoin arginine naphthylamine) to detect arginine specific proteases liberated by some periodontopathic organisms (e.g. *P. gingivalis, B. forsythus, T. denticola*)

- molecular studies using principles of DNA hybridization to detect specific pathogens.

However, these tests are useful only if the identified organisms are definitively known to cause the disease, and if samples can be collected accurately from the site of disease (i.e. probably the base of the periodontal pocket). As this stage has not yet been reached, doubt exists as to the value of these tests in diagnosis. Sampling for the presence of *A. actinomycetemcomitans* in agressive periodontitis is the only microbiological test that is likely to contribute to the treatment of chronic periodontal diseases at present. A positive test would suggest that tetracycline therapy should be used as an adjunct to root instrumentation.

KEY FACTS

- Periodontal disease can be broadly categorized into **gingivitis** and **periodontitis**
- Clinical features of plaque-related **gingivitis** are **redness, oedema** and **bleeding**
- *Periodontitis usually develops from a pre-existing gingivitis; however, not every gingivitis develops into periodontitis*
- Periodontitis can be classified into two main groups: chronic and aggressive. The chronic form is by far the most prevalent disease globally
- The aggressive form of periodontitis includes those previously categorized as juvenile (localized or generalized), rapidly progressive and prepubertal periodontitis
- Currently recognized key Gram-negative **periodontopathogens** include *Porphyromonas gingivalis, Prevotella intermedia, Bacteroides forsythus, Actinobacillus actinomycetemcomitans, Fusobacterium nucleatum* and *Capnocytophaga* species
- *Disease activity in periodontal disease may range from slow, chronic progressive destruction to brief and acute 'episodic bursts' with varying intensity and duration (in different sites in the same mouth); hence microbiological sampling for diseased sites or activity is extremely difficult*
- In adult periodontitis the microflora changes from aerobic,

non-motile, Gram-positive cocci to anaerobic, motile, Gram-negative bacilli

- *Localized or generalized aggressive periodontitis is strongly associated with* Actinobacillus actinomycetemcomitans, *either alone or synergistically with* Capnocytophaga spp. *and* Porphyromonas gingivalis
- *Necrotizing ulcerative gingivitis is a specific, anaerobic, polymicrobial infection due to the combined activity of* Fusobacterium nucleatum *and oral spirochaetes (* Treponema spp.*): the fusospirochaetal complex*
- *In the developing world (e.g. sub-Saharan Africa), an extremely severe, tissue-destructive sequel of acute necrotizing ulcerative gingivitis (ANUG) called noma or cancrum oris is seen, mainly in children*
- *Microbiological tests used in the management of periodontal disease help identify sites of active tissue destruction, monitor efficacy of therapy, and decide recall intervals*
- *The presence of putative periodontopathogens could be detected by (a) direct microscopy, (b) microbial cultures, (c) enzymes liberated by organisms and (d) DNA/RNA probes*
- *Periodontal diseases can be treated by plaque control, root surface debridement, periodontal surgery and the prudent use of antimicrobial agents*

FURTHER READING

Armitage, GC (1999). Development of a classification system for periodontal disease. *Annals of Periodontology* 4, 1–6.

Haffajee, AD, and Socransky, SS (1994). Microbial aetiologic agents of destructive periodontal disease. *Periodontology 2000* 5, 78–111.

Marsh, PD, and Marin, MV (1999). *Oral microbiology* (4th edn). Butterworth-Heinemann, London.

Meyer, DH, and Fives-Taylor, PM (1997). The role of *Actinobacillus actinomycetemcomitans* in the pathogenesis of periodontal diseases. *Trends in Microbiology* 5, 224–228.

Socransky, SS, and Haffajee, AD (1997). Microbiology of periodontal disease. In Lindhe, J, Karring, T, and Lang, NP (eds) *Clinical periodontology and implant dentistry* (3rd edn), Ch. 4. Munksgaard, Copenhagen.

Slots, J (1997). Microflora of the healthy gingival sulcus of man. *Scandinavian Journal of Dental Research* 85, 247–254.

Zambon, JJ (1996). Periodontal diseases: microbial factors. *Annals of Periodontology* 1, 879–925.

34 Dentoalveolar infections

Dentoalveolar infections can be defined as pus-producing (or **pyogenic**) infections associated with the teeth and surrounding supporting structures, such as the periodontium and the alveolar bone. Other terms for these conditions include periapical abscess, apical abscess, chronic periapical dental infection, dental pyogenic infection, periapical periodontitis and dentoalveolar abscess. The clinical presentation of dentoalveolar infections depends on the **virulence** of the causative microorganisms, the **local** and **systemic defence** mechanisms of the host, and the **anatomical features** of the region. Depending on the interactions of these factors, the resulting infection may present as:
- an abscess localized to the tooth that initiated the infection
- a diffuse cellulitis which spreads along fascial planes
- a mixture of both.

SOURCE OF MICROORGANISMS

Endogenous oral commensals, usually from the apex of a necrotic tooth or from periodontal pockets as a result of either caries or periodontal disease (Fig. 34.1).

DENTOALVEOLAR ABSCESS

A dentoalveolar abscess usually develops by the extension of the initial carious lesion into dentine, and spread of bacteria to the pulp via the dentinal tubules (Fig. 34.1). The pulp responds to infection either by rapid **acute inflammation** involving the whole pulp, which quickly becomes necrosed, or by development of a **chronic localized abscess** with most of the pulp remaining viable. Other ways in which microbes reach the pulp are:
- by traumatic tooth fracture or pathological exposure due to tooth wear
- by traumatic exposure during dental treatment (iatrogenic)
- through the periodontal membrane (periodontitis and pericoronitis) and accessory root canals
- rarely by **anachoresis**, i.e. seeding of organisms directly into pulp via the pulpal blood supply during bacteraemia (e.g. tooth extraction at a different site).

Sequelae

Once pus formation occurs, it may remain **localized** at the root apex and develop into either an **acute** or a **chronic** abscess; develop into a **focal osteomyelitis**; or spread into the surrounding tissues (Fig. 34.2).

Direct spread

1. Spread into the superficial soft tissues may:
   - **localize** as a soft-tissue abscess (Fig. 34.3)
   - extend through the overlying oral mucosa or skin, producing a **sinus** linking the main abscess cavity with the mouth or skin
   - extend through the soft tissue to produce a **cellulitis**.
2. Spread may occur into the adjacent fascial spaces, following the **path of least resistance**; such spread is dependent on the anatomical relation of the original abscess to the adjacent tissues (Table 34.1). Infection via fascial planes often spreads rapidly and for some distance from the original abscess site, and occasionally may cause severe respiratory distress as a result of occlusion of the airway by oedema (e.g. Ludwig's angina).
3. Infection may extend into the deeper medullary spaces of alveolar bone, producing a spreading osteomyelitis.

Indirect spread

Other sequelae entail indirect spread via:
- **lymphatic routes**, to regional nodes in the head and neck region (submental, submandibular, deep cervical, parotid and occipital). Usually the involved nodes are tender, swollen and painful, and rarely may suppurate, requiring drainage
- **haematogenous** routes: to other organs such as the brain (rare).

Clinical features

Clinical signs and symptoms depend on the:
- site of infection
- degree and mode of spread
- virulence of the causative organisms
- efficiency of the host defences.

Clinical features may include a non-viable tooth with or without a carious lesion, a large restoration, evidence of trauma, swelling, pain, redness, trismus, local lymph node enlargement, sinus formation, raised temperature and malaise. The latter two symptoms are a direct consequence of increased levels of systemic inflammatory cytokines such as

Table 34.1   Sites of contiguous spread of dentoalveolar infection (see also Fig. 34.2)

Site of spread	Maxillary teeth	Mandibular teeth
Palate	Palatal roots of premolars and molars; also lateral incisors with a palatally curved root	—
Buccal space	Canines, premolars and molars	Canines, premolars and molars
Infraorbital/periorbital region	Canines mainly	—
Maxillary sinus	Canines, premolars and molars	—
Upper lip	Central and lateral incisors	—
Masseteric space, pterygomandibular space, lateral pharyngeal space	—	Lower third molars
Lower lip	—	Incisors and canines
Submandibular space	—	Root apices below insertion of mylohyoid — usually molars but can also be premolars
Submental space	—	Incisors and canines
Sublingual space	—	Root apices above mylohyoid/geniohyoid — usually incisors, canines and premolars; rarely molars

interleukins and tumour necrosis factor in response to bacterial products such as lipopolysaccharides (i.e. endotoxins).

Microbiology

Microbiologically, the dentoalveolar abscess is characterized by the following features:

- infection is usually **polymicrobial** (endogenous), with a mixture of three or four different species
- monomicrobial (endogenous) infection (i.e. with a single organism) is unusual
- strict anaerobes are the predominant organisms and the viridans group streptococci are less common than once thought.

The common species isolated from dentoalveolar abscesses are *Prevotella*, *Porphyromonas* and *Fusobacterium* spp., and anaerobic streptococci; facultative anaerobes are the second largest group, e.g. *Streptococcus milleri* (Table 34.2). There is evidence that some strictly anaerobic bacteria, especially

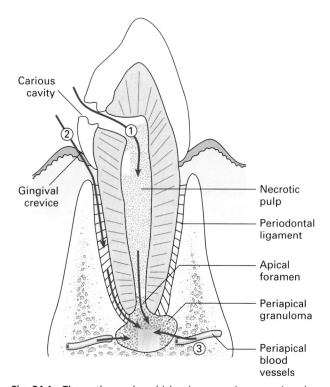

Fig. 34.1 The pathways by which microorganisms may invade the pulp and periapical tissues: (1) from the apical foramen, (2) via the periodontal ligament, (3) via the bloodstream (anachoresis).

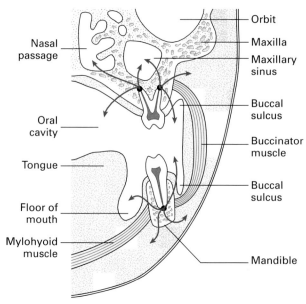

Fig. 34.2 Pathways by which pus may spread from an acute dentoalveolar abscess (coronal section, at first molar tooth level).

Porphyromonas gingivalis and *Fusobacterium* spp., are more likely to cause severe infection than other species, and that synergistic microbial interactions play an important role in the severity of dentoalveolar abscesses.

Collection and transport of pus samples

1. Wherever possible, pus should be collected by **needle aspiration**, or in a sterile container after external incision. Care must be exercised during recapping the syringe after needle aspiration and a safety device must be used. Also, it is important to drain the residual pus, once the aspirate has been obtained via an appropriate incision (see Ch. 6).
2. If swabs must be used then strict aseptic collection technique is required (because of the indigenous flora on mucosal surfaces it is difficult, if not impossible, to collect uncontaminated samples when intraoral swabs are used for pus collection). When the pus sample is contaminated with saliva or dental plaque during collection, this information must be recorded on the request form.

Management

The specific treatment for any given individual will vary. The major management guidelines entail:
1. **Draining** the pus.
2. **Removing** the source of **infection**.
3. Prescribing **antibiotics**; probably not required for the majority of localized abscesses, although it may be necessary:
   - when drainage cannot be established immediately
   - if the abscess has spread to the superficial soft tissues
   - when the patient is febrile.

Standard antibiotics include:
- phenoxymethylpenicillin (penicillin V) or short-course, high-dose amoxicillin (amoxycillin)
- in penicillin-hypersensitive patients: erythromycin or metronidazole (as most infections are due to strict anaerobes).

LUDWIG'S ANGINA

Ludwig's angina is a spreading, bilateral infection of the sublingual and submandibular spaces.

Table 34.2 Bacteria commonly isolated from dentoalveolar abscesses

Facultative anaerobes
  Streptococcus milleri
  Streptococcus sanguis
  Actinomyces spp.

Obligate anaerobes
  Peptostreptococcus spp.
  Porphyromonas gingivalis
  Prevotella intermedia
  Prevotella melaninogenica
  Fusobacterium nucleatum

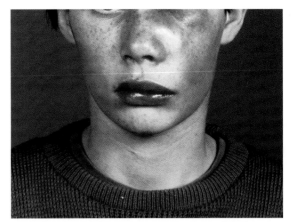

Fig. 34.3 Extension of periapical infection from the left upper canine tooth to the infraorbital region in a teenager.

Aetiology

In the vast majority of cases (about 90%) Ludwig's angina is precipitated by dental or post-extraction infection; uncommon sources of infection include submandibular sialadenitis, infected mandibular fracture, oral soft-tissue laceration, and puncture wounds of the floor of the mouth. The infection is essentially a **cellulitis** of the **fascial spaces** rather than true abscess formation.

Clinical features

The infection of sublingual and submandibular spaces raises the floor of the mouth and tongue and causes the tissues at the front of the neck to swell. The brawny swelling has a characteristic board-like consistency which can barely be indented by the finger. There is severe systemic upset with fever.

Complications include:
- airway obstruction due to either oedema of the glottis or a swollen tongue blocking the nasopharynx
- spread of infection to the masticator and pharyngeal spaces
- death due to asphyxiation is a certainty without immediate intervention.

Surgical drainage may yield little pus.

Microbiology

Oral commensal bacteria are common agents, especially *Porphyromonas* and *Prevotella* spp., fusobacteria and anaerobic streptococci; i.e. it is a **mixed endogenous infection**. Because of the severity of the condition, samples for microbiology assessment should always be obtained, if possible.

Management

1. Ensure that the patient's **airway** remains open (surgically, if necessary).
2. Maintain **fluid balance**.
3. Institute **high-dose, empirical antibiotic therapy** (usually intravenous penicillin, with or without metronidazole) immediately.

4. Collect a sample of pus before antibiotic therapy, if the patient's condition permits, or immediately afterwards.
5. Change the prescribed antibiotic if necessary, once the bacteriological results are available.
6. Institute surgical drainage as soon as possible.
7. Eliminate the primary source of infection (e.g. a non-vital tooth).

PERIODONTAL ABSCESS

A periodontal abscess is caused by an acute or chronic destructive process in the periodontium, resulting in localized collection of pus communicating with the oral cavity through the gingival sulcus and/or other periodontal sites (and not arising from the tooth pulp).

Aetiology

The abscess probably forms by occlusion or trauma to the orifice of a periodontal pocket, resulting in the extension of infection from the pocket into the supporting tissues. These events might result from **impaction of food** such as a fish bone, or of a detached toothbrush bristle; or **compression of the pocket wall** by orthodontic tooth movement or by unusual occlusal forces. Normally the abscess remains localized in the periodontal tissues, and its subsequent development depends on:
- the virulence, type and number of the causative organisms
- the health of the patient's periodontal tissues
- the efficiency of the specific and non-specific defence mechanisms of the host.

Clinical features

1. Onset is sudden, with swelling, redness and tenderness of the gingiva overlying the abscess.
2. Pain is continuous or related to biting and can be elicited clinically by percussion of the affected tooth.
3. There are no specific radiographic features, although commonly associated with a deep periodontal pocket.
4. Pus from the lesion usually drains along the root surface to the orifice of the periodontal pocket; in deep pockets pus may extend through the alveolar bone to drain through a sinus which opens on to the attached gingiva.
5. Because of intermittent drainage of pus, infection tends to remain localized and extraoral swelling is uncommon.
6. Untreated abscesses may lead to severe destruction of periodontal tissues and tooth loss.

Microbiology

Endogenous, subgingival plaque bacteria are the source of the microorganisms in periodontal abscesses; infection is polymicrobial, with the following bacteria being commonly isolated:
- anaerobic Gram-negative rods, especially black-pigmented *Porphyromonas* and *Prevotella* spp., and fusobacteria
- streptococci, especially haemolytic streptococci and anaerobic streptococci
- others such as spirochaetes, *Capnocytophaga* spp. and *Actinomyces* spp.

Treatment

1. Make a thorough clinical assessment of the patient, including a history of systemic illnesses (e.g. diabetes).
2. If the prognosis is poor, owing to advanced periodontitis or recurrent infection, and it is unlikely that treatment will achieve functional periodontal tissues, then extract the tooth. If the abscess is small and localized, extraction may be carried out immediately; otherwise extraction should be postponed until acute infection has subsided.
3. Drainage should be encouraged and gentle subgingival scaling performed to remove calculus and foreign objects.
4. Irrigate the pocket with warm 0.9% sodium chloride solution and prescribe regular hot saline mouthwashes.
5. If pyrexia or cellulitis is present, antibiotics should be prescribed: penicillin, erythromycin or metronidazole are the drugs of choice.

SUPPURATIVE OSTEOMYELITIS OF THE JAWS

Suppurative osteomyelitis is a relatively rare condition which may present as an acute or chronic infection, depending on a variety of factors.

Definition

An inflammation of the medullary cavity of the mandible or the maxilla, with possible extension of infection into the cortical bone and the periosteum as a sequel.

Aetiology

Osteomyelitis of the head and neck region is much rarer than dentoalveolar infections, probably because of the good vascular supply to the bone. Conditions that tend to reduce the vascularity of bone predispose to osteomyelitis, e.g. radiation, osteoporosis, Paget's disease, fibrous dysplasia and bone tumours. A wide range of organisms have been associated with osteomyelitis of the jaws, including endogenous bacteria (described below) and rarely exogenous organisms such as *Treponema pallidum* and *Mycobacterium tuberculosis*.

1. The source of infection is usually a **contiguous focus**, or **haematogenous seeding** of bacteria may occur infrequently.
2. Bacteria multiply in bony medulla and elicit an acute inflammatory reaction.
3. This results in increased intramedullary pressure leading to venous stasis, ischaemia and pus formation.
4. Pus spreads through the haversian canal system, breaching the periosteum, with resultant **sinus formation** and appearance of **soft-tissue abscesses** on the oral mucosa or skin.
5. If there is no intervention, chronic osteomyelitis results, with new bone (**involucrum**) formation and separation of fragments of necrotic bone (**sequestra**).

Clinical features

Acute osteomyelitis

Clinical features include pain, mild fever, paraesthesia or anaesthesia of the related skin; loosening of teeth; and exudation of pus from gingival margins or through sinuses or fistulae in the affected skin.

Chronic osteomyelitis

In chronic osteomyelitis there is minimal systemic upset; chronic sinuses with little pus, and tender and indurated skin.

Microbiology

As the majority of osteomyelitis cases begin as a dentoalveolar infection, the causative organisms of both diseases are similar. **Anaerobes** are the most common isolates, e.g. *Bacteroides*, *Prevotella* and *Porphyromonas* spp., fusobacteria and anaerobic streptococci; rarely **enterobacteria** may be present. *Staphylococcus aureus*, the most common agent of osteomyelitis in long bones, is infrequently isolated from jaw lesions.

Treatment

The management of osteomyelitis is complex. The main principles are:
1. Rapid diagnosis of the disease.
2. Empirical prescription of antibiotics (to prevent further bone destruction and surgical intervention).
3. Collection of a pus sample, if feasible, for investigations: collect pus with care when it is exuding from the gingival sulcus, to prevent contamination with commensal bacteria; aspirate pus from contiguous soft-tissue lesions.
4. Send the sample immediately to the laboratory in anaerobic transport medium for identification and sensitivity testing of causative bacteria.
5. Drugs of choice are penicillin, penicillinase-resistant penicillins (e.g. flucloxacillin), and in penicillin-allergic patients, clindamycin and erythromycin.
6. Other treatment options include tooth extraction, sequestrectomy, and resection and reconstruction of the jaws.

CERVICOFACIAL ACTINOMYCOSIS

Actinomycosis (see Ch. 13) is an endogenous, granulomatous disease which may occur in the following sites:
- cervicofacial region — most common (60–65%)
- abdomen (10–20%)
- lung
- skin.

Aetiology

In humans the main infecting organism is *Actinomyces israelii*, which is a common oral commensal present in plaque, carious dentine and calculus. Trauma to the jaws, tooth extraction, and teeth with gangrenous pulps may precipitate infection (e.g. calculus or plaque becoming impacted in the depths of a tooth socket at the time of extraction).

Clinical features

Predominantly a disease of younger people, although all ages may be affected, the infection can present in an **acute, subacute** or **chronic form**. There is usually a history of trauma, such as a tooth extraction or a blow to the jaw. Most infections start as an acute swelling indistinguishable on clinical grounds from a dentoalveolar abscess. The chronic form of the disease follows, due to either inadequate or no therapy, or subacute infection related to trauma.

Swelling is common, and is either localized or diffuse; if untreated, it may progress into discharging sinuses. Classically, this discharge of pus contains visible granules which may be gritty to touch, yellow and are known as '**sulphur granules**' (a descriptive term, as sulphur is not found in the granules). These granules in pus are almost pathognomonic of the disease.

The submandibular region is most commonly affected; rarely the maxillary antrum, salivary glands and tongue may be involved. Pain is a variable feature. Other features, depending on the site of infection, are multiple discharging sinuses, trismus, pyrexia, fibrosis around the swelling, and the presence of infected teeth.

Microbiology

The most common agent is *Actinomyces israelii*, although *A. bovis* and *A. naeslundii* may occasionally be isolated. In a minority *Actinobacillus actinomycetemcomitans* may be isolated in mixed culture with *Actinomyces israelii*.

Laboratory diagnosis

If a fluctuant abscess is present, collect fluid pus by aspiration using a syringe, or in a sterile container if drainage by external incision is performed. Examine the pus for the presence of 'sulphur granules'; Gram films are made from any part with a lumpy or granular appearance. The granules are washed and crushed in tissue grinders and cultured on blood agar under anaerobic conditions at 37°C for 7 days. Colonies often produce a typical 'molar tooth' morphology. Pure cultures are then identified using biochemical techniques (see Fig. 13.1). A Gram film of a colony will reveal moderate to large clumps of Gram-positive branching filaments.

Management

Acute lesions

1. Removal of any associated dental focus.
2. Incision and drainage of facial abscess.
3. A short (2–3 weeks) course of antibiotics; penicillin is the drug of choice.

Subacute or chronic lesions

1. Surgical intervention, as in (1) and (2) above.
2. A *longer* antibiotic course, 5–6 weeks on average.

If penicillin cannot be given because of hypersensitivity, erythromycin, tetracycline and clindamycin are good alternatives. The latter drugs penetrate bony tissues well.

KEY FACTS

- Dental caries is the main cause of pulpal and periapical infection; other routes include periodontal pocket and rarely, **anachoresis** (i.e. haematogenous seeding)
- **Dentoalveolar infections** are usually **polymicrobial** in nature and **endogenous** in origin, with a predominance of strict anaerobes
- *Ideally, an aspirated sample of pus should be collected for microbiological examination of a dentoalveolar abscess in the head and neck region*
- *Drainage of pus is the mainstay of treatment of dentoalveolar and periodontal abscesses; elimination of the infective focus and antibiotic therapy should be considered on an individual basis*
- Ludwig's angina is a spreading, bilateral infection of the sublingual and submandibular spaces; it is a a life-threatening infection
- *Prompt intervention and maintenance of the airway is of critical importance in the management of Ludwig's angina; high-dose, empirical, systemic antibiotic therapy is also essential*

- **Periodontal abscess**: an acute or chronic destructive process in the periodontium, resulting in localized collection of pus communicating with the oral cavity through the gingival sulcus and/or other periodontal sites (and not arising from the tooth pulp)
- **Periodontal abscess** is an **endogenous, polymicrobial** infection with a predominantly anerobic, periodontopathic flora
- *Suppurative osteomyelitis of the jaws is uncommon; it is mostly seen in immunocompromised patients. Usually a polymicrobial infection, it requires both medical and surgical intervention*
- *Cervicofacial actinomycosis: an endogenous granulomatous disease, usually presenting at the angle of the mandible and related to trauma or a history of tooth extraction, mainly caused by* Actinomyces israelii; *'sulphur granules' may be present in pus*
- *Actinomycoses are managed by surgical drainage and long-term antibiotics, preferably penicillin*

FURTHER READING

Brook, I, Frazier, IH, and Gher, ME (1996). Microbiology of periapical abscess and associated maxillary sinusitis. *Journal of Periodontology* 67, 608–610.

Dahlen, G, and Moller, AJR (1992). Microbiology of endodontic infections. In Slots, J, and Taubman, MA (eds) *Comtemporary oral microbiology and immunology*, Ch. 24. Mosby Year Book, St Louis.

Lewis, MAO, MacFarlane, TW, and McGowan, DA (1990). A microbiological and clinical review of the acute dentoalveolar abscess. *British Journal of Oral and Maxillofacial Surgery* 28, 359–366.

Marsh, PD, and Martin, MV (1999). *Oral microbiology* (4th edn). Butterworth-Heinemann, London.

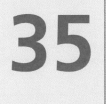

35 Oral mucosal and salivary gland infections

ORAL MUCOSAL INFECTIONS

The oral mucosa, which covers a significant proportion of the oral cavity, is affected by a number of infectious diseases. The majority of these are of fungal (candidal) and viral origin and are similar to infections seen in other superficial mucosal surfaces of the body, such as the vagina. In this section candidal infections are discussed first, followed by viral infections.

Oral candidiasis

Oral candidiasis or candidosis is caused mainly by the yeast *Candida albicans*, although other *Candida* species may cause infection in some. All forms of oral candidiasis are considered to be opportunistic infections, and the epithet '**disease of the diseased**' has been applied to these infections, which are seen mainly in the '**very young, the very old and the very sick**'.

Classification

Oral candidiases can be classified as follows (Fig. 35.1):
1. **Primary oral candidiases**: **localized** candidal infections present **only** in the oral and perioral tissues.
2. **Secondary oral candidiases**: candidal infections that manifest in a **generalized** manner **both in the oral cavity and in other mucous and cutaneous surfaces** (systemic mucocutaneous candidal infections). These are due to rare disorders (except perhaps in candidiasis of HIV infection) such as thymic aplasia and chronic endocrine diseases.

The classic **triad** of both the primary or secondary oral candidiases are:
- pseudomembranous variant
- erythematous (atrophic) variant
- hyperplastic variant.

Pseudomembranous candidiasis (thrush)

Pseudomembranous candidiasis, classically termed 'thrush' (Fig. 35.2), is an acute infection but may persist intermittently for many months or even years in patients using corticosteroids topically or by aerosol, in HIV-infected individuals, and in other immunocompromised patients. It may also be seen in neonates and in the terminally ill, particularly in association with serious underlying conditions such as leukaemia.

Clinical features. Characterized by **white membranes** on the surface of the oral mucosa, tongue and elsewhere. The lesions develop to form confluent plaques that resemble milk curds and can be wiped off to reveal a raw, **erythematous** and sometimes **bleeding base**.

Microbiology and pathology. The white patches consist of necrotic material and desquamated parakeratotic epithelium, penetrated by yeast cells and hyphae which invade as far as the stratum spinosum. Oropharyngeal thrush may sometimes spread into the adjacent mucosa, particularly that of the upper respiratory tract and the oesophagus. The combination of oral and oesophageal candidiasis is particularly prevalent in HIV disease.

Treatment. Topical antifungal preparations, mainly containing the polyene drugs nystatin and amphotericin, are given as lozenges or pastilles.

Erythematous (atrophic) candidiasis

Erythematous candidiasis is a poorly understood condition associated with corticosteroids, topical or systemic broad-spectrum antibiotics, or HIV disease. It may arise as a consequence of persistent acute pseudomembranous candidiasis when the pseudomembranes are shed, or may develop de novo. Erythematous candidiasis of the palate is a common *Candida*-associated lesion frequently observed in elderly people wearing full dentures (*Candida*-associated denture stomatitis; see below).

Clinical features. The clinical presentation is of one or more asymptomatic erythematous areas, generally on the dorsum of the tongue, palate or buccal mucosa (Fig. 35.3). Lesions on the dorsum of the tongue present as depapillated areas; red areas are often seen on the palate in HIV disease. There can be associated angular stomatitis, especially in candida-associated denture stomatitis.

Microbiology. Not much is known of the role of yeasts in this condition, although antifungal therapy leads to resolution of the lesions.

Treatment. Topical antifungal treatment, mainly nystatin and amphotericin, is given as lozenges or pastilles. Azole group agents, such as oral fluconazole tablets, are useful in HIV disease.

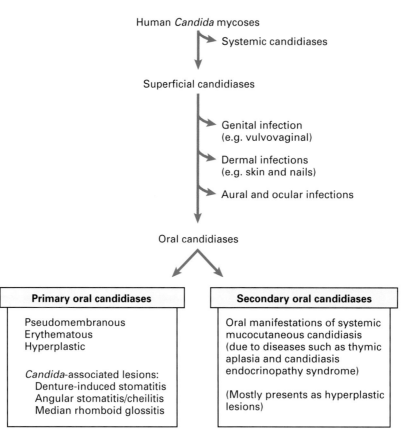

Human *Candida* mycoses

Systemic candidiases

Superficial candidiases

Genital infection
(e.g. vulvovaginal)

Dermal infections
(e.g. skin and nails)

Aural and ocular infections

Oral candidiases

Primary oral candidiases	Secondary oral candidiases

Pseudomembranous
Erythematous
Hyperplastic
 	
Candida-associated lesions:
  Denture-induced stomatitis
  Angular stomatitis/cheilitis
  Median rhomboid glossitis
	Oral manifestations of systemic
	mucocutaneous candidiasis
	(due to diseases such as thymic
	aplasia and candidiasis
	endocrinopathy syndrome)
	
	(Mostly presents as hyperplastic
	lesions)

Fig. 35.1 Classification of oral candidiasis.

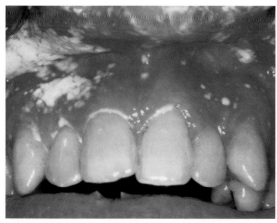

Fig. 35.2 Multiple white plaques of pseudomembranous candidiasis (thrush) in an HIV-infected individual.

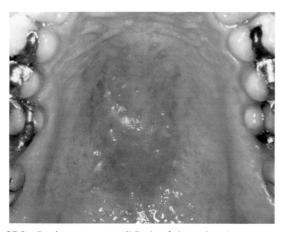

Fig. 35.3 Erythematous candidiasis of the palate in an HIV-infected individual.

Hyperplastic candidiasis (candida leukoplakia)

The lesions in hyperplastic candidiasis present as chronic, discrete raised areas that vary from small, palpable, translucent, whitish areas to large, dense, opaque plaques (Fig. 35.4), hard and rough to the touch (plaque-like lesions). Homogeneous areas or speckled areas that do not rub off (nodular lesions) can also be seen. The lesions are often asymptomatic and usually occur on the inside surface of one or both cheeks (retrocommissural area). Oral cancer supervenes in 9–40% of cases of hyperplastic candidiasis, as compared with the 2–6% risk of malignant transformation cited for oral white patches in general. Therefore, patients with recalcitrant hyperplastic candidal lesions resistant to therapy should be kept under regular surveillance.

Microbiology and histopathology. Parakeratosis and epithelial hyperplasia occur, with candidal invasion restricted to the upper layers of the epithelium (Fig. 35.5). The condition has been associated in a minority with iron and folate deficiencies and with defective cell-mediated immunity. Biopsy is important as the condition is premalignant and shows varying degrees of dysplasia.

Treatment. Topical antifungal treatment, mainly nystatin and amphotericin, is given as lozenges or pastilles. Azole group agents, such as oral fluconazole tablets, may help resolve chronic infections. Because of the possibility of malignant transformation, patients should be followed up if the condition is chronic.

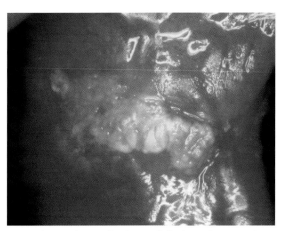

Fig. 35.4 Chronic hyperplastic candidiasis at the commissures of the mouth.

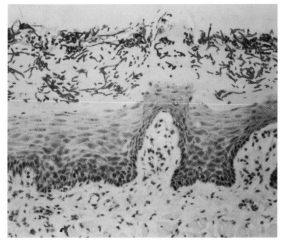

Fig. 35.5 Histopathological section of a chronic hyperplastic candidiasis lesion showing numerous candidal hyphae infiltrating the superficial layers of the oral epithelium.

Candida-associated lesions

Candida-*associated denture stomatitis*

Candida-associated denture stomatitis, also called denture sore mouth or chronic atrophic candidiasis, is one of the most common ailments in wearers of full dentures; in some areas such as Scandinavia 60% of wearers over 60 years old were reported to suffer from the condition. It is also associated with patients wearing orthodontic appliances or obturators for cleft palate. The characteristic presenting signs are erythema and oedema of the mucosa that is in contact with the fitting surface of the upper denture. The mucosa below the lower dentures is hardly ever involved.

Clinical features. The patient may occasionally experience slight soreness but is usually free from symptoms; the only presenting complaint is sometimes an associated angular stomatitis. Depending on the severity of inflammation, the lesions may appear as:

- **pinpoint erythema** of the denture-bearing mucosa (Newton's type 1)
- diffuse and **confluent erythema** and oedema of the denture-bearing mucosa (Newton's type 2; Fig. 35.6)
- **papillary hyperplasia** and inflammation, commonly involving the central part of the hard palate and the alveolar ridge (Newton's type 3; Fig. 35.7).

Aetiology
1. **Local factors**: poor denture hygiene, ill-fitting dentures, traumatic dentures, carbohydrate-rich diets, xerostomia (e.g. Sjögren's syndrome).
2. **Systemic factors**: iron and folate deficiency, diabetes mellitus, immune defects.

Microbiology and histopathology. Generally considered to be due to accumulation of microbial plaque with yeasts and bacteria on the fitting surface of the denture and the underlying mucosa. In the papillary hyperplastic variety, *Candida* species do not invade the epithelium. Other aetiological factors such as mechanical irritation or an allergic reaction to the denture base material may be involved.

Treatment. The condition is treated by:
- scrupulous denture hygiene and removal of dentures at night (these measures alone, without antifungals, are adequate in a majority of cases)
- regular disinfection of dentures by steeping them in sodium hypochlorite or chlorhexidine to eradicate the reservoir of candidal cells in the prosthesis
- review of the denture fitness to relieve trauma, if any
- a diet with a low content of fermentable carbohydrates
- polyene antifungals — nystatin, amphotericin (lozenges, pastilles, etc.).

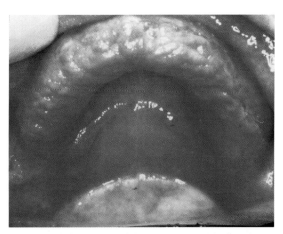

Fig. 35.6 *Candida*-associated denture stomatitis showing the erythematous and oedematous denture-bearing (palatal) mucosa (Newton's type 2 lesion).

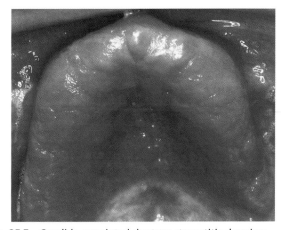

Fig. 35.7 *Candida*-associated denture stomatitis showing palatal papillary hyperplasia (Newton's type 3 lesion).

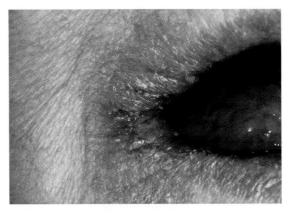

Fig. 35.8 Angular cheilitis in a denture wearer. Note the yellow crusting due to staphylococcal infection.

Angular stomatitis (perleche, angular cheilitis)

The lesions of angular stomatitis are seen in one or both angles of the mouth (Fig. 35.8), especially as a complication of *Candida*-associated denture stomatitis.

Clinical features. Characterized by soreness, erythema and fissuring, this condition is commonly associated with denture-induced stomatitis. Both yeasts and bacteria (especially *Staphylococcus aureus*) are involved as interacting predisposing factors. However, angular stomatitis is very occasionally an isolated initial sign of anaemia or vitamin deficiency, such as vitamin B₁₂ deficiency, and resolves when the underlying disease has been treated. The condition is also seen in HIV-associated disease (Fig. 35.9).

Microbiology. Candida spp. are present with or without co-infection with *Staphylococcus aureus*. The presence of yellow crusting may indicate staphylococcal infection.

Treatment
1. Elimination of the intraoral reservoir of infection in concurrent denture stomatitis.
2. Adjustment of vertical dimension of the dentures to prevent saliva retention, and moisture at the angles of the mouth (*note*: moist surfaces encourage the growth of *Candida*).
3. Topical antifungal therapy with nystatin, amphotericin or miconazole (miconazole has both antifungal and antistaphylococcal activity and is useful for mixed infections); antistaphylococcal preparations (dictated by

microbiological investigation) include fusidic acid and neomycin/chlorhexidine.
4. Investigate for possible underlying disease: iron or vitamin B₁₂ deficiency; HIV infection.

Median rhomboid glossitis

Midline glossitis, or glossal central papillary atrophy, is characterized by an area of papillary atrophy which is elliptical or rhomboid in shape and symmetrically placed centrally at the midline of the tongue, anterior to the circumvallate papillae. Occasionally median rhomboid glossitis presents with a hyperplastic exophytic or even lobulated appearance. The condition frequently shows a mixed bacterial–fungal microflora.

Candidiasis and immunocompromised hosts

A few patients have chronic candidiasis from an early age, sometimes with a definable immune defect; e.g. chronic mucocutaneous candidiasis (Figs 35.10, 35.11). Candidal infections in these patients are seen in the oral mucosa, skin and other body parts. These secondary oral candidal infections have increased recently because of the high prevalence of attenuated immune response, consequential to diseases such as HIV infection, haematological malignancy and treatment protocols including aggressive cytotoxic therapy.

Oral candidiasis in HIV disease

Candidal infections, with oral thrush and oesophagitis as frequent clinical manifestations, are the most common opportunistic infections encountered in acquired immune deficiency syndrome (AIDS). It has also been shown that the occurrence of an otherwise unexpected mycosis (typically oral candidiasis) in an HIV-infected individual is a poor prognostic indicator of the subsequent development of full-blown AIDS (see also Ch. 30).

Systemic candidiasis

Candidiasis is usually restricted to the skin and mucous membranes but may occasionally spread and manifest systemically (multisystem involvement). Systemic forms of candidiasis may affect only one organ or be disseminated (candidal septicaemia, candidaemia). This occurs mainly in compromised patients, e.g. up to 30% of all patients with acute leukaemia die with systemic candidal infections.

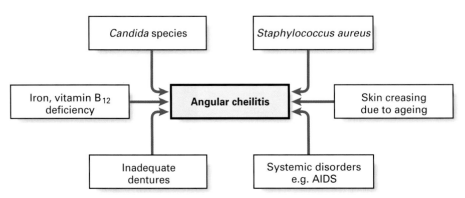

Fig. 35.9 The aetiological factors implicated in angular cheilitis.

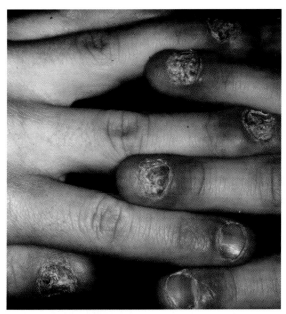

Fig. 35.10 Candidal paronychia in a patient with chronic mucocutaneous candidiasis (*note*: this patient also had scalp and oral involvement).

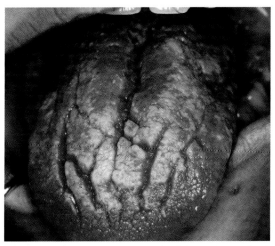

Fig. 35.11 Chronic mucocutaneous candidiasis: hyperplastic lesions of the tongue in the same patient shown in Figure 35.10.

Laboratory diagnosis

A summary of the specimens required for the laboratory diagnosis of oral candidal infections is given in Table 35.1.

ORAL MANIFESTATIONS OF SYSTEMIC MYCOSES

A number of systemic fungal infections may manifest as oral ulcerations or granulomas. Many of these are caused by dimorphic fungi and are uncommon in the West, but are seen in developing countries. These oral lesions are usually secondary diseases, the primary lesions being confined to the lungs and/or the skin. Because the primary lesion is internal, it may go unnoticed until the secondary oral lesion presents as the apparently initial manifestation of the infection (e.g. histoplasmosis). Usually the lesions heal without causing illness, but in progressive disease, sometimes related to lung cavitation, infection can disseminate to skin, mucosae and

internal organs. In a majority of patients the initial lesion heals, often asymptomatically, and delayed hypersensitivity develops, with a positive skin test reaction to the appropriate antigen. Almost all these infections present in the oral cavity as ulcerations.

Diagnosis

Direct demonstration of yeast-like forms of the fungi in exudate, sputum or biopsy specimens; isolation in appropriate culture media and/or serology.

Treatment

Almost all dimorphic fungi are sensitive to amphotericin; fluconazole may be an alternative.

Some examples of these infections are given below:

Examples of systemic fungal infections

Histoplasmosis

Agent. *Histoplasma capsulatum*, a dimorphic fungus.

Main oral sites affected. Oral mucosa, tongue, palate, gingiva, periapical region.

Clinical features. Nodular indurated or granular masses and ulceration; tissue destruction with bone erosion.

Frequency of oral infection. In 40–50% of cases.

Paracoccidioidomycosis

Agent. *Paracoccidioides brasiliensis*, a dimorphic fungus (more common in Western countries than in Asia).

Main oral sites affected. Tongue, hard and soft palate, gingiva.

Clinical features. Papules or vesicles leading to ulceration.

Table 35.1 Specimens required for the laboratory diagnosis of oral candidal infections

Disease	Smear	Swab	Biopsy
Pseudomembranous candidiasis	+	+	−
Erythematous candidiasis	±	+	−
Denture stomatitis:			
palate	+	+	−
denture	+	+	−
Hyperplastic candidiasis	+	±	+
Angular cheilitis	+	+	−
Median rhomboid glossitis	+	+	−

+, useful; ±, may be useful; −, inappropriate.
Note: an oral rinse (with 10 mL of saline) for 1 min is required to evaluate the oral carriage of *Candida* in terms of colony forming units/mL (CFU/mL).

Frequency of oral infection. Common.

Penicilliosis

Agent. *Penicillium marneffei*, a dimorphic fungus, common in South-East Asia.

Main oral sites affected. Palate, gingiva, labial mucosa, tongue, oropharynx.

Clinical features. Erosions or shallow ulcers covered with a white slough.

Frequency of oral infection. Very common.

ORAL VIRAL INFECTIONS

The majority of virus infections of the oral mucosa are due to the herpes group of viruses. Occasionally other viruses, such as coxsackieviruses, papillomaviruses and paramyxoviruses (which cause measles and mumps), may manifest with oral symptoms (see Ch. 21).

Primary herpes simplex infection: herpetic stomatitis (HHV-1, HHV-2)

Herpetic stomatitis is the most common viral infection to affect the mouth; it is caused by human herpesviruses 1 and 2 (HHV-1, HHV-2). The incubation period is about 5 days and the virus is transmitted by contact with skin lesions or infected saliva. Children may carry the virus asymptomatically, or as convalescent carriers, in saliva for several months, but the virus is rarely isolated from adults once the primary lesion heals. The early childhood infection is usually subclinical, frequently dismissed as 'teething', but if the infection occurs in adults the symptoms are obvious and severe. In countries with high standards of hygiene, there is an increasing frequency of adults presenting with primary herpes.

Clinical features

In the initial stages there is mild to severe fever and enlarged lymph nodes, with pain in the mouth and throat; then a variable number of vesicles develop haphazardly on the oral mucosa, the tongue and gingivae. These vesicles rupture quickly to form small round or irregular superficial ulcers with erythematous haloes and greyish-yellow bases. The gingivae are inflamed and the infection may be confused with acute necrotizing ulcerative gingivitis (ANUG) of bacterial origin. In some, ANUG may develop secondary to primary herpetic stomatitis. The mouth is very painful and eating and swallowing may be difficult. The lesions resolve without scarring within 5–10 days.

Secondary herpes simplex infection: herpes labialis (HHV-1, HHV-2)

About a third of the patients who have had primary infection develop herpes labialis (cold sore) in later life as a result of **reactivation of the latent virus**, which usually resides in the trigeminal ganglion. The stimulus for reactivation could be:

- stress
- trauma
- exposure to sunlight
- menstruation
- debilitating disease.

The lesion develops at the mucocutaneous junction of the lip or on the skin adjacent to the nostrils. Characteristically the lesions are preceded, some 24 hours before, by a premonitory sign of itching, prickling or a burning sensation. Blisters then develop, enlarge, coalesce, rupture, become encrusted and heal within 10–14 days (see Fig. 21.3).

Intraoral recurrent herpetic infections are infrequent; they involve the hard palate, alveolar ridges and gingiva. These lesions develop in a similar manner to those of the lips, and appear as a cluster of small, shallow ulcers with red, irregular margins. Pain is not a common feature and the intraoral lesions may or may not recur intermittently for years.

Herpetic dermatitis and herpetic whitlow (HHV 1 and 2)

Primary herpetic dermatitis is localized and characterized by pruritus, burning and pain. Multiple vesicles appear, persist for 4–5 days and burst, with resultant crusting scabs which heal within 2–3 weeks. Dentists who escaped exposure in childhood may contract herpetic dermatitis from patients who have either primary or secondary herpes. Infection may take the form of a herpetic whitlow on the finger, resulting in an intensely painful lesion (see Fig. 21.2). Herpetic whitlow may recur, but less frequently than the perioral infection.

Laboratory diagnosis of herpetic infection

See also Chapter 6.

Direct examination. Smears should be stained with monoclonal fluorescent antisera to herpes simplex virus type 1 or 2 (HHV-1 or -2). This technique is specific and rapid.

Culture. Herpes simplex virus is readily isolated from samples of oral lesions in a variety of tissue culture systems.

Serology. In primary infection a fourfold or greater increase in antibody titre between the acute and convalescent sera is indicative of recent infection with herpes simplex virus. The demonstration of IgM antibodies by immunofluorescence techniques in a single sample can also be used in diagnosis.

Management

Moderate to severe primary herpetic stomatitis is treated with oral and topical aciclovir, together with symptomatic measures. However, the use of aciclovir in recurrent herpetic infections should be limited to immunocompromised patients and those who have a past history of severe, extensive or frequently recurring lesions. The patients should apply the drug *before* vesicles form to obtain the best results.

Varicella and zoster (HHV-3)

Primary infection with the varicella–zoster virus causes chickenpox. Zoster or shingles is the **secondary** (syn. post-primary, reactivation) **infection** due to the reactivation of the virus hiding in the latent form in sensory ganglia (e.g. the trigeminal ganglion for the facial region; see Fig. 21.3).

Chickenpox

Chickenpox is a common infectious disease and is usually contracted in childhood.

Oral manifestations. Before the typical skin rash develops, lesions may be found in the mouth, especially on the hard palate, pillars of the fauces and uvula, although any area of the oral mucosa may be involved. The characteristic skin rash, which is centripetal, and progresses from macular to papular, vesicular and pustular forms before scabbing, helps to differentiate chickenpox from other causes of oral ulceration. The oral lesions consist of small ulcers surrounded by an area of erythema. The vesicles are quickly ruptured in the mouth and therefore rarely noticed. The lesions may be painful in adults, but children rarely complain of discomfort.

Shingles (zoster)

Shingles is a localized eruption due to the reactivation of the herpes zoster virus. It involves an area of skin supplied by one or more sensory ganglia in which the virus is residing. In some 10% of cases zoster reflects an underlying immunedeficiency state, possibly a neoplasm such as lymphoma or HIV disease.

Oral manifestations. The trigeminal nerve is affected in about 15% of cases, with the ophthalmic, maxillary and mandibular divisions involved in that order of precedence. The lesions of shingles may be found on the skin, on the oral mucosa, or both. Severe localized oral pain often precedes the rash and mimics the pain of toothache. The most common intraoral sites affected are the anterior half of the tongue, the soft palate and the cheek. The vesicles break down intraorally within a few hours to give very painful ulcerated areas with a yellowish-grey surface and erythematous borders. The oral lesions heal more quickly than the skin lesions and rarely scar.

Laboratory diagnosis of chickenpox and shingles

The clinical presentation is characteristic, but in unusual circumstances the disease can be confirmed in the laboratory by submitting:
- vesicle fluid for electron microscopy and virus isolation
- smears from an ulcer for immunofluorescence
- acute or convalescent sera to test for the presence of specific IgM antibodies by immunofluorescence.

Management

Chickenpox is self-limiting; but an effective vaccine is available to prevent infection. For zoster, high-dose aciclovir (800 mg five times daily) should be prescribed as soon as possible, especially in immunocompromised patients.

Epstein–Barr virus infections (HHV-4)

Epstein–Barr virus is the agent of a number of infections including infectious mononucleosis, nasopharyngeal carcinoma, Burkitt's lymphoma, and oral hairy leukoplakia and post-transplant lymphoproliferative diseases.

Infectious mononucleosis

Infectious mononucleosis is an acute infectious disease, mainly of children and young adults. The agent, the Epstein–Barr virus, is present in the oropharyngeal secretions of patients suffering or convalescing from infectious mononucleosis; the disease is transmitted by kissing. The virus has also been demonstrated in the oropharynx of healthy carriers.

Oral manifestations. At the onset the throat is painful and congested but exudate is absent. An enanthem consisting of clusters of fine petechial haemorrhages may be seen at the junction of the hard and soft palates (these lesions are also found in other virus infections of the respiratory tract). Subsequently, a white pseudomembrane may develop on the tonsil and on other parts of the oral mucosa, and oral ulceration may occur. Other presenting signs may be submandibular lymphadenitis and mild fever.

Laboratory diagnosis. The diagnosis of infectious mononucleosis may be possible on the typical clinical presentation. Laboratory tests required to confirm the diagnosis include:
- **haematology**: differential white blood cell count to demonstrate the lymphocytosis and atypical mononuclear cells (20%)
- **serology**:
  - testing an acute serum sample for the presence of IgM antibodies to the Epstein–Barr virus capsid antigen (using an immunofluorescence technique)
  - the monospot or Paul–Bunnell tests.

Hairy leukoplakia

See Chapter 30.

Oral manifestations of other herpesviruses (HHV 5–8)

Other herpesvirus infections are generally of minor consequence, except for Kaposi's sarcoma caused by HHV-8 (see Ch. 21).

Coxsackievirus infections

Two diseases caused by group A coxsackieviruses produce oral signs and symptoms:
- **hand, foot and mouth disease**, caused mainly by coxsackievirus A16 and less commonly by types A4, A5, A9 or A10
- **herpangina**, caused by coxsackieviruses A2, A4, A5, A6 and A8.

Oral manifestations of herpangina

This febrile disease is characterized by sore throat, dysphagia, anorexia and occasionally a stiff neck. Accompanying oral signs and symptoms are small, papulovesicular lesions about 1–2 mm in diameter, with a greyish-white surface surrounded by red areolae, especially in the palate. The disease lasts for about 3–4 days, the fever abates and the oral lesions heal promptly.

Paramyxovirus infections

Measles, mumps, parainfluenza and respiratory syncytial viruses are categorized as paramyxoviruses. Of these, measles and mumps are of concern in dentistry as they commonly manifest with oral signs or symptoms. Measles is discussed in Chapter 21; mumps is described later under salivary gland infections.

ORAL MANIFESTATIONS OF BACTERIAL INFECTIONS

Syphilis

Primary syphilis

Chancre is the characteristic sign of primary syphilis and normally appears in the genitalia, but extragenital lesions, mostly in the oral cavity, occur in some 10% of cases. The common sites affected are the lips and tongue, and to a lesser extent the gingival and tonsillar area. The lesions heal spontaneously about 5 weeks after appearing. The regional lymph nodes are usually enlarged.

Secondary syphilis

Oral manifestations are slightly raised, greyish-white glistening patches on the mucosa — the so-called '**mucous patches**' of the tonsils, soft palate, tongue and cheek (Fig. 35.12); gingivae are rarely involved. The surface membrane covering the lesions is grey and easily removed, and contains many spirochaetes. The mucous patches may later coalesce to produce a serpiginous lesion ('**snail-track' ulcer**). The cer-

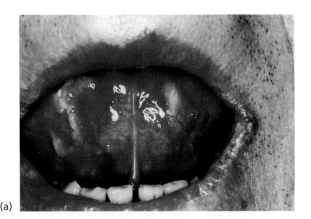
(a)

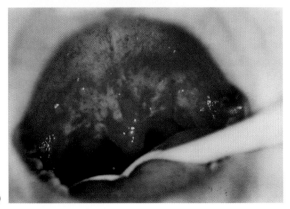
(b)

Fig. 35.12 Mucous patches of secondary syphilis on the tongue (a) and soft palate (b).

Table 35.2 Oral manifestations and infectivity of syphilis

Stage	Orofacial manifestations	Infectivity
Primary	Chancre of lip, tongue, gingiva	+++
Secondary	Mucous patches on tonsil, tongue, soft palate, cheek; 'snail-track' ulcers; rubbery, enlarged cervical lymph nodes	++
Tertiary	'Gumma' of palate; rarely osteomyelitis; syphilitic leukoplakia leading to carcinoma	±
Congenital	Hutchinson's incisors; 'mulberry' molars; facial deformities with open bite or dish face	−

vical lymph nodes are enlarged and rubbery in consistency. The lesions heal spontaneously 2–6 weeks after appearing. However, typical lesions may not always be present because of unrelated antibiotic therapy.

Tertiary syphilis

The characteristic sign of this stage is the **gumma**. The most common oral site of gumma formation is the hard palate, but the soft palate, lips and tongue may be involved (Table 35.2). The lesion starts as a small, pale, raised, painless area which ulcerates and rapidly progresses to a large, necrotic zone with exposure of bone, and in the case of the palate may eventually perforate into the nasal cavity. The palatal lesions are usually midline; in rare cases the soft palate may be involved. No spirochaetes are found in gummata.

Atrophic or interstitial glossitis is another oral manifestation of tertiary syphilis. Clinically there is atrophy of the filiform and fungiform papillae, which results in a smooth, sometimes wrinkled, lingual surface. Subsequent leukoplakia may develop.

Late and quaternary syphilis

The quaternary stage of syphilis, which may develop 10–20 years after primary syphilis, is characterized by two main clinical forms; cardiovascular syphilis and neurosyphilis. No specific oral manifestations are seen at this stage.

Congenital syphilis

The dental lesions are a result of infection of the developing tooth germ by *Treponema pallidum*. The deciduous teeth are minimally affected; the permanent teeth may be malformed or fail to develop. The most common dental manifestations of congenital syphilis are **Hutchinson's incisors** and '**mulberry**' **molar** teeth. In the former, upper central incisors are mostly involved; the teeth are barrel-shaped and have a crescentic notch at the incisal edge. In the latter the first permanent molar teeth have a roughened dirty, yellow, hypoplastic occlusal surface, with poorly developed cusps resembling the surface of a mulberry. Other manifestations of congenital syphilis include frontal bossing and saddle nose.

Tuberculosis

Oral lesions of tuberculosis are usually secondary to primary infection elsewhere, commonly the lung. Primary infections of the oral mucosa by *Mycobacterium tuberculosis* are rare. In the case of secondary infection the sources of infection are contaminated sputum or blood-borne bacilli. Lesions are found more commonly in the posterior area of the mouth and it has been suggested that this may be due to the relative propensity of lymphoid tissue in this region. The major oral lesions are:

- oral ulceration
- tuberculous lymphadenitis
- periapical granulomas and bone infections.

Oral ulceration

There is a wide spectrum of tuberculous lesions of the oral mucosa, including indolent **ulcers**, diffuse inflammatory lesions, **granulomas** and **fissures**; pain may be mild or absent. The tongue is most commonly affected but lesions have been noted on the buccal mucosa, gingivae, floor of the mouth, lips, and the hard and soft palates. Primary tuberculosis of the oral mucosa is more common in children and adolescents than in adults and usually presents as a single, painless indolent ulcer, commonly on the gingiva, with enlarged cervical lymph nodes, or as a white patch.

Tuberculous lymphadenitis

The cervical glands are most commonly affected, and in patients with pulmonary tuberculosis the route of infection is probably by lymphatic or haematogenous spread, or via an abrasion of the mouth. In patients with no evidence of systemic infection the route is probably via the tonsils or oral mucosa. The typical presentation is a lump in the neck, which may be painful. The size may vary and in the early stages the swelling is firm but mobile. Later the mass becomes fixed, with the formation of an abscess and sinus — a **cold abscess**. The lesions may be unilateral, bilateral, single or multiple.

Periapical granuloma and bone infections

In patients with active tuberculosis, tubercle bacilli are seen in periapical granulomas. Tooth extraction may lead to delayed healing of the socket, which fills with '**tuberculous granulations**'.

Bone infections are not uncommon in tuberculosis: secondary tuberculous osteomyelitis may involve the maxilla or mandible. Here the bacilli may gain access to the bone by:

- haematogenous spread
- direct spread from an oral lesion
- infected saliva entering an extraction socket or fracture.

Tuberculous osteomyelitis of the jaws is chronic in nature, usually with severe pain and the production of bony sequestra.

Tuberculosis of the salivary glands

See below.

Leprosy

Leprosy, a granulomatous disease caused by *Mycobacterium leprae*, is of two main types, the tuberculoid and the lepromatous variants (see Ch. 19).

Tuberculoid leprosy

Tuberculoid leprosy does not directly affect the oral mucosa but the associated neurological features may affect the mouth and face. Such manifestations vary from loss of eyebrows to nodular involvement of all facial cutaneous and subcutaneous structures. If the trigeminal nerve is involved, **hyperaesthesia** or **paraesthesia** of the face, lips, tongue, palate, cheeks or gingiva may be present; secondary **ocular changes** may occur, with subsequent corneal and conjunctival sensory loss. The facial lesions of tuberculoid leprosy comprise dry, hairless, anaesthetic plaques, with a well-defined and raised border, which are red on white skin and hypopigmented on dark skin.

Lepromatous leprosy

In lepromatous leprosy *M. leprae* is present in many tissues of the body, and multiple, erythematous, bilateral and symmetrical lesions are found on the skin of the face, arms and legs. The lesions are anaesthetic. The nasomaxillary complex is the primary area of destruction in the facial region. Facial skeletal changes, such as saddle nose, atrophy of the anterior nasal spine and premaxillary bone recession, are common, with or without tooth loss (see Fig. 19.2). Dental deformities are limited to a pink discoloration of the upper incisors due to invasion of the pulp by infected granulomatous tissue, which can produce pulpitis and pulp death.

The incidence of oral lesions in lepromatous leprosy varies from 10% to 60%. Intraoral nodules have been described as yellowish-red, soft to hard, sessile, single or confluent lesions which tend to ulcerate. Healing is by secondary intention with fibrous scars. The sites most commonly involved are the premaxillary gingivae, the hard and soft palates, the uvula and tongue. Tongue lesions, particularly on the anterior two-thirds, consist of single or multiple nodules, giving a 'cobblestone' appearance, or in some instances may resemble a geographic tongue. As the saliva of patients with oral lesions commonly contains *M. leprae*, this could be a possible source of infection.

SALIVARY GLAND INFECTIONS

Inflammation of the salivary glands (**sialadenitis**) due to infective causes is not an uncommon phenomenon. Sialadenitis can be:

- viral (in the majority)
- bacterial (in the minority).

The parotid glands are more commonly infected than the submandibular glands, and infections of the accessory salivary glands are very rare (Table 35.3). Apart from mumps, the majority of salivary gland infections are seen in adults.

Pathogenesis

Initiation and progression of salivary gland infections depend on the **decrease in host resistance** to infection:

- **general**: debility, dehydration
- **local**: obstruction of ducts due to sialoliths (salivary stones), strictures or other pathology

Table 35.3 Classification of salivary gland infections

Type of infection	Gland usually affected	Predisposing factor(s)
Mumps (endemic parotitis)	Parotid	No prior exposure to virus
Acute suppurative parotitis	Parotid	Severe xerostomia (e.g. Sjögren's syndrome), localized and diffuse abnormalities of the salivary glands
Obstructive sialadenitis	Submandibular	Sialoliths, foreign bodies, ductal strictures, mucus plugs
Suppurative and chronic recurrent parotitis of childhood	Parotid	Congenital or acquired abnormality of ductal system
Rare miscellaneous disorders, e.g. tuberculosis, actinomycosis and fungal infections	Parotid or submandibular	Systemic infection by specific agents, e.g. *Mycobacterium tuberculosis*

and the **virulence** of the causative organism. Factors important in salivary gland infections are shown in Figure 35.13.

Viral infections of salivary glands

Mumps (endemic parotitis)

Mumps is caused by an RNA paramyxovirus, which infects circulating lymphocytes, especially activated T cells. These spread in the blood, 'targeting' salivary duct epithelial cells and replicating in them, leading to acinar disintegration, periductal oedema and a mononuclear infiltrate (Fig. 35.14). Subsequently the virus is shed in saliva and spreads into the bloodstream, causing a viraemia.

Epidemiology. The disease is frequently seen in winter and spring. Clinical or subclinical infection may occur at all ages but is most common in childhood.

Incubation period and infectivity. Approximately 14–28 days; the saliva of patients incubating mumps (during the prodromal period) is infectious for a few days before parotitis develops and up to 2 weeks after the onset of clinical symptoms. Mumps is transmitted by direct contact with saliva and by droplet spread, and hence the disease may be contracted in the dental clinic environment.

Clinical features. These include:
- pyrexia, sore throat, furred tongue, trismus and earache, commonly

- pain on chewing and/or pain and tenderness on upward pressure beneath the angle of the lower jaw (pain may be acute during salivation)
- reddening of the opening of the parotid duct
- increase in glandular size, and varying consistency of the gland from normal to very hard
- low salivary flow rate leading to non-specific stomatitis and halitosis
- trismus and earache due to parotid involvement
- either one or both parotid glands may be involved, with a delay of up to 5 days in between; salivary glands other than the parotid may be enlarged in some 10% of cases
- the clinical course of mumps varies widely, from a mild upset lasting a day or two to a severe illness with high fever lasting up to 2 weeks; complete recovery is usual.

Complications. Complications are due to involvement of other glands or tissues, leading to meningoencephalitis (30%) and orchitis (25% of adult males); rarely thyroiditis, neuritis, myocarditis and nephritis.

Diagnosis. Diagnosis is normally made on clinical grounds. On unusual clinical presentation, laboratory investigations may be required and include:
- **serology**: demonstrate of antibodies to mumps virus antigens using serological tests, e.g. the detection of IgM antibodies using immunofluorescence
- **electron microscopy**: saliva (pure parotid saliva collected by cannulation) may be examined for typical virus particles.

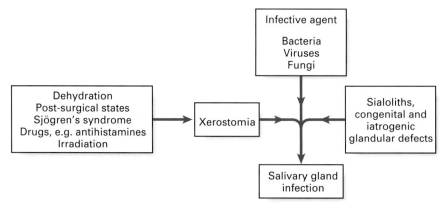

Fig. 35.13 Factors important in the pathogenesis of salivary gland infections.

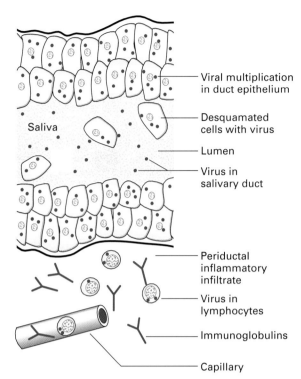

Saliva

Viral multiplication
in duct epithelium

Desquamated
cells with virus

Lumen

Virus in
salivary duct

Periductal
inflammatory
infiltrate

Virus in
lymphocytes

Immunoglobulins

Capillary

Fig. 35.14 Mumps virus multiplication in salivary duct and shedding into saliva.

Salivary gland disease in HIV infection

Salivary gland disease may occur in a minority of HIV-infected individuals. **Xerostomia** and/or **enlargement** of the major salivary glands are the two main presentations: xerostomia is present in some 10% of cases, while major gland enlargement may be accompanied by illness resembling Sjögren's syndrome.

The histological picture is variable, with lymphocytic sialadenitis, hyperplasia of salivary lymph nodes, Kaposi's sarcoma or lymphoma. The aetiology of HIV-induced salivary gland disease is not clear.

Other viral infections

Mumps is the most common viral cause of sialadenitis, but a member of the herpesvirus group, cytomegalovirus, can also cause a clinical disease, **cytomegalic inclusion disease** (salivary gland inclusion disease), which affects newborns, children and adults and has multiple systemic manifestations, including salivary gland enlargement. The disease is so called because of the large, doubly-contoured **'owl eye' inclusion bodies** seen within the nucleus or cytoplasm of duct cells of the parotid gland.

Rarely, other viruses such as parainfluenza virus types 2 and 3, echoviruses and coxsackieviruses have been implicated in non-suppurative sialadenitis.

Bacterial infections of salivary glands

Acute suppurative parotitis (bacterial sialadenitis)

Acute suppurative parotitis is seen mostly in adults with salivary gland abnormalities. In the past it was primarily a disease of dehydrated or postoperative patients, but with the introduction of proper fluid balance and antibiotic prophylaxis, suppurative parotitis in these groups is now rare.

Aetiology and pathogenesis. In health, potential oral pathogens cannot ascend the salivary ducts and invade the glandular tissue because of the flushing action of saliva. However, if the flow of saliva is greatly reduced or stopped, a retrograde infection via the salivary duct may ensue. Predisposing factors include:

- drugs that reduce salivary flow, e.g. diuretics, certain antihistamines, tranquillizers and anticholinergics
- localized salivary gland abnormalities, e.g. calculus, mucus plug or benign strictures
- generalized sialectasis, e.g. in patients who become dehydrated after gastrointestinal surgery or patients with Sjögren's syndrome (a progressive degenerative disease affecting salivary gland tissue).

Clinical features

1. Unilateral or bilateral swelling of the parotid glands may be present for days or weeks. Swelling may be limited to the gland or, in more severe infections, extend locally, involving the pre- and postauricular areas. The ear lobes may be displaced laterally.
2. Purulent salivary secretions occur at the duct orifice.
3. Trismus results from pain and swelling.
4. Usually there are no systemic symptoms, but occasionally fever, chills and leucocytosis may be seen.
5. In chronic infection, recurrent bouts of acute exacerbation of infection followed by periods of remission may lead to replacement fibrosis.

Investigations

- If possible pus should be aspirated through a fine, small-bore, polythene catheter attached to a syringe, or collected aseptically on a cotton-wool swab by 'milking' the duct, and sent immediately to the laboratory. The ductal orifice and the subjacent mucosa should be decontaminated with an antiseptic such as chlorhexidine prior to swab collection of pus.
- Catheter collection of pus should not be performed during the acute stage.
- Pus should be collected before antibiotics are prescribed.

Microbiology. Both monomicrobial and polymicrobial infections may occur. The organisms most commonly isolated are α-haemolytic streptococci; the frequency of isolation of *Staphylococcus aureus* is gradually diminishing (Table 35.4).

Treatment. The treatment of choice is **parenteral antibiotic therapy**, guided by culture of pus and sensitivity tests. Amoxicillin is the agent of choice, or erythromycin in patients hypersensitive to penicillins. A Gram-stained smear of the pus is useful in deciding initial antibiotic therapy.

Thorough oral hygiene is extremely important. Salivation should be encouraged by increased fluid intake (rehydration) and the use of **sialagogues** (e.g. lemon juice). In severe cases, consider surgical drainage of pus.

Once the acute condition has resolved, the patient should be referred for sialographic investigation of the affected gland or glands to identify correctable salivary gland abnormalities

Table 35.4   Bacteria commonly isolated from bacterial parotitis

Common isolates[a]
Alpha-haemolytic streptococci
Staphylococcus aureus

Less common isolates
Haemophilus spp.
Eikenella corrodens
Bacteroides spp.
Anaerobic streptococci

Rare isolates
Neisseria gonorrhoeae
Mycobacterium tuberculosis
Actinomyces spp.
Treponema pallidum

[a] Polymicrobial infections are common.

(e.g. mucus plugs, benign strictures and calculi) which lead to recurrence of infection. *Note:* sialography should never be attempted during the acute phase of the illness.

Subsequent treatment options include duct dilation, removal of ductal obstructions or surgical revision of ducts.

Sequelae. If acute bacterial parotitis is untreated, severe complications may ensue, especially in debilitated patients. These are:

- extension of inflammation and oedema into the neck and resultant respiratory obstruction
- cellulitis of the face and neck
- osteomyelitis of adjacent facial bones
- rarely, septicaemia and death.

Submandibular sialadenitis

Submandibular sialadenitis is less common than acute suppurative bacterial parotitis. Most bacterial infections of the submandibular glands are associated with obstructive ductal disease (e.g. sialoliths and ductal strictures). The aetiology, microbiology and management of submandibular (submaxillary) sialadenitis are similar to those of bacterial parotitis.

Neonatal suppurative parotitis and recurrent parotitis of childhood

These rare diseases, with unknown aetiology, are confined to the first decade of life. In recurrent parotitis, the child experiences repeated, acute episodes of painful parotid gland enlargement. The suggested predisposing factors include congenital abnormalities of the ductal system, preceding mumps, and foreign bodies in the parotid duct. Management includes removal of the aetiological agent, symptomatic therapy and antibiotics, if necessary.

Rare bacterial infections of salivary glands

Salivary gland infections by organisms such as *Treponema pallidum*, *Neisseria gonorrhoea*, *Actinomyces israelii* and *Mycobacterium tuberculosis* have been rarely described. These may be due to:

- endogenous, ascending infection via salivary ducts (e.g. *A. israelii*)
- infection via an adjacent, contiguous focus (e.g. *T. pallidum*)
- reactivation of an old lesion (e.g. *M. tuberculosis*).

KEY FACTS

- **Oral candidiasis**, an opportunistic infection, is the most common oral fungal infection in humans, and is usually seen in the **very young, the very old and the very sick**
- *Oral candidiasis, classified as a superficial (as opposed to systemic) mycosis can be broadly subdivided into* **primary** *and* **secondary disease**: *primary infection is strictly confined to the oral cavity whereas the secondary disease is present both in the oral and other superficial body sites*
- *The classic disease triad of oral candidiasis comprises* **pseudomembranous (thrush)**, **erythematous** *and* **hyperplastic** *variants*
- Other common *Candida*-associated lesions are denture stomatitis, angular cheilitis and median rhomboid glossitis
- **Herpesviruses** (eight are now recognized) cause the majority of oral viral infections
- *In general,* **herpes simplex viruses types 1 and 2 (HHV-1, HHV-2)** *cause infections above and below the belt, respectively (i.e. oral and genital infections)*
- *Herpetic gingivostomatitis is the primary infection and herpes labialis the reactivation infection caused by HHV-1*
- *Varicella–zoster virus (HHV-3) causes chickenpox (primary infection) and zoster/shingles (reactivation infection) affecting well-defined dermatomes ('belt of roses from hell')*

- *Epstein–Barr virus (HHV-4) causes* **infectious mononucleosis** *or* **glandular fever**, *common in young adults*
- *Group A coxsackieviruses cause* **hand, foot and mouth disease** *of children and* **herpangina**; *oral lesions are papulovesicular, small and greyish-white*
- **Oral manifestations of syphilis** are chancre (primary syphilis), **mucous patches** and **snail-track ulcers** (secondary), and **gumma** and **interstitial glossitis** (tertiary)
- **Mulberry (moon) molars** and **Hutchinson's incisors** can be seen in congenital syphilis, due to infection of the tooth germ by *Treponema pallidum*; other manifestations are frontal bossing and saddle nose
- *Oral ulceration, lymphadenitis, and periapical granulomas and bone infection are the common* **oral manifestations of tuberculosis**; *these are secondary to primary infection of the lungs*
- *Leprosy, a chronic granulomatous disease, manifests as* **tuberculous** *and* **lepromatous** *variants; intraoral nodules, which ulcerate and heal with fibromatous scars, and gross facial disfiguration are seen in the lepromatous variant*
- The **most common salivary gland infection** is caused by the **mumps virus**; bacterial infections of salivary glands are relatively uncommon

KEY FACTS (continued)

- *Mumps* *is characterized by enlargement and inflammation of one or both parotid glands, reddening of the parotid duct orifice, pyrexia and (sometimes) earache*

- **Xerostomia** and **enlargement of major salivary glands** are seen in **HIV infection**

- *Acute suppurative parotitis,* *caused mainly by* α-*haemolytic streptococci and* Staphylococcus aureus, *is exquisitely painful*

- *Management* *of bacterial parotitis entails* **antibiotic therapy,** *good* **oral hygiene, rehydration, sialagogues** *and, if necessary, surgical drainage*

- Less commonly, salivary gland infections are caused by *Mycobacterium tuberculosis,* *Actinomyces* spp., *Neisseria gonorrhoeae* and *Treponema pallidum*

FURTHER READING

Kibber, CC, MacKenzie, DWR, and Odds, FC (eds) (1996). *Principles and practice of clinical mycology*. John Wiley, Chichester.

Lamey, PJ, Boyle, MA, MacFarlane, TW, and Samaranayake, LP (1987). Acute suppurative parotitis in out-patients: microbiological and post-treatment sialographic findings. *Oral Surgery, Oral Medicine, Oral Pathology* 63, 37–41.

Lewis, MAO, and Lamey, PJ (1993). *Clinical oral medicine*. Wright, London.

Odds, FC (1988). *Candida and candidosis* (2nd edn). Baillière Tindall, London.

Reichart, P, Samaranayake, LP, and Philipsen, HP (2000). Pathology and clinical correlates in oral candidiasis and its variants: a review. *Oral Diseases* 6, 85–91.

Samaranayake, LP, and MacFarlane, TW (eds) (1990). *Oral candidosis*. Wright, London.

Scully, C, El-Kabir, M, and Samaranayake, LP (1994). *Candida* and oral candidosis: a review. *Critical Reviews in Oral Biology and Medicine* 5, 125–157.

Scully, C, Flint, SR, and Porter, SR (1996). *Oral diseases* (2nd edn). Martin Dunitz, London.

Cross-infection and control

Part 6

The theoretical and practical aspects described here will undoubtedly regulate the daily infection control regimen of any dental practice. Thus the student is strongly advised to be thoroughly conversant with this subject matter, and to supplement this section with further reading from the lists of recommended books and articles.

- Principles of infection control
- Infection control procedures in dentistry

36 Principles of infection control

CROSS-INFECTION

Cross-infection may be defined as the transmission of infectious agents between patients and staff *within a clinical environment*. Transmission may result from person-to-person contact or via contaminated objects (fomites) (Fig. 36.1). Organisms capable of causing cross-infection in humans are derived from:

- other human sources (the most important)
- animal sources (less important)
- inanimate sources (of least importance).

Principles of infection transmission

Transmission of infection from one person to another requires:

1. A **source** of infection — the person with the infection is called the **index case**.
2. A **mode** or **vehicle** by which the infective agent is transmitted, e.g. blood, droplets of saliva, instruments contaminated with blood, saliva and tissue debris. (Animals or insects may act as vehicles or vectors of transmission, for example in malaria, but are not described here.)
3. A **route** of transmission, e.g. inhalation, ingestion.

Source of infection

The sources of infection in clinical dentistry are mainly human; they include:

1. **People with overt infections** who liberate large numbers of organisms into the environment (e.g. droplets and discharges from the mouth or other portals; wounds, ulcers and sores on the skin). Fortunately, in routine clinical dentistry few patients with acute diseases are seen.
2. **People in the prodromal stage of certain infections.** During the prodrome or the incubating period the organisms multiply without evidence of infection; although the patient is healthy at this stage, he or she is highly infectious. Viral infections, such as measles, mumps and chickenpox, easily spread in this manner.
3. **People who are healthy carriers of pathogens** and can be classified as:
   - convalescent carriers
   - asymptomatic carriers.

Convalescent carriers are those who suffer an illness and apparently recover, although blood and secretions of the individual act as persistent reservoirs of infective organisms. For example, following diphtheria or streptrococcal sore throat, the organisms may persist in the throat for some time and infect others; or in the case of hepatitis B the patient may recover fully, although he or she may carry the infectious agent in the blood for a considerable period. The latter are called **chronic carriers**.

Asymptomatic carriers give no past history of infection as they may have unknowingly had a non-apparent or subclinical infection (recognized merely because of the presence of specific antibodies in the person's blood). Nevertheless, these individuals may carry infective microbes in saliva, blood and other body secretions.

Hepatitis B is a classic example of a disease that may manifest with or without symptoms, and thus the clinician may be faced with either convalescent or asymptomatic carriers of hepatitis B virus. *Note*: a convalescent carrier can be identified from the past history of infection, as opposed to an asymptomatic carrier who cannot be diagnosed in this way.

UNIVERSAL INFECTION CONTROL

From the foregoing it is clear that it is impossible to ascertain whether the patient who attends for dental treatment is a carrier of infectious agents. Therefore, each patient should be treated as if he or she were a reservoir of pathogens. The infection control procedures involved in such treatment are termed **universal precautions** and all clinical procedures performed on **any patient** should be conducted using **universal infection control**. The corollary of this is that no additional infection control precautions should be necessary when a patient who is a carrier of infection such as HIV disease attends the clinic. The importance of this concept cannot be overemphasized and should be noted by all who practise dentistry.

There is however, one exception where universal infection control measures have to be modified. This is the case of potential carriers of **transmissible spongiform encephalopathy** (TSE), a disease caused by a group of very short proteins called **prions** that can multiply without the DNA machinery of the host cell. Prions cannot be destroyed using the routine sterilization protocol, hence when TSE patients are treated special sterilization procedures are required, or alternatively all instruments need to be disposable (see Ch. 4). Fortunately, patients with this disorder are

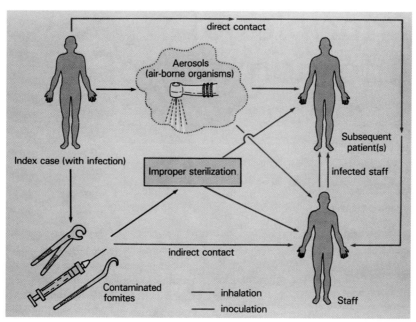

Fig. 36.1 Routes and modes by which infection may spread in the dental clinic.

rare and the disease condition is usually diagnosed post-mortem, but progressive loss of muscular and cognitive function may lead to a presumptive diagnosis.

MODE OF TRANSMISSION

Transmission of infection may occur by:
- **direct contact** of tissues with secretions or blood; this is the least common mode (e.g. an ungloved practitioner with a cut on the finger performing an extraction)
- **droplets** containing infectious agents
- **contaminated sharps** and instruments that have been improperly sterilized (Fig. 36.1).

Some of the infectious agents of concern in dentistry and their possible routes of transmission are given in Table 36.1.

Airborne infection

Airborne infective organisms in the form of infectious aerosols may be inhaled, causing diseases such as influenza, the common cold and tuberculosis. When aerosols are created, for example by high-speed instruments, different sizes of droplets are produced. Their fate depends on their size. Droplets greater than 100 µm in diameter are called **spatter** and settle very quickly on surfaces as a result of gravitational pull; they contaminate whatever is immediately in front of and below the patient. Small droplets of less than 100 µm in diameter account for the majority of droplets created (Table 36.2). They evaporate instantaneously and remain suspended or **entrained** in the air for many hours as **droplet nuclei**, which consist of dried salivary or serum secretions and any organisms they may contain. Eventually they fall to the ground. In practical terms this underscores the importance of adequate ventilation of the clinical environment, particularly during the use of aerosol-creating instruments and the routine disinfection of surgery surfaces.

Table 36.1 Some infectious agents of concern in dentistry and their routes of transmission

Microorganism	Major transmission route
Viruses	
Cytomegalovirus	Inhalation
Hepatitis viruses	
Hepatitis B	Inoculation
Hepatitis C	Inoculation
Delta hepatitis (hepatitis D)	Inoculation
Herpes simplex virus types 1 and 2	Inoculation
Human immunodeficiency virus (HIV)	Inoculation
Measles and mumps viruses	Inhalation
Respiratory viruses	
Influenza virus	Inhalation
Rhinovirus	Inhalation
Adenovirus	Inhalation
Rubella virus	Inhalation
Bacteria	
Neisseria gonorrhoeae	Inoculation
Treponema pallidum (syphilis)	Inoculation
Mycobacterium tuberculosis	Inoculation/inhalation
Streptococcus pyogenes	Inhalation

Table 36.2 Characteristics of aerosols produced by high-speed instrumentation

	Particles	Droplet nuclei
Diameter	> 100 µm	< 100 µm
Time spent airborne	Minutes	Hours
Penetration into respiratory tract	Unlikely	Possible
Possible mode of transmission	Direct contact or from dust	Inhalation

Infection via sharps and needlestick injuries

The major route of cross-infection in the dental surgery is through the skin or mucosa due to accidents involving sharps or needlestick injuries (Fig. 36.1). There is evidence that hepatitis B transmission from patient to dentist and vice versa has occurred by this means.

MODE OF ENTRY

Transmission of the pathogen to the new host is sometimes by **direct contact** but is more often an **indirect process** involving various vehicles of infection, dealt with above. Once the organism has approached the new host it may gain ingress via a number of portals:

- inhalation
- inoculation or injection
- ingestion (e.g. diarrhoeal diseases, see Ch. 26)
- transplacental (e.g. congenital syphilis or HIV acquired in utero).

Inhalation, inoculation and rarely, direct contact are the modes by which the pathogens gain access to the host tissues in the dental clinic environment.

INFECTION CONTROL PROCEDURES

From the foregoing it is evident that the number of infectious diseases that dental personnel may be exposed to during the working day could be fairly substantial. Several measures are available to dental personnel (dentists, dental hygienists, dental surgery assistants, school dental nurses, dental laboratory technicians and radiology technicians) to break this chain of cross-infection; these may be categorized as:

- patient evaluation
- personal protection
- sterilization and disinfection
- safe disposal of waste
- laboratory asepsis.

These subjects are dealt with in detail in the next chapter.

KEY FACTS

- Cross-infection may be defined as the transmission of infectious agents between patients and staff **within a clinical environment**
- The **animate** (e.g. insects, humans) and **inanimate** sources that carry and transmit infection are called **vectors** and **fomites**, respectively
- **Transmission of infection** from one person to another requires a **source** of infection (the index case), a **mode** or **vehicle** of transmission (e.g. vectors and fomites) and a **route** of transmission (e.g. inhalation, percutaneous)
- **Transmission of infection in dentistry** could occur by **direct contact, airborne spread** or via contaminated **sharps**

- The **sources** of infection in clinical dentistry are mainly humans and constitute those (a) with **overt infections,** (b) in the **prodromal stage** of infections, and (c) who are healthy **carriers** of pathogens
- The infective agents may gain entry into the body by **inhalation, inoculation** (or injection) or **ingestion**
- **Healthy carriers** of pathogens are of two types: **convalescent** carriers and **asymptomatic** carriers
- *Universal infection control upholds the concept of treating every patient as a potential carrier of infectious disease. All patients in dentistry, irrespective of whether they carry apparent infections or not, should be treated under a universal infection control protocol*

FURTHER READING

Cottone, JA, Terezhalmy, GT, and Molinari, JA (1991). *Practical infection control in dentistry.* Lea & Febiger, Philadelphia.

Mims, C, Playfair, J, Roitt, I, Wakelin, D, and Williams, R (1998). Hospital infection, sterilization and disinfection. In *Medical microbiology* (2nd edn), Ch. 34. Mosby, London.

Samaranayake, LP (1989). Cross infection prevention in dentistry. Part I: general concepts and surgery attire. *Dental Update* 16, 58–63.

Samaranayake, LP, Scheutz, F, and Cottone, J (1991). *Infection control for the dental team.* Munksgaard, Copenhagen.

37 Infection control procedures in dentistry

Implementation of **universal infection control** in dentistry (also termed **standard precautions**) entails prevention of infection transmission within the dental clinic environment, and **assumes that ALL patients are carriers of infectious diseases**. Such a policy protects both patients and staff, reduces staff concerns and prevents discrimination against patients. In this chapter, the major features reflecting the best current practice of universal infection control are outlined, but the reader is strongly advised to keep up to date with the literature because of the rapidity of changes that occur in this area.

PRACTICE MANAGEMENT AND STAFF DEVELOPMENT

All staff who join a practice should undergo a **formal education programme** that includes the theory and practice of infection control in dentistry. In addition, a written **infection control protocol** specific for the practice should be available for inspection by patients and other interested parties.

An **in-service training** programme, updating techniques and material, should be provided for the staff. This may take the form of regular attendance at local scientific meetings and access to current information such as journals and the internet.

INFECTION CONTROL: SPECIFIC PRACTICAL FEATURES

There are a number of elements in a comprehensive infection control protocol:
- patient evaluation
- personal protection
- instrument cleaning, sterilization and storage
- use of disposables
- disinfection
- laboratory asepsis
- disposal of waste
- staff training including continuing education.

Patient evaluation

A thorough medical history should be taken from each patient and updated at each recall visit. It is not only a good clinical practice but may reveal disease that is important in relation to cross-infection and relevant to the dental procedure to be undertaken. If a questionnaire is used for this purpose, it should always be supported by direct discussions with the patient. The medical history should not be used to categorize patients as high or low risk, as was the procedure prior to the introduction of universal infection control. In taking a history the practitioner should identify the infectious disease of concern, and relevant questions should be asked in an environment conducive to the disclosure of sensitive personal information. It is also important that:
- all staff are trained in the **proper management of records**, including keeping them away from the public view in the front office, safe storage, and maintenance with due regard to appropriate data protection legislation
- a written **policy on confidentiality** should be signed by all staff members
- personal **medical or dental details are not disclosed** to other health-care workers without the consent of the patient.

Personal protection

This subject is dealt with under the following headings:
- personal hygiene
- clinic clothing
- barrier protection (gloves, eye shield, face masks, rubber dam isolation)
- immunization procedures.

Personal hygiene

The personal hygiene of all members of staff who are either directly or indirectly in contact with patients should be scrupulous. A rigidly followed code of hygiene will greatly reduce cross-infection in the dental clinic. In general, when working with patients, dental personnel should observe the following precautions:
- Refrain from touching anything not required for the particular procedure. Specifically, staff should keep their hands away from their eyes, nose, mouth and hair, and avoid touching sores or abrasions.
- Cover cuts and bruises on fingers with dressings because they serve as easy portals for pathogens.
- Hair should be kept short or tied up, or a hair net worn.

Hand care. Fingers are the most common vehicles of infection transmission. Hence the whole dental team should pay attention to meticulous hand care.

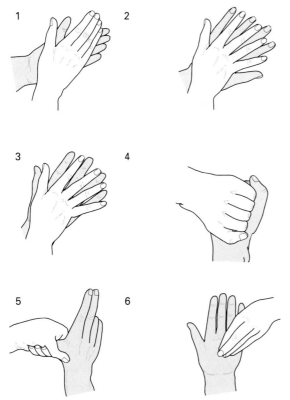

Fig. 37.1 A suggested hand-washing technique, showing the six movements required for a satisfactory wash: 1, the palms; 2, the webs between the fingers; 3, the webs again with altered grip; 4, palms to knuckles of opposing hands; 5, thumbs clasped in opposing palm; 6, tips of fingers against palms of opposing hand (4, 5, 6 repeated for each hand in turn). Continue washing hands and wrists for 1 minute. Rinse and dry thoroughly.

- A dedicated clean sink should be provided in the clinic for hand-washing, and the taps should be operated by elbow or foot controls or sensors (no-touch technique).
- Keep fingernails short and clean. Jewellery such as rings should be removed as they tend to entrap organisms and damage gloves.
- Thoroughly wash the hands before and after treating each patient using a proprietary antimicrobial handwash (e.g. chlorhexidine gluconate) before putting on gloves. Hands should also be washed before leaving the surgery for any purpose, and upon return.
- A good hand-washing technique, as shown in Figure 37.1, should be developed by all staff so that all areas of the hands are washed consistently (Fig. 37.2).
- Any obvious cuts or abrasions must be covered with adhesive waterproof dressings.
- Liquid (not bar) soap should be used for routine hand-washing, and antimicrobial liquids for hand-washing prior to surgical procedures.
- Hands should be dried thoroughly using disposable paper towels, and gloves should be worn as the last step before treatment commences.
- Moisturizing cream should be used as a routine at the end of each treatment session.

Clinic clothing

A freshly laundered uniform or overgarment should be worn by all clinical personnel. Garments should be changed at least daily, and more frequently if they become visibly con-taminated. Renewable overgarments should be washed at an appropriate temperature in a well-maintained washing machine. Grossly contaminated clothing should be dealt with separately.

Wear overgarments *only* in the clinic premises, not in corridors, canteens or lifts. An additional waterproof vinyl apron could be worn to protect the overgarment when working in the instrument cleaning area or the laboratory (e.g. denture trimming).

Barrier protection

Personal hygiene measures reduce the level of possible pathogens on our bodies and clothes, although they do not completely eliminate them. In order to further minimize the spread of organisms from staff to patients (and vice versa), the following protective barriers should be used:
- gloves
- eye shields
- face masks
- rubber dam isolation.

Gloves. All dentists and close support personnel should routinely wear **disposable latex** or **vinyl gloves**. The main aim of wearing gloves in routine dentistry is not to achieve consistent surgical sterility but to establish **reasonable standards of hygiene** in order to safeguard both the dental personnel and the patient.

The efficacy of gloves greatly diminishes if they are perforated. As gloves may perforate during surgical procedures it is advisable to change gloves at least **hourly** during long operative procedures on the same patient. Gloves should be checked for visible defects immediately after wearing them, and immediately changed when breaches occur; never wash and re-use gloves. Rarely, **allergic reactions** to gloves may develop in staff or patients. Skin creams, a spray-on microfilm on the skin or a cotton glove liner may help these individuals.

There are three main types of gloves used in dentistry: their different uses should be clear:
- clean, high-quality, **protective latex gloves** should be used whenever examining a patient's mouth or providing routine dental treatment when no blood-letting procedures are undertaken

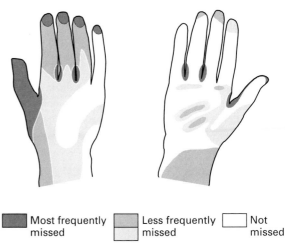

| Most frequently missed | | Less frequently missed | | Not missed |

Fig. 37.2 Areas of the hand that are not thoroughly washed owing to poor hand-washing technique.

- **sterile gloves** should be used for surgical procedures or procedures that may lead to blood-letting
- **heavy-duty utility gloves** should be used for cleaning instruments or surfaces or handling chemicals.

Care should be taken to prevent contact between gloves and incompatible material (e.g. some impression materials) or naked flames.

Gloves should be removed as soon as patient contact is over. The hands should then be washed, rinsed thoroughly and hand cream applied to prevent excessive drying of the skin. In addition, dental personnel should wash their hands with an antimicrobial handwash before leaving the clinic. Dental personnel with **exudative lesions** or **weeping dermatitis** should refrain from all direct patient care and from handling equipment until the condition resolves.

A new pair of gloves should be worn for each patient. Gloves should **never be reused**, as this will result in defects which will diminish their value as an effective barrier, and adequate removal of previous patients' pathogens cannot be guaranteed. Treat gloves as surgical waste and dispose of them accordingly.

Eye shields. Eye shields should be worn by dentists and close support personnel during all procedures to protect the conjunctivae from spatter and debris generated by high-speed handpieces, scaling (manual or ultrasonic), and polishing and cleaning of instruments.

- eyewear and face shields should be cleaned regularly, and when visibly soiled
- it is preferable to use eyewear with side protection
- a supine patient's eyes should always be protected.

Face masks. Wearing a face mask, such as a surgical mask, is a necessary hygienic measure, particularly during high-speed instrumentation, as it prevents inhalation of contaminated aerosols which might lead to both upper and lower respiratory tract infections. The **filtration efficacy** of such aerosols depends upon:

- the **material** used for mask manufacture (paper masks are inferior to glassfibre and polypropylene types)
- the **length of time** the mask is worn: the useful life of a mask is thought to be about 30–60 minutes, particularly if the mask is wet. Thus a clean mask should be worn for each patient.

Always ensure that masks are well adapted so that the nose and the mouth are completely covered. Masks with metal inserts are preferable as they can be tailored to fit the individual's profile.

Masks should not be touched with gloves during treatment or worn outside the treatment zone; they should be worn beneath face shields as the latter provide only minimal protection from aerosols.

Rubber dam isolation. As far as possible rubber dam should be used in operative procedures to minimize saliva and blood-contaminated aerosol production. Use of rubber dam during operative procedures:

- provides a **clear visual field** as the tissues are retracted
- minimizes instrument contact with the mucosa (thus minimizing tissue injury and subsequent bleeding)

- reduces **aerosol formation**, as saliva pooling does not occur on the rubber dam surface.

A chlorhexidine gluconate mouthwash (0.1–0.2%) prior to treatment is recommended by some, to reduce the intraoral microbial load and hence the number of airborne pathogens.

Aspiration and ventilation. Routine use of efficient high-speed aspirators with external vents and good ventilation will minimize cross-infection from aerosols. Aspirator tips should be sterilized and the lines regularly cleaned according to the manufacturer's instructions.

Handling sharps and related injuries

Numerous objects with sharp edges are used in dentistry (e.g. needles, blades, burs, endodontic files, orthodontic wires and matrix bands). A list of all the types of sharps used in the practice should be kept, identifying those that are disposable and those that may be reused and hence need to be processed. **Sharps containers** of approved type should be used in each working area and kept as close as possible to the point of use. They should not be overfilled and must be properly closed to prevent tampering, and they must be disposed of as clinical waste, ideally by **incineration**.

Extreme care should be taken when **re-capping** needles; a single-handed 'bayonet technique' or a resheathing device (Fig. 37.3) should be used for this purpose. The dental team should be conversant with all sharps handling procedures, which should be an integral part of ongoing staff education.

Sharps injury protocol. All sharps injuries should be recorded in a designated register and followed up. A standard protocol for sharps injury should be displayed clearly and at least one staff member assigned the responsibility for providing **post-injury counselling**, in the first instance. However, detailed counselling should be provided by a specialist in this field, to allay any residual concerns. Guidelines for the management of sharps injuries are shown in Table 37.1.

Imunization procedures

Practitioners should have a written policy on the vaccination (including administration of boosters) of all staff, and maintain an up-to-date immunization record of themselves and their staff which should be kept confidential. Staff who refuse vaccination and follow-up tests should be counselled regarding the implications of this course of action, and a signed acknowledgement to the effect kept on file. A list of vaccines that are available to dental health-care workers is shown in

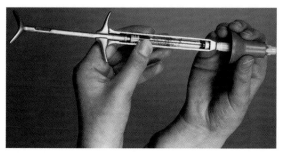

Fig. 37.3 A needle resheathing device.

Table 37.1 Principles guiding the management of sharps injuries

First aid
- Wash puncture site thoroughly with soap and warm water; antiseptics may be used in addition
- Encourage bleeding by squeezing the injured area
- Dry aseptically and report to supervisor according to the local regulations

Further action
- Review hepatitis B, C, and HIV risk of source patient
- Inform source patient of the incident and counsel patient regarding HIV test, if indicated
- Arrange venesection of the patient
- Contact Occupational Health Authority, as per local regulations

Action by Occupational Health Authority
- Record in detail circumstances of the sharps injury (i.e. demographic information of the exposed worker, details of the exposure)
- Check hepatitis B vaccination status of staff. If unvaccinated, commence *immediately* hepatitis B vaccination procedure together with intramuscular hepatitis B immunoglobulin
- Offer counselling to the recipient with regard to HIV risk
- Arrange venesection of the recipient for baseline serum antibody levels
- Arrange follow-up antibody testing at 6 months, or earlier if the recipient is anxious
- Return details to the Occupational Health Authority and the infection control team as appropriate

Chapter 10 (Table 10.2). In the UK, vaccination against hepatitis B virus, tuberculosis and rubella (for women) has been recommended for clinical dental staff, in addition to routine immunization against tetanus, poliomyelitis and diphtheria. In the USA, immunization against all the conditions listed, except tuberculosis and influenza, is recommended. A brief outline of vaccines available to dental personnel is given below.

BCG vaccine

Organism. Active against *Mycobacterium tuberculosis*. The vaccine contains live *M. bovis* (termed bacille Calmette–Guérin) attenuated by propagation in a bile–potato medium. Killed vaccines do not produce the cell-mediated immune response essential for protection against tuberculosis.

Indications. In the UK, all children between their 10th and 14th birthdays, if tuberculin test indicates no reaction.

Administration. Single dose intradermally in the deltoid muscle.

Poliomyelitis vaccine

Organism. Live poliovirus types 1, 2 and 3 — Sabin vaccine (used in UK) or killed poliovirus — Salk vaccine (used in developing countries and Scandinavia).

Indications. All infants, after 3 months.

Administration. Oral: three spaced doses result in multiplication of the innocuous organisms in the gut and resultant gut IgA and serum IgG production. Booster doses at school entry and school leaving.

Protection. Excellent for both vaccines.

Measles–mumps–rubella (MMR) vaccine

Organism. Live-attenuated strains of measles, mumps and rubella viruses.

Indications. All children in the second year of life, to prevent complications of common childhood fevers, such as respiratory tract infection and encephalitis associated with measles, meningitis associated with mumps, and congenital infections associated with rubella. The last is especially relevant for women of childbearing age working in dentistry.

Administration. One dose by the intramuscular route.

Protection. Good.

Triple vaccine: diphtheria–tetanus–pertussis (DTP)

Organism. Three-in-one vaccine for prevention against diphtheria caused by *Corynebacterium diphtheriae*, whooping cough caused by *Bordetella pertussis* and tetanus caused by *Clostridium tetani*. Contains killed *Bordetella pertussis* and diphtheria and tetanus toxoid.

Indications. All infants.

Administration. Three spaced doses by injection; subsequent booster doses of diphtheria and tetanus toxoids only.

Protection. Effective, but booster doses of tetanus and diphtheria are required to maintain immunity.

Tetanus toxoid

Organism. The toxin of *Clostridium tetani* which has been formol treated.

Indications. Active immunization of the entire population. Although the disease is rare, tetanus can develop after very trivial wounds.

Administration. Three spaced injections in infancy, as a component of the triple vaccine. Booster doses at 5 years, and in the event of injury.

Protection. Excellent.

Hepatitis B vaccine

Organism. The surface antigen of the hepatitis B virus, HBsAg (see Ch. 29), manufactured in yeasts by genetic recombination and absorbed on to aluminium salt. Successful vaccination also offers protection against delta hepatitis (hepatitis D).

Indications. All health-care workers who are at special risk, including dentists, dental hygienists, dental surgery assistants, medical laboratory workers and those handling blood products. In countries in South-East Asia where the disease is endemic, blanket vaccination programmes of all infants have been introduced in the hope of eradicating the disease.

Administration. Three doses (two doses at an interval of 1 month, followed by a third 6 months later) intramuscularly in the deltoid.

Protection. About 95% response rate. If antibody levels are suboptimal then a fourth (booster) dose may be given. Individuals having the initial course of vaccination should undergo pre- and post-immunization tests, and those who fail to seroconvert should be followed up as appropriate.

There is controversy over the necessity for booster doses. Some authorities in the UK advocate boosters after 3–5 years, depending on the degree of initial antibody production, whereas others, especially in the USA, contend that booster doses are unnecessary because of the anamnestic response of the immune system.

Passive immunization with hepatitis B immunoglobulin. Passive immunization with HBIG should be instituted **within 48 hours** if an **unprotected** health-care worker sustains an accident with blood or saliva containing hepatitis B antigens. This should be followed by a complete course of the hepatitis B vaccine, the first dose of which may be administered immediately or within 7 days of the accident. If the person declines the vaccine then a second dose of HBIG should be administered 1 month after the first dose.

Influenza vaccine

Organism. Usually contains two of the influenza A virus strains which are currently circulating, together with the influenza B strain. It is important to recognize that because of the phenomenon of antigenic 'drift' and 'shift' seen in influenza viruses, the vaccine composition needs to be reviewed and altered each year, which is a formidable task. The vaccine contains partially purified, disrupted virus particles or the surface antigens (haemagglutinin and neuraminidase).

Indications. Normally indicated for elderly individuals with respiratory diseases and those in residential facilities or long-stay hospitals, but elderly health-care personnel, including dental workers, may require vaccination in the event of an imminent outbreak.

Administration. One dose by injection, repeated each winter, which is the usual period of outbreak.

Protection. Relatively short (approximately a year).

Instrument sterilization

All instruments and appliances used in dentistry should ideally be **sterilized**, although some items of equipment and certain surfaces (e.g. bracket tables attached to the dental chair) do pose problems. In such circumstances the best alternative is to **disinfect** the items or surfaces concerned.

- **sterilization** is a process that kills or removes all organisms (and their spores) in a material or an object
- **disinfection** is a process that kills or removes pathogenic organisms in a material or an object, **excluding bacterial spores**, so that they pose no threat of infection
- **antisepsis** is the application of a chemical agent externally on a live surface (skin or mucosa) to destroy organisms or to inhibit their growth. Thus, all antiseptics could be used as disinfectants, but all disinfectants cannot be used as antiseptics because of toxicity.

In general, sterilization involves extensive treatment of equipment and materials, and is costly and labour-intensive. It is dependent on:

- knowledge of the death curves of bacteria or spores when they are exposed to the inactivation process; spores vary in their resistance to sterilizing agents: spores of *Bacillus stearothermophilus* are used to test the efficacy of steam autoclaves, while *B. subtilis* spores are used to test the efficacy of ethylene oxide sterilization
- the penetrating ability of the inactivating agent: steam penetrates more effectively than dry heat
- the ability of the article to withstand the sterilizing process, with no appreciable damage to instruments and other materials (e.g. corrosion of sharp, cutting edges of instruments)
- a procedure that is simple but efficient and relatively quick (so that there is a readily available supply of sterile instruments and materials): thus the temperature of sterilization is of crucial importance, as is the period for which the instrument or material is held at a given temperature — both these factors dictate the efficacy of the chosen sterilization method
- the effects of organic matter, such as saliva and blood, which enhance the survival of bacteria and interfere with the sterilization process. All articles must be clean before sterilization.

Sterilization can be divided into four stages:
1. Presterilization cleaning.
2. Packaging.
3. The sterilization process.
4. Aseptic storage.

Presterilization cleaning

The removal of contaminated instruments and equipment from the treatment area should follow a set routine, avoiding cross-contamination between the soiled and sterilized instruments. Once an effective method of instrument or equipment flow has been worked out, this method should be strictly adhered to. Heavy-duty household utility gloves must be used when cleaning instruments; eye protection and face masks are also desirable. Instruments should be cleaned as soon as possible after use. Sharps should be handled very carefully during scrubbing to prevent injury to the hands. Uncapped needles should never be left on the instrument tray, and after use these and other sharps should be placed directly in puncture-resistant containers.

In dentistry. Presterilization cleaning of instruments in dentistry can be achieved by **manual scrubbing** or **ultrasonic cleaning**. Ultrasonic cleaning is more desirable than manual cleaning because of:

- increased cleaning efficacy
- reduced danger of aerosolization of infectious particles
- reduced incidence of sharps injuries
- reduction in manual labour.

Packaging

After cleaning, instruments should be packaged to suit the appropriate clinical procedures. Instruments used in dentistry may be packaged for sterilization using:

- an open tray system sealed with a see-through sterilization bag
- perforated trays with fitted covers wrapped with sterilization paper
- individual packaging in commercially available sterilization bags.

The sterilization process

In dentistry, sterilization is usually achieved by one of three methods:

- moist heat (steam under pressure in an autoclave)
- dry heat (hot-air oven)
- gaseous chemicals (chemiclave).

Other sterilization methods, not used in dentistry, are ethylene oxide gas and gamma irradiation (employed by commercial suppliers of plastic goods), and filtration (used for sterilization of injectable drugs).

Moist heat sterilization (steam under pressure). Steam is a very effective sterilizing agent as it:

- liberates latent heat when it condenses to form water, potentiating microbicidal activity
- contracts in volume during condensation, thus reinforcing penetration.

When water is heated in a closed environment, its boiling point is raised, together with the temperature of the generated steam; for example at 104 kPa (15 p.s.i.) the steam temperature is 121°C (Table 37.2). This phenomenon is utilized

Table 37.2 Time-temperature combinations required for sterilization with an autoclave

Temperature (°C)	Pressure		Minimum hold time (min)	Overall cycle time[a] (min)
	p.s.i.	kPa		
134–138	30	207	3[b,c]	20
126–129	20	138	10	30
121–124	15	104	15[c]	40
115–118	10	69	30	50

[a] Maximum with empty chamber.
[b,c] Options recommended for dental instruments ([b] UK, [c] USA).

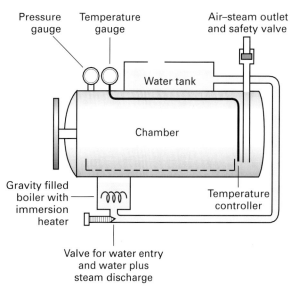

Fig. 37.4 Principal features of a small autoclave used in dentistry.

in steam sterilization by the **autoclave** (Fig. 37.4). Put simply, an autoclave is a glorified domestic pressure cooker with a double-walled or jacketed chamber; steam circulates under high pressure inside the chamber, in which the objects for sterilization (the load) have been placed. Once the sterilization cycle is complete, drying the load is accomplished by evacuating the steam. Drying can be accelerated by the suction of warm, filtered air into and through the chamber. It is important to expel the air in the chamber at the beginning of a sterilization cycle because:

- the temperature of an air–steam mixture at a given pressure is lower than that of pure steam
- air pockets interfere with steam penetration.

There are two types of autoclave:

1. **High-vacuum autoclaves** (porous load autoclaves) in which air is evacuated from a metal chamber by vacuum suction. These are mainly used in central sterile supply units in hospitals.
2. **Downward displacement autoclaves** are small, automatic bench-top autoclaves, very popular in dentistry. They work on the principle of downward displacement of air as a consequence of steam entering at the top of the chamber. The efficacy of this type of autoclave is low. Hence, recently introduced, bench-top, vacuum autoclaves are desirable for routine dentistry.

The time–temperature combinations required for sterilization with an autoclave are shown in Table 37.2. Of the options given, a sterilization cycle of 134°C for 3 minutes at 207 kPa is recommended for both wrapped and unwrapped dental instruments.

The sterilization cycle. The sterilization cycle (either in an autoclave or a hot-air oven) can be divided into three periods (Fig. 37.5): the **heating-up period**, the **holding period**, and the **cooling period**. For the bench-top autoclave (routinely used in dentistry) this entails:

1. Downward displacement of air by incoming steam while the chamber is heated to the selected temperature.
2. 'Holding' the load, which is sterilized, for the appropriate period at the selected temperature and pressure.

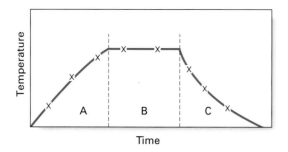

A = Heat up   B = Holding time   C = Cooling time

Fig. 37.5 The stages of a full sterilization cycle.

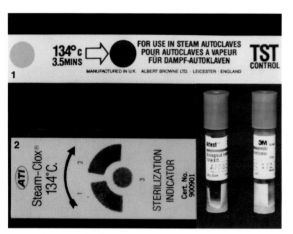

Fig. 37.6 Process indicators (1, 2) and a biological indicator (3) used for autoclave monitoring.

3. Drying the load to its original condition by a partial vacuum (this is assisted by the heat from the jacket).
4. Restoration of the chamber to atmospheric pressure by rapid exhaustion of steam.

Notes on the proper use of bench-top autoclaves

● Autoclaves should not be overloaded with instruments.
● The water reservoir should be checked daily and the water replaced according to manufacturer's instructions, to prevent build-up of residues or lubricant.
● Autoclaves should be serviced annually, and a log book of autoclave maintenance and defects kept.
● The mechanical indicators of the autoclave should be monitored routinely as a quality control exercise.
● A drying cycle should be used for bagged instruments.

Sterilization with dry heat. Dry heat penetrates less well and is less effective than moist heat; consequently, higher temperatures and longer times are required for sterilization. The total time for heating up, holding and cooling may be several hours. It is therefore essential that hot-air ovens should have a **time lock** on the door so that items cannot be added or removed during the cycle, and a **fan** to distribute the heat evenly.

Chemical vapour sterilization (chemiclave). A combination of formaldehyde, alcohols, acetone, ketones and steam at 138 kPa serves as an effective sterilizing agent. (The premixed chemicals must be purchased from the manufacturers as their balance is critical.) Microbial destruction results from the dual action of the toxic chemicals and the heat. In general, chemical vapour units sterilize more slowly than autoclaves (30 min versus 15–20 min, for packaged instruments) but are faster than hot-air ovens. The usual temperature and pressure combinations are 127–132°C at 138–176 kPa for a period of 30 minutes, once the correct temperature has been attained.

This process cannot be used for materials or objects that can be altered by the chemicals or are made of heat-sensitive material. Rusting is unusual if instruments are dried before sterilization as there is relatively low (7–8%) humidity throughout the process.

The major advantages of the chemiclave are that it is faster than dry heat sterilization, it does not corrode instruments or burs, and dry instruments are available as soon as the cycle is over. Adequate ventilation must be provided in order to dispel the residual fumes released on opening the chamber at the end of the cycle.

The advantages and disadvantages of sterilization using autoclave, chemiclave and hot-air oven are summarized in Table 37.3.

Monitoring sterilization. Achievement of the requisite temperature and pressure, as indicated by the gauges of the autoclave (or any other sterilizer), does not guarantee that the entire load has been sterilized. All sterilization procedures must therefore be carefully and regularly monitored so that failures are detected and sterility is assured. The indicators used for checking sterility are (Fig. 37.6):
● mechanical indicators (i.e. the temperature and pressure gauges of the autoclave)
● process indicators (chemical indicators)
● biological indicators/monitors.

Table 37.3 Advantages and disadvantages of sterilization with the autoclave, chemiclave and hot-air oven

	Autoclave	**Chemiclave**	**Hot-air oven**
Sterilization cycle	Short (3–30 min)	Intermediate (30–45 min)	Long (> 60 min)
Residual moisture	Present[a]	Present[a]	Nil
Long-term effect on instruments	Possible corrosion or rust	Minimal corrosion or rust	Affects temper and brittleness of sharp edges
Cycle interruption	Not possible	Not possible	Possible
Other hazards	None	Chemical hazards, possible	Spontaneous combustion of paper > 175°C

[a] Unless a drying cycle is available.

Process indicators are materials (either liquid or paper) that change colour on exposure to the appropriate sterilization cycle, indicating that the load has been processed. Note that process indicators **do not prove** sterilization but merely verify that the items have been subjected to the processing conditions; thus the main function of a process indicator is to assure the operator that the material has gone through a sterilization cycle. At least one process indicator should be cycled with every sterilization load and the results documented in a sterility control file.

In contrast to process indicators, **biological monitors** are designed to **prove** sterilization. The indicators used in this system are bacterial spores (see above), which require high temperatures for extended periods to lose their viability (the corollary is that if the spores are killed, then less-resistant microbes are killed more readily and sterility is achieved).

Biological monitoring or **spore tests** should be used on a **weekly basis** in dentistry. The monitor should be placed in the sterilizer at a point where sterilization is most difficult to achieve (e.g. inside bags or trays). After cycling, each strip should be sent for culture or cultured in the clinic according to the manufacturer's instructions. The results of biological monitoring should be routinely recorded and kept in a sterility control file. Spore tests should also be done when commissioning a new autoclave, after servicing or repairs, and as part of the training of new staff.

Storage and care of sterile instruments

Once sterilized, the instruments or items should be maintained in a sterile state until they are used again. The proper storage of sterile instruments is therefore as important as the sterilization process itself; improper storage would break the 'chain of sterility'.

The expected shelf-life of a sterile package depends on where it is stored and the material used for packaging. A closed, protected area of the clinic with a minimal air flow, such as a cabinet or drawer, that can easily be disinfected is preferable to an open stacking system. Packages of sterile instruments should be stored away from areas where splashing may occur, and checked for integrity before use.

DISINFECTION

Methods of disinfection consist of:
- heat (pasteurization; boiling in water)
- physical methods (ultrasonics)
- chemical methods.

Disinfection by heat

Pasteurization

Named after Louis Pasteur's discovery that mild heating prevents the spoilage of wine by selective killing of unwanted microbes. A similar treatment is now applied to milk to delay souring due to microbial activity. Milk is raised to a temperature of either 63–66°C for 30 minutes or (in the flash method) to 72°C for 15 seconds. This procedure renders the milk safe from contamination with *Mycobacterium tuberculosis*, *Campylobacter* and other pathogens. It should be noted that pasteurization is not a sterilization process.

Boiling water

If the boiling period is short, bacterial spores can survive; boiling water is therefore inadequate for sterilization of dental instruments.

Physical methods: ultrasonics

Ultrasound is an effective way of disrupting microbial cell membranes and is used for removing debris before autoclaving.

Chemical methods

Choosing a chemical disinfectant should be done carefully because a disinfectant used for one purpose may not be equally effective for another. Further, the antimicrobial activity of a chemical disinfectant falls drastically in the presence of organic debris. Products that usually disinfect items or surfaces may not do so when there is heavy contamination, particularly with resistant microbes in large numbers. The residual levels of organisms following disinfection may still represent an infection risk to unusually susceptible patients.

Mode of action of chemical disinfectants

The chemicals used as disinfectants generally behave as 'protoplasmic poisons' in three different ways:
1. Membrane-active disinfectants **damage the bacterial cell membrane** with resultant egress of the cell constituents; examples are chlorhexidine, quaternary ammonium compounds, alcohols and phenols.
2. **Fixation** of the cell membrane and blockage of egress of cellular components appears to be the mode of action of formaldehyde and glutaraldehyde.
3. Oxidizing agents **oxidize** cellular constituents; examples are halide disinfectants such as hypochlorite and bromides (the former is more active than the latter).

Conditions determining the effectiveness of a disinfectant

Spectrum of activity. Disinfectants vary widely in their activity, e.g. some are more active against Gram-positive than Gram-negative bacteria (Table 37.4).

Satisfactory contact. All contaminated surfaces should come into contact with the disinfectant for the specified period. Organic debris, air and greasy material may prevent this, hence the importance of thorough cleaning of the material or instrument before disinfection.

Concentration. Adequate concentration of disinfectants is essential and they should always be accurately dispensed. It is important to use the manufacturer's stated dilution of the disinfectant.

pH. The activity of a disinfectant is often pH–dependent (e.g. glutaraldehydes act only at alkaline pH, whereas phenols work best at acid pH).

Neutralization. A wide range of substances, including hard water, soaps and detergent, may neutralize the disinfectant.

Table 37.4 Properties of disinfectants used in dentistry

Disinfectant	Activity against				Inactivated by		Corrosive action
	GPC	GNB	Spores	TB	Protein	Soap	
Glutaraldehyde	++	++	++	++	±	–	+
Chlorine compounds	++	++	++	+	++	–	++ or ±Θ
Iodophors	++	++	± or –	+	+	–	–
Phenolics	++	++	–	+	±	–	+ or ±
Alcohol (70%)	++	++	–	+	++	–	–
Chlorhexidine	++	+	–	–	+	++	–

Θ, Buffered solutions; GPC, Gram-positive cocci; GNB, Gram-negative bacilli; TB, tubercle bacilli.
++, High; +, moderate; ±, low; –, nil.

Stability. Not all disinfectants are stable, especially when diluted, and may deteriorate with age or storage. Solutions should be freshly prepared for use and marked with an expiry date.

Speed of action. In general, disinfectants act slowly, and their activity depends on the concentration used. Hypochlorites have a rapid action, but are corrosive at high concentrations. Glutaraldehyde is slow-acting but is an effective sporicidal agent.

Absence of odour and toxicity. These attributes are desirable for disinfectants used in dentistry.

Cost. This is an important factor when choosing a disinfectant, although inexpensive disinfectants should not be used at the expense of those with desirable properties.

Biodegradability and environmental impact

Potency of disinfectants and their uses

Disinfectants can be generally categorized as having **high, intermediate** or **low potency**, depending on their ability to kill various groups of organisms.
- **high-level disinfectants** are active against Gram-positive and Gram-negative bacteria, spores and *Mycobacterium tuberculosis* (Table 37.4)
- **intermediate-level disinfectants** destroy *M. tuberculosis*, vegetative bacteria, most viruses and fungi, but few, if any spores
- **low-level disinfectants** kill most bacteria and most fungi, but not *M. tuberculosis* or spores.

A rough guide to the use of these three categories of disinfectants is given below.

Step 1. **Categorize** the items that require disinfection or sterilization into three groups:
- **critical items** are those that penetrate the skin or mucosa and/or touch exposed tissues including bone (e.g. scalpel blades, burs)
- **semi-critical items** are those that touch but do not penetrate the mucosal surface

- **non-critical items** come into contact with skin (e.g. surfaces of sinks, etc.)

Step 2. **Use** the appropriate technique:
- sterilization for all critical items
- sterilization or high-potency disinfectants for semi-critical items
- intermediate or low-potency disinfectants for non-critical items.

Disinfectant and antiseptic agents commonly used in dentistry

Alcohols

Ethyl alcohol or propyl alcohol (70%) in water is useful for skin antisepsis prior to cannulation, injection and surgical hand-scrubbing. Alcohol combined with aldehydes is used in dentistry for surface disinfection, but authorities in the USA do not recommend alcohol for this purpose as it evaporates relatively quickly, and leaves no residual effect. Other disadvantages are its flammability, limited sporicidal activity and ready inactivation by organic material. Yet, alcohols are still popular because they are cheap, readily available and water-soluble.

Aldehydes

Glutaraldehyde is perhaps the most popular disinfectant used in dentistry in some regions, whereas it is banned in others. It is both a skin irritant and a sensitization agent, which results in both long-term and short-term health effects. It is mainly used for so-called 'cold sterilization' or the high-level disinfection of equipment (such as fibreoptic instruments) that does not withstand autoclaving procedures. All aldehydes are high-potency disinfectants.

The free aldehyde groups of glutaraldehyde react strongly with the free amino groups of proteins in a pH-dependent manner. This leads to the effective microbicidal activity, sensitization of skin and incidentally, cross-linking with proteins such as collagen when used as a component of dentine bonding systems. Hence, as the pH decreases the activity of glutaraldehyde declines while its stability increases. Conversely, when the pH is alkaline, the activity is higher and it becomes less stable. Hence, in practice glutaraldehyde is commercially available as a 2% acidic solution, to which an 'activator' has to be added to bring the solution to the 'in-use' alkaline pH of 8.0. Although the activated solution has a shelf-life of up to 14 days, this should be interpreted with caution as the solution may become prematurely ineffective due to other factors.

Bisguanides

Chlorhexidine is an example of a bisguanide disinfectant; it is widely used in dentistry as an antiseptic and a plaque-controlling agent. For example, a 0.4% solution in detergent is used as a surgical scrub (Hibiscrub); 0.2% chlorhexidine gluconate in aqueous solution is used as an antiplaque agent (Corsodyl); and at a higher concentration (2%) it is used as denture disinfectant. It is a cationic bisguanide molecule, usually prepared as salts of acetate, digluconate, hydrochloride and nitrate.

As chlorhexidine has two positive charges at its polar ends it is highly active against both Gram-positive and Gram-negative organisms. (*Note*: all bacteria possess negatively charged cell walls in nature.) It also kills *Candida* (but not *M. tuberculosis*). Due to ingress of the disinfectant the cell membrane permeability is altered with resultant leakage of cell contents, precipitation of the cytoplasm leading to cell death. Its **substantivity** (i.e. prolonged persistence) in the oral cavity is mainly due to absorption on to hydroxyapatite and salivary mucus.

Halogen compounds

Hypochlorites and povidone–iodine are oxidizing agents and act by releasing halide ions. Although cheap and effective, they readily corrode metal and are quickly inactivated by organic matter. (Examples of proprietary preparations are Chloros, Domestos and Betadine.) *Note*: available chlorine is a measure commonly used to indicate the oxidizing capacity of hypochlorite agents and is expressed as the equivalent amount of elemental chlorine. Thus, the equivalence of 1% available chlorine corresponds to 10 000 p.p.m. available chlorine.

Phenolics

Phenolic disinfectants are either clear, soluble or black/white fluids (latter not used in dentistry). They do not irritate skin, and are used for gross decontamination because they are not easily degraded by organic material. They are poorly virucidal and sporicidal. As most bacteria are killed by these agents they are used widely in hospitals and laboratories. Examples are Clearsol and Stericol.

Chloroxylenol is also a non-irritant phenolic used universally as an antiseptic; it has poor activity against many bacteria and its use is limited to domestic disinfection (e.g. Dettol).

A sterilization and disinfection guide for items commonly used in dentistry is given in Table 37.5.

Dental unit water lines: disinfection and management

The question of the quality of water in dental unit water lines (DUWL) has been debated recently. The source of water to the dental unit is either from the municipal supply or wells,

Table 37.5 Sterilization and disinfection guide for items commonly used in dentistry

	Steam autoclave	Dry-heat oven	Chemiclave	Chemical disinfection/ sterilization	Disposable
Angle attachments	+	+	+	+	*
Burs					
Carbon steel	–	+	+	–	++
Steel	+	+	+	–	++
Tungsten-carbide	+	++	+	+	*
Condensers	++	++	++	+	*
Dapen dishes	++	+	+	+	*
Endodontic instruments (broaches, files, reamers)	+	++	++	—	*
Stainless steel handles	++	++	++	+	*
Non-stainless, metal handles	—	++	++	—	*
Stainless with plastic handles	–	–	–	+	*
Fluoride gel trays					
Heat-resistant plastic	++	—	—	—	*
Non-heat-resistant plastic	—	—	—	—	++
Glass slabs	++	++	++	+	*
Hand instruments					
Carbon steel	–	++	++	–	*
Stainless steel	++	++	++	+	*
Handpieces					
Autoclavable	++	–	–	—	*
Contra-angles	–	–	–	+	*
Non-autoclavable	–	–	–	+	*
Prophylaxis angles	+	+	+	+	*

Table 37.5 *Continued*

	Steam autoclave	Dry-heat oven	Chemiclave	Chemical disinfection/ sterilization	Disposable
Impression trays					
Aluminium metal:					
chrome-plated	++	++	++	+	*
Custom acrylic resin	—	—	—	+	*
Plastic	—	—	—	+	++
Instruments in packs	++	+	++	*	*
Instruments tray setups					
Restorative or surgical	+	+	+	*	*
Mirrors	–	++	++	+	*
Needles	—	—	—	—	++
Orthodontic pliers					
High-quality stainless	++	++	++	+	*
Low-quality stainless	–	++	++	–	*
With plastic parts	—	—	—	+	*
Pluggers	++	++	++	+	*
Polishing wheels and discs					
Garnet and cuttle	—	–	–	—	+
Rag	++	–	+	—	*
Rubber	+	–	–	+	+
Prostheses, removable	–	–	–	+	*
Rubber dam equipment					
Carbon steel clamps	–	++	++	–	*
Metal frames	++	++	++	+	*
Plastic frames	–	–	–	+	*
Punches	–	++	++	+	*
Stainless steel clamps	++	++	++	+	*
Rubber items					
Prophylaxis cups	+	–	–	+	++
Saliva evacuators, ejectors					
Low-melting plastic	–	–	–	+	++
High-melting plastic	++	+	+	+	*
Stones					
Diamond	+	++	++	+	*
Polishing	++	+	++	–	*
Sharpening	++	++	++	–	*
Surgical instruments					
Stainless steel	++	++	++	+	*
Ultrasonic scaling tips	+	—	—	+	*
Radiographic equipment					
Plastic film holders	–	–	–	–	++
Collimating devices	–	—	–	+	*

+, Effective and preferred method; ++, effective and acceptable method; –, effective method, but risk of damage to materials; —, ineffective method with risk of damage to materials. * Not applicable.
(Adapted from ADA Accepted Therapeutics and Dentists' Desk Reference Materials, Instruments and Equipment.)

and after entering the unit it passes through a multichannel control box which distributes the water to hoses feeding various attachments such as the high-speed handpiece, the air/water syringe and the ultrasonic scaler. The lines have a very small bore and hence bacteria tend to form **biofilms** on the internal surfaces unless they are regularly cleaned and disinfected. Although it has been questioned whether these innocuous saprophytic bacteria that live in water reservoirs are truly pathogenic, legislation has provided guidelines for the upper limits of bacteria and hence the quality of the water resources that service the DUWL. Generally, the water enter- ing the DUWL contains a very few organisms: 0–100 colony forming units (CFU)/mL. However, water exiting the hand- piece may contain up to 100 000 CFU/mL, mainly because of the organisms that are picked up from the bacterial biofilms growing within the lines.

The guidelines of the American Dental Association are that the water delivered to patients from DUWL during **non-surgical** dental procedures should not contain more than 200 CFU/mL of aerobic, mesophilic, heterotrophic bacteria at any point. The Association also stipulates that all dental units in future should contain a separate water reservoir independent of the public water supply, allowing dentists to have better control over the quality of the water used in patient care.

Recommendations on care of water lines

- All DUWL should be flushed for 2 minutes at the beginning of each day, prior to commencing treatment.
- The DUWL should be flushed for 30 seconds between patients to reduce temporarily the microbial count, as well as to clean the handpiece water line of materials that may have entered from the patient's mouth.
- All DUWL should be fitted with non-retractable devices, to prevent suck-back of material.
- Water from DUWL should **never** be used as an irrigant in procedures involving breaches of the mucosa and bone exposure.

Recommendations on care of handpieces

Different types of handpieces are used in dentistry and they should all be sterilized prior to use. The handpiece surface should be cleaned and the internal elements cleaned and lubricated according to the manufacturer's instructions before sterilization. Following sterilization, the handpiece should be stored as appropriate and run to remove excess lubricant immediately before use on patients.

LABORATORY ASEPSIS

Dental practitioners regularly send clinical material to the laboratory: impression material, dentures sent to the technology laboratory, or pathological samples such as pus or biopsy specimens referred to pathology laboratories, for example. The dentist is obliged to deliver all such items in a manner that obviates infectious hazards, whether during transport or within the laboratory. Blood and saliva must be carefully cleaned from the impressions and denture work, etc., by washing under running water and disinfection, and, if appropriate, placed in plastic bags before transport to the laboratory. Proprietary disinfectant sprays may be useful in decontaminating the microbes retained on impression surfaces.

The dental laboratory itself should be regarded as a clean (not a contaminated) area, and appropriate protocols for disinfection of surfaces and material, as well as regular and timely renewal of disinfectant solutions, should be established. Smoking and eating should be prohibited.

Microbiological specimens sent to the laboratory should be securely bagged to avoid contamination of personnel who handle the items. The request form should be separately enclosed to prevent contamination. Biopsy specimens should be put in a sturdy container with a secure lid to prevent leakage during transport. Care should be taken when collecting specimens to avoid contamination of the external surface of the container.

OFFICE/SURGERY DESIGN AND MAINTENANCE

Proper office or surgery design is the cornerstone of an effective infection control programme (Fig. 37.7). Major features of such a design are:

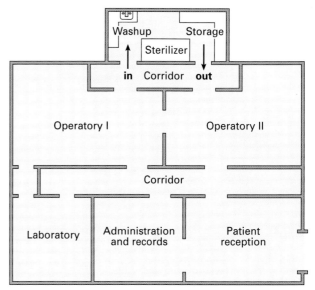

Fig. 37.7 Floor plan of a dental clinic designed to minimize cross-infection.

1. There is a clear demarcation between the **contaminated** and **clean zones**, i.e. the surgery and the sterilizing and storage areas, respectively.
2. Treatment areas and the laboratory should have few, if any, wood surfaces, porous or heavy draperies, or textured wall coverings, in order to facilitate cleaning and disinfection.
3. No eating or smoking is allowed in contaminated zones.
4. Carpets should not be used in the treatment areas, where flooring should be covered with seamless, disinfectant-resistant vinyl in order to minimize dust and microbial burden and to withstand frequent cleaning.
5. Ideally ventilation in the surgical and peripheral areas should be centrally controlled (air renewal three changes per hour) and planned to minimize cross-currents of air from one area to another. The air filter, if any, should be periodically changed and special venting installed to scavenge noxious chemical vapour.

Infection control requirements should always be borne in mind when selecting new equipment.

Instrument recirculation and office design

In order to conduct an efficient and routine sterility programme it is important to organize the various arms of the infection control programme outlined above in the most effective manner. Therefore it is essential to design the dental office and instrument recirculation areas (washing up, sterilizing and storage) to achieve this aim. The instrument recirculation area should be organized in order to:

- separate contaminated objects from sterile or clean objects
- store sterile items until required
- facilitate easy cleaning and disinfection
- facilitate a smooth flow of items between contaminated to clean zones.

A suitable instrument recirculation profile is shown in Figure 37.8. Other noteworthy points are:

- if possible, the instrument recirculation centre should be close to the clinic for ease of use

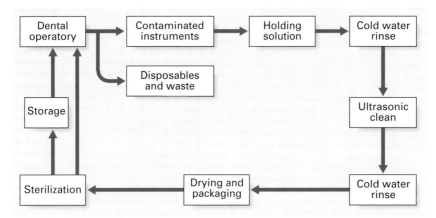

Fig. 37.8 A suggested scheme for instrument recirculation.

- the work surfaces of the area should be smooth, non-porous and seamless
- an air evacuation system (low volume) with continuous movement of air upward from the working surface should be operational to reduce airborne microbes and noxious chemical vapour (these should be regularly serviced and filters replaced as appropriate).

DISPOSAL OF WASTE

Any waste material that has been in contact with human sources is contaminated with potentially pathogenic microbes or will possibly support their growth. All sharp items (especially needles), tissues or blood should be considered as particularly dangerous and should be handled and disposed of with special precautions. Disposable needles, scalpels or other sharp items **must** be placed intact into puncture-resistant containers before disposal. Clinical waste should never be mixed with domestic waste as this is a dangerous practice; it may also lead to litigation.

KEY FACTS

- *The policy of **universal infection control** (also termed **standard precautions**), which assumes that **ALL** patients are potential carriers of infectious diseases, should be the norm in dental practice*
- The main features in a **comprehensive infection control protocol** are patient evaluation, personal protection, instrument cleaning, sterilization and storage, use of disposables, cleaning and disinfection of surfaces, laboratory asepsis, disposal of waste and staff training, including continuing education
- *Personal protection should incorporate appropriate clinic clothing, personal hygiene, barrier protection (gloves, eye shield, face masks, rubber dam isolation) and immunization procedures*
- As far as possible **rubber dam** should be used in operative procedures to minimize saliva/blood-contaminated aerosol production
- Use of efficient high-speed **aspirators** will minimize cross-infection from aerosols
- *To avoid sharps injuries, be conversant with all **sharps handling procedures**, which should be an integral part of staff education*
- *Have a written policy on the vaccination of all staff and maintain a confidential, up-to-date immunization record for all staff members*
- **Sterilization** is a process that kills or **removes all** organisms (and their spores) in a material or an object
- **Disinfection** is a process that kills or removes **pathogenic organisms** in a material or an object, **excluding bacterial spores**, so that they pose no threat of infection
- **Antisepsis** is the application of a chemical agent externally on a **live surface** (skin or mucosa) to destroy organisms or to inhibit their growth (all antiseptics are disinfectants but not vice versa)
- Sterilization can be divided into four stages: **presterilization cleaning, packaging, the sterilization process** and **aseptic storage**
- In dentistry, sterilization is usually achieved by **moist heat** (steam under pressure in an autoclave; most popular), **dry heat** (hot-air oven) or **gaseous chemicals** (chemiclave; least popular)
- The sterilization cycle (either in an autoclave or a hot-air oven) can be divided into the **heating-up period**, the **holding period** and the **cooling period**
- *The indicators that must be routinely used for checking sterility are **mechanical indicators** (i.e. the temperature and pressure gauges of the autoclave), **process** or **chemical indicators**, and **biological** indicators/monitors*
- *The key modes of disinfection are **heat** (boiling in water; pasteurization), **physical** (ultrasonics) and **chemical** methods (most used in dentistry)*
- Disinfectants can be generally categorized as having **high, intermediate** or **low potency**, depending on their ability to kill various groups of organisms
- Water in dental unit water lines for *non-surgical* procedures should not contain more than **200 CFU/mL** of aerobic, heterotrophic bacteria
- *Deliver all clinical **material sent to the laboratory** to obviate **infectious hazards** either during transport or within the laboratory*
- *Dispose of **clinical waste**, including sharps, in a **safe manner***
- **Proper office/surgery design** is the cornerstone of an effective infection control programme

FURTHER READING

ADA Council on Scientific Affairs and ADA Council on Dental Practice (1996). Infection control recommendations for the dental office and the dental laboratory. *Journal of the American Dental Association* 127, 672–680.

Beltramy, EM, Williams, IT, Shapiro, CN, and Chamberland, ME (2000). Risk and management of blood-borne infections in health care workers. *Clincial Microbiology Reviews* 13, 385–407.

Lowbury, EJL, Ayliffe, GAJ, Geddes, AM, and Williams, JF (eds) (1992). *Control of hospital infection* (3rd edn). Chapman & Hall, London.

Miller, CH (1996). Infection control. *Dental Clinics of North America* 40, 437–456.

Russell, AD, Hugo, WB, and Ayliffe, GAJ (1992). *Principles and practice of disinfection, preservation and sterilization* (2nd edn). Blackwell, Oxford.

Samaranayake, LP (1989). Cross infection prevention in dentistry. Part II: practical procedures. *Dental Update* 16, 108–112.

Samaranayake, LP, Scheutz, F, and Cottone, J (1991). *Infection control for the dental team.* Munksgaard, Copenhagen.

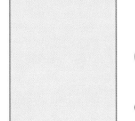

Glossary of terms and abbreviations

abscess A localized collection of pus (see pus)

acidophile An organism that prefers acidic environments; such an organism is said to be acidophilic

acquired immune deficiency syndrome (AIDS) The final stage of infection with the human immunodeficiency virus in which the patient has a low count of CD4$^+$ T cells and suffers from opportunistic infections, opportunistic malignancies and/or encephalitis/dementia

acquired immunity Immunity or resistance acquired at some point in an individual's lifetime

active acquired immunity Immunity or resistance acquired as a result of the active production of antibodies and activated T-cells

active immunization Stimulation of the immune system by intentional vaccination with foreign antigens

acute disease A disease having a sudden onset and short duration

acute-phase proteins Proteins whose concentration rises rapidly in body fluids following tissue injury or infection and which reduce inflammatory tissue damage

adaptive immunity The development of specifically activated B and/or T cells following exposure to antigen

adhesion molecule Cell surface molecule that enhances inter-cellular interactions

adjuvant A substance that enhances the immune response to an antigen

aerotolerant anaerobe An organism that can live in the presence of oxygen, but grows best in an anaerobic environment (one that contains no oxygen)

affinity maturation Introduction of point mutations into IgV genes which increases the strength of binding of antibody to antigen

agammaglobulinaemia Absence of, or extremely low levels of, the gamma fraction of serum globulin; sometimes used to denote the absence of immunoglobulins

agglutination The clumping of particles (including cells and latex beads) in solution

agglutination test Laboratory procedure that results in agglutination, usually following reaction with antibodies and antigenic determinants on particles

AIDS Acquired immunedeficiency syndrome

allergen An antigen to which one may become allergic

allergy Immediate hypersensitivity reaction in susceptible persons caused by release of pharmacological mediators from mast cells and basophils following interaction of surface-bound IgE with allergen

α_1-antitrypsin An acute-phase protein which neutralizes proteases released by bacteria or damaged tissue

$\alpha\beta$ T cells T lymphocytes bearing TCRs consisting of α and β chains

alternative pathway Complement activation independent of antibody, often induced by bacterial products such as endotoxin and lipopolysaccharide

amino acids The basic units or building blocks of proteins

anaerobe An organism that does not require oxygen for survival; can exist in the absence of oxygen

anamnestic response An immune response following exposure to an antigen to which the individual is already sensitized; also known as a secondary response or memory response

anaphylactic shock Severe immune reaction mediated by IgE which may be fatal owing to constriction of bronchial smooth muscles

anaphylatoxin Complement split products C3a, C4a and C5a which directly cause smooth muscle contraction and mast cell degranulation

anaphylaxis An immediate, severe, sometimes fatal, systemic allergic reaction

anergy Non-responsiveness to antigen. T cells may become specifically anergic when exposed to antigen in the absence of activation signal 2

angioedema Collections of fluid (oedema) in the skin, mucous membrane or viscera due to overproduction of anaphylatoxins

angstrom A unit of length, equivalent to 0.1 nanometre; roughly the diameter of an atom

antagonism The killing, injury, or inhibition of one microorganism by products of another

antibiotic A substance produced by a microorganism that inhibits or destroys other microorganisms

antibody Immunoglobulin (a glycoprotein) molecule produced by B lymphocytes in response to an antigen; binds specifically to the antigen that induced its secretion; often protective

antibody-dependent cell-mediated cytotoxity Killing of antibody-coated target cells by polymorphs, monocyte/macrophages or NK cells which have surface receptors for the Fc portion of IgG

anticodon The trinucleotide sequence that is complementary to a codon; found on a transfer RNA molecule

antigen Any molecule which can induce an immune response; sometimes called an immunogen

antigen presentation Display of short peptides bound to MHC molecules on antigen-presenting cells for recognition by T cells

antigen-presenting cells (APCs) Cells that are able to present peptides on MHC molecules to T cells and activate them

antigen processing Digestion of complex antigen molecules into short peptides, assembly of peptide–MHC complexes and transport of complexes to the cell surface of antigen-presenting cells

antigenic determinant The smallest part of an antigen capable of stimulating the production of antibodies or activating T-cells (see also 'epitope')

antigenic disguise Binding of normal, non-immunogenic, self molecules to the surface of a parasite so that its foreignness is masked

antigenic drift Minor structural changes of viral antigens due to point mutations

antigenic modulation Loss of antigen from cell surfaces following binding of antibody

antigenic shift Exchange of large segments of genetic material between viruses resulting in major changes in antigenicity

antigenic variation Modification of the structure of pathogen antigens

anti-idiotype vaccine Anti-anti-pathogen antibody with immunostimulating properties similar to those of the pathogen

anti-idiotypic antibody Antibody against V regions of antibodies, B-cell or T-cell receptors

antimicrobial agent A drug, disinfectant or other substance that kills microorganisms or suppresses their growth

antisepsis Prevention of infection by inhibiting the growth of pathogens

antiseptic An agent or substance capable of effecting antisepsis; usually refers to a chemical disinfectant that is safe to use on living tissues

antiserum Serum containing a particular antibody or antibodies; also called immune serum

antisialagogue Substance that prevents salivation

antitoxin An antibody produced in response to a toxin; often capable of neutralizing the toxin that stimulated its production

273

APC antigen-presenting cell

apicectomy An operation in which the apex of a tooth is removed

apoptosis A form of programmed cell death in which products of cell disintegration are packaged as membrane-bound particles which are readily phagocytosed

approximal Surface between adjacent teeth

aseptic technique Measures taken to ensure that living pathogens are absent

asymptomatic disease A disease having no symptoms

asymptomatic infection The presence of a pathogen in or on the body, without any symptoms of disease

atrophy Shrinkage in size of an organ or tissue by reduction in size of its cells

attenuated live vaccine Live vaccine containing organism of reduced virulence due to culturing under unfavourable conditions

autochthonous population A characteristic member of the microbial community of a habitat

autoclave An apparatus used for sterilization by steam under pressure

autogenic succession Bacterial succession influenced by microbial factors; for example, the metabolism of pioneer species lowers the redox potential during plaque development; this allows obligate anaerobes to colonize

autoimmune disease A disease in which the body produces antibodies directed against its own tissues

autoimmunity Diseases caused by pathogenic immune reactions against self antigens

autoradiography Exposure of a gel or blot to radiographic film to identify the position of a radioactive probe

autotroph An organism that uses carbon dioxide as its sole carbon source

avirulent Not virulent

axial filament An organelle of motility possessed by spirochaetes

B7 Molecules (B7.1 and B7.2) present on 'professional' APCs which bind to CD28 (to signal for activation) or CTLA-4 (to signal for inactivation) on T cells

bacillus (pl. **bacilli**) A rod shaped bacterium; also a member of the genus *Bacillus* (aerobic, Gram-positive, spore-forming rods)

bacteraemia The presence of bacteria in the bloodstream

bacteria (sing. **bacterium**) Primitive, unicellular, prokaryotic microorganisms

bacterial succession Pattern of development of a microbial community

bactericidal agent A chemical agent or drug that kills bacteria; a bactericide

bacteriocins Proteins produced by certain bacteria (those possessing bacteriocinogenic plasmids) that can kill other bacteria

bacteriophage A virus that infects a bacterium; also known simply as a phage

bacteriostatic agent A chemical agent or drug that inhibits the growth of bacteria

bacteriuria The presence of bacteria in the urine

basophil Type of polymorphonuclear leucocyte with granules that stain with basic dyes

B cell See B lymphocyte

B-cell receptor (BCR) Surface Ig molecules on B cells which recognize and bind antigens

bcl-2 An inhibitor of programmed cell death

β2-microglobulin A polypeptide associated with MHC-I molecules

binary fission A method of reproduction whereby one cell divides to become two cells

B lymphocyte Bone marrow derived lymphocyte responsible for production of antibodies

blotting Transfer of proteins on to nitrocellulose following electrophoresis

bone marrow Primary lymphoid organ, the site of production and development of blood cells

botulinum toxin The neurotoxin produced by *Clostridium botulinum*; causes botulism

candidiasis Infection with, or disease caused by, a yeast in the genus *Candida* — usually *Candida albicans*; formerly called moniliasis; also called candidosis

candidosis See Candidiasis (pl. candidoses or candidiases)

capnophile An organism that grows best in the presence of increased concentrations of carbon dioxide

capsid The external protein coat or covering of a virion

capsomeres The protein units that make up the capsid of some virions

capsule An organized layer of glycocalyx, firmly attached to the outer surface of the bacterial cell wall

cariogenic Dental caries-inducing (e.g. bacteria, carbohydrate-rich diets, etc.)

carrier An individual with an asymptomatic infection that can be transmitted to other susceptible individuals

CD28 Surface molecule on T cells which binds to B7 on 'professional' APCs to transmit T-cell activation signal 2

CD3 A group of proteins associated with the TCR that help transmit activation signals following engagement of TCR by MHC-peptide

CD4 Surface molecule on a subset of T cells that binds to MHC-II molecules during antigen recognition. The receptor for HIV

CD40 Surface molecule on 'professional' APCs that binds to CD40L on T helper cells to transmit B-cell activation signal 2

CD40 ligand (CD40L) Molecule present on T helper cells which binds to CD40 on 'professional' APCs and can transmit signal 2 for activation

CD45RA A molecule found on naive T helper cells

CD45RO A molecule found on memory T helper cells

CD8 Surface molecule on a subset of T cells that binds to MHC-I molecules during antigen recognition

cell membrane The protoplasmic boundary of all cells; controls permeability and serves other important functions

cell wall The outermost rigid layer of the cell (bacterial, fungal and plant cells)

cellulitis Spreading infection of subcutaneous tissues

centriole Tubular structure thought to play a role in nuclear division (mitosis) in animal cells and the cells of lower plants

cervicitis Inflammation of the neck of the uterus, the cervix uteri

chemokine One of a family of low-molecular-weight cytokines involved in lymphocyte trafficking

chemotaxis Migration of cells, especially phagocytes, towards a high concentration of a chemotactic factor

chitin A polysaccharide found in fungal cell walls, but not found in the cell walls of other microorganisms

chromatin The genetic material of the nucleus; consisting of DNA and associated proteins; during mitotic division, the chromatin condenses and is seen as chromosomes

chromosome A condensed form of chromatin; the location of genes; bacterial cells usually contain only one chromosome, which divides to become two just prior to binary fission

chronic disease A disease of slow progress and long duration

cilia (sing. **cilium**) Thin, hair-like organelles of motility

cistron The smallest functional unit of heredity; a length of chromosomal DNA associated with a single biochemical function; a gene may consist of one or more cistrons; sometimes used synonymously with gene

classical pathway Activation of complement by antigen–antibody complexes

climax community Stable complex microbial community that develops by, and is the final product of, the process of bacterial succession

clonal selection The process whereby an antigen induces proliferation of a single antigen-specific lymphocyte to produce large numbers of identical antigen-reactive daughter cells

coaggregation The attachment of a cell to a preattached organism by specific molecular interactions

coagulase A bacterial enzyme that causes plasma to clot or coagulate

coccus (pl. **cocci**) A spherical bacterium

codon A sequence of three nucleotides in a strand of messenger RNA that provides the genetic information (code) for a certain amino acid to be incorporated into a growing protein chain

coenzyme A substance that enhances or is necessary for the action of an enzyme; several vitamins are coenzymes; a type of cofactor

collagenase A bacterial enzyme that causes the breakdown of collagen

colonization resistance The ability of the resident microflora to prevent colonization by exogenous species

colony stimulating factor Cytokines that stimulate haematopoiesis

commensalism An interbacterial interaction beneficial to one population but with a neutral effect on the other

communicable disease A disease capable of being transmitted

community-acquired infection Any infection acquired outside of a hospital setting

competition Rivalry among bacteria for growth-limiting nutrients

complement An enzyme cascade consisting of over 25 components (including Cl through C9); involved in inflammation, chemotaxis, phagocytosis and lysis of microorganisms

conjugation As used in this book, the union of two bacterial cells, for the purpose of genetic transfer; not a reproductive process

convalescent carrier A person who no longer shows the signs of a particular infectious disease, but continues to harbour and transmit the pathogen during the convalescence period (e.g. hepatitis B)

co-stimulator molecule Molecule that stimulates second signals for activation

C-reactive protein An acute-phase protein which promotes phagocytosis of bacteria

C region Constant region of an antibody, BCR or TCR polypeptide

cross-reactivity Binding of antibody, BCR or TCR with antigen other than the one that induced activation

CTLA-4 Like CD28, binds to B7, but unlike the former induces T-cell inactivation

cyst A fluid-filled pathological cavity lined by epithelium

cytokine Soluble hormone-like messenger of the immune system (e.g. lymphokines, monokines)

cytoplasm The portion of a cell's protoplasm that lies outside the nucleus of the cell

cytotoxic Detrimental or destructive to cells

cytotoxin Toxic substance that inhibits or destroys cells (e.g. verocytotoxin of *E. coli*)

demineralization Dissolution of enamel or cementum by acid

dendritic cell A type of 'professional' antigen-presenting cell present in secondary lymphoid tissues which expresses high levels of MHC-I and -II molecules

dental caries Localized dissolution of the enamel or root surface by acid derived from the microbial degradation of dietary carbohydrates

dental plaque Tenacious deposit on the tooth surface comprising bacteria, their extracellular products and polymers of salivary origin

deoxyribonucleic acid (DNA) A macromolecule containing the genetic code in the form of genes

dermatophyte Fungal organism causing superficial mycosis of the skin, hair or nails

diplococci Cocci arranged in pairs

disinfect To destroy pathogens in or on any substance or to inhibit their growth and vital activity

disinfectant A chemical agent used to destroy pathogens or inhibit their growth; usually refers to a chemical agent used on inanimate material

disinfection A process that kills or removes pathogenic organisms in a material or an object, excluding bacterial spores so that they pose no threat of infection

diversity (D) gene Selectable V-region genes of BCR H chains, TCR β chains and TCR δ chains which contribute to the diversity of B- and T-cell repertoires

DNA Deoxyribonucleic acid

ecology The branch of biology concerned with interrelationships among living organisms; encompassing the relationships of organisms to each other, to the environment, and to the entire energy balance within a given ecosystem

ecosystem An ecological system that includes all the organisms and the environment within which they occur naturally

empirical therapy Therapy (usually antibiotics) prescribed without the benefit of laboratory tests

encephalitis Inflammation or infection of the brain

encephalomyelitis Inflammation or infection of the brain and spinal cord

endemic disease A disease that is always present in a particular community or region

endogenous processing The processing of intracellular proteins, including those of intracellular pathogens, on to MHC-I molecules for recognition by cytotoxic T cells

endoplasmic reticulum The network of cytoplasmic tubules and flattened sacs in a eukaryotic cell

endospore A resistant body formed within a bacterial cell

endotoxin The lipid portion of the lipopolysaccharide found in the cell walls of Gram-negative bacteria; intracellular toxin

enriched medium Culture medium that enables isolation of fastidious organisms from samples or specimens and growth in the laboratory

enterotoxin A bacterial toxin specific for cells of the intestinal mucosa

eosinophil Type of polymorphonuclear leucocyte with granules that stain with acidic dyes such as eosin

epidemic disease A disease occurring in a higher than usual number of cases in a population during a given time interval

epidemiology The study of relationships between the various factors that determine the frequency and distribution of diseases

episome An extrachromosomal element (plasmid) that may either integrate into the host bacterium's chromosome or replicate and function stably when physically separated from the chromosome

epitope The portion of an antigen that binds to the V region of an antibody, BCR or TCR

erythrogenic toxin A bacterial toxin that produces redness, usually in the form of a rash

eukaryotic cell A cell containing a true nucleus; organisms having such cells are referred to as eukaryotes

exogenous processing Processing of endocytosed extracellular proteins on to MHC-II molecules for recognition by T helper cells

exotoxin A toxin that is released from the cell; an extracellular toxin (opposite of endotoxin)

exudate Any fluid (e.g. pus) that exudes (oozes) from tissue, often as a result of injury, infection or inflammation

fastidious bacterium A bacterium that is difficult to isolate or grow in the laboratory owing to its complex nutritional requirements

Fc receptors Cell surface molecules on phagocytes and NK cells which bind to antibody-coated target cells

fermentation An anaerobic biochemical pathway in which substances are broken down and energy and reduced compounds are produced; oxygen does not participate in the process

fimbria (pl. fimbriae) Fine short, hair-like filaments that extend from the bacterial cell surface; synonymous with pili (see pili)

flagellum (pl. flagella) A whip-like organelle of motility

fomite An inanimate object or substance capable of absorbing and transmitting a pathogen (e.g. bed linen, towels)

fungus (pl. fungi) Eukaryotic, non-photosynthetic microorganism that is saprophytic or parasitic

fungicidal agent A chemical agent or drug that kills fungi; a fungicide

γδ T cells T cells using γ and δ instead of α and β TCR genes Probably important in defence against bacteria

GALT Gut-associated lymphoid tissue

gene A functional unit of heredity that occupies a specific space (locus) on a chromosome; capable of directing the formation of an enzyme or other protein

generalized infection An infection that has spread throughout the body; also known as a systemic infection

generation time The time required for a cell to split into two cells; also called the doubling time

genetic vaccines Pathogen-specific RNA or DNA segments capable of inducing pathogen protein expression and both humoral and cell-mediated immunity

genotype The complete genetic constitution of an individual; all of that individual's genes

genus (pl. genera) The first name in binomial nomenclature; contains closely related species

germinal centre The site of B-cell activation and differentiation in secondary lymphoid tissue

gingival crevice Protected habitat formed where the teeth rise out of the gum

gingival crevicular fluid Serum-like exudate bathing and flushing the gingival crevice. It has a considerable influence on the ecology of this region by introducing (1) nutrients for the microbial community and (2) components of the immune system and other host defences

gingivitis Inflammation or infection of the gingiva (gums)

glycocalyx Extracellular material that may or may not be firmly attached to the outer surface of the cell wall (e.g. capsule, slime layers)

gnotobiotic animal Germ-free animal deliberately infected with a known bacterial population or microflora

gp120 A component of the envelope of HIV, responsible for binding to CD4

gp41 A component of the envelope of HIV, responsible for fusion with target cell membranes

Gram stain A differential staining procedure named for its developer, Hans Christian Gram, a Danish bacteriologist; differentiates bacteria into those that stain purple (Gram-positive) and those that stain pink/red (Gram-negative)

granulocyte A granular leucocyte; neutrophils, eosinophils, and basophils are examples

granuloma Collection of macrophages, epithelioid cells, giant cells and fibroblasts formed in response to chronic immune stimulation, e.g. following persistent infection of macrophages

granzymes Granular proteases found in cytotoxic T cells and NK cells

growth curve A graphic representation of the change in size of a bacterial population over a period of time; includes a lag phase, a log phase, a stationary phase and a death phase

gut-associated lymphoid tissue (GALT) Accumulations of secondary lymphoid tissue associated with the gastrointestinal tract

haematopoietic stem cell Multipotent progenitor of all types of blood cells

haemolysin A bacterial enzyme capable of lysing erythrocytes, and releasing their haemoglobin

haemolysis Destruction of red blood cells (erythrocytes) in such a manner that haemoglobin is liberated into the surrounding environment

hapten A small, non-antigenic molecule that becomes antigenic when combined with a large molecule

HBV Hepatitis B virus; the aetiologic agent of serum hepatitis

HCV Hepatitis C virus; the aetiologic agent of hepatitis C

HDV Hepatitis D virus; the aetiologic agent of hepatitis D or delta hepatitis

hepatitis Inflammation of the liver

heterotroph An organism that uses organic chemicals as a source of carbon; sometimes called an organotroph

HGV Hepatitis G virus; the aetiologic agent of hepatitis G

HIV Human immunodeficiency virus; the aetiologic agent of AIDS

HLA Human leucocyte antigen

hopanoids Sterol-like molecules present in bacterial plasma membranes

host The organism on or in which a parasite lives

human immunodeficiency virus (HIV) The virus that causes AIDS

human leucocyte antigen (HLA) Product of the MHC in humans

hyaluronic acid A gelatinous, mucopolysaccharide that acts as an intracellular cement in body tissue

hyaluronidase A bacterial enzyme that breaks down hyaluronic acid; sometimes called diffusing or spreading factor, because it enables bacteria to invade deeper into tissue

hybridoma Hybrid cell produced by fusing an antibody-producing cell with a myeloma cell; hybridomas are immortal and produce monoclonal antibody

hyperimmune globulin Preparation containing specific antibodies used to prevent disease after exposure to a pathogen

hyperplasia Increase in the size of an organ by increase in the number of cells

hypersensitivity A condition in which there is an exaggerated or inappropriate immune reaction that causes tissue destruction or inflammation

hypha (pl. hyphae) Long, branching, thread-like tubes containing the fungal cytoplasm and its organelles; intertwining structural units of moulds

hypogammaglobulinaemia Decreased quantity of the gamma fraction of serum globulin, including a decreased quantity of immunoglobulins

ICAM Intercellular adhesion molecule

idiotype Antibody, BCR and TCR V regions

IFN Interferon

IgA Immunoglobulin class with the major function of protecting mucosal surfaces against pathogens

Igα, Igβ Proteins asociated with the BCR which help transmit B-cell activation signals

IgD Immunoglobulin class found on mature B-cell surfaces

IgE Immunoglobulin class that protects against helminths and is responsible for symptoms of allergy

IgG Major antibody class of the secondary immune response

IgM Major antibody class of the primary immune response

IL Interleukin

immune complex Complex of antigen with antibody

immune deviation Suppression of an ongoing immune response by a switch from type 1 to type 2 or type 2 to type 1 cytokine production

immunocompetent Able to produce a normal immune response

immunocompromised The state of being susceptible to infection by virtue of impairment or malfunction of the immune system

immunodeficiency A state in which the immune system is deficient in a particular type of immune response

immunodiagnostic procedures Diagnostic test procedures that utilize the principles of immunology; used to detect either antigen or antibody in clinical specimens

immunoglobulin Proteins, consisting of two light polypeptide chains and two heavy chains which function as antibodies

immunological synapse The signalling complex formed between an APC and a T cell

immunostimulating complex (ISCOM) Preparation of antigen combined with saponin, cholesterol and phosphatidylcholine that induces strong T- and B-cell immune responses

immunosuppression A condition in which a person is unable to mount a normal immune response owing to suppression or depression of their immune system

in vitro In an artificial environment, such as a laboratory setting

in vivo In a living organism; used in reference to what occurs within a living organism

inactivated vaccine Killed whole organisms, products of organisms or subunits of organisms that induce protective immune responses

inclusion body Distinctive structure frequently formed in the nucleus and/or cytoplasm of cells infected with certain viruses

indigenous microflora Microorganisms that live on and in the healthy body; also called indigenous microbiota, normal flora

infective endocarditis Infection of the lining of the heart (endocardium)

inflammation A pathologic process comprising a dynamic complex of cytologic and histologic reactions induced by injury or abnormal stimulation by physical, chemical or biological agents

innate immunity The natural protective mechanisms present before contact with antigen

intercellular adhesion molecule (ICAM) Molecule that interacts at cell surfaces to promote cell–cell contact

interferon (IFN) A class of small, antiviral glycoproteins, produced by cells infected with an animal virus; cell-specific and species-specific, but not virus-specific. Interferons are mediators that increase resistance to viral infection: IFNα is produced by leucocytes, IFNβ by fibroblasts and IFNγ by activated T cells and NK cells; IFNγ has numerous effects in modulating immune responses

interleukin (IL) A mediator involved in signalling between cells of the immune system

intravenous immunoglobulin Pooled antibodies from normal donors used to provide passive protection against infection in patients with antibody deficiencies

invariant chain A molecule that stabilizes 'empty' MHC-II molecules which can be replaced by antigenic peptides

ISCOM See Immunostimulating complex

isotype Immunoglobulin class, dependent on the type of heavy chain C gene used

isotype switching The change from expression of a 5′ Ig C_H gene by a B cell to expression of a downstream C_H gene

joining (J) gene Selectable V region genes of BCRs and TCRs which contribute to diversity of B- and T-cell repertoires

κ (kappa) light chain One of two types of Ig light chain

lag phase That part of a bacterial growth curve during which multiplication of the organisms is very slow or scarcely appreciable; the first phase in a bacterial growth curve

λ (lambda) light chain One of two types of Ig light chain

latency Incorporation of viral genes into those of the host cell without overt production of virions

latent infection An asymptomatic infection capable of manifesting symptoms under particular circumstances or if activated

lecithin A name given to several types of phospholipids that are essential constituents of animal and plant cells

lecithinase A bacterial enzyme capable of breaking down lecithin

leucocidin A bacterial enzyme capable of destroying leucocytes

leucocyte function-associated antigen (LFA) Molecule that interacts at cell surfaces to promote cell–cell contact

lipopolysaccharide A macromolecule of combined lipid and polysaccharide, found in the cell walls of Gram-negative bacteria

log phase Logarithmic phase; a bacterial growth phase during which maximal multiplication is occurring by geometrical progression; plotting the logarithm (log) of the number of organisms against time produces a straight upward-pointing line; the second phase in a bacterial growth curve; also known as the exponential growth phase

lophotrichous bacteria Bacteria possessing two or more flagella at one or both ends (poles) of the cell

lymphadenitis Inflammation of a lymph node or lymph nodes

lymphadenopathy A disease process affecting a lymph node or lymph nodes

lymph node Secondary lymphoid tissue which drains fluids from the tissues and concentrates foreign antigens on to APCs

lymphocyte Cell that expresses immunological specificity and is responsible for adaptive immune responses

lymphocytosis An increased number of lymphocytes in the blood

lymphokines Soluble protein mediators released by sensitized lymphocytes; examples include chemotactic factors and interleukins; lymphokines represent one category of cytokines

lymphotoxin Pro-inflammatory cytokine, also known as tumour necrosis factor β

lyophilization Freeze-drying; a method of preserving microorganisms and foods

lysogenic conversion Alteration of the genetic constitution of a bacterial cell due to the integration of viral genetic material into the host cell genome

lysosome Membrane-bound vesicle found in the cytoplasm of eukaryotic cells, containing a variety of digestive enzymes, including lysozyme

lysozyme A digestive enzyme found in lysosomes, tears and other body fluids; especially destructive to bacterial cell walls

lytic cycle Process occurring when a virus takes over the metabolic machinery of the host cell, reproduces itself and ruptures (lyses) the host cell to allow the newly assembled virions to escape

MAC See Membrane attack complex

macrophage A large phagocytic cell that arises from a monocyte

major histocompatibility complex (MHC) A complex genetic system coding for cell surface molecules which bind peptides for presentation to T cells

malaise A generalized feeling of discomfort or unease

MALT Mucosa-associated lymphoid tissue

mast cell Cells which bind IgE and release mediators of inflammation and allergy

membrane attack complex (MAC) The final stage of complement activation which can result in target cell lysis

memory The survival of certain T and B cells after initial encounter with antigen which are able to produce an accelerated and enhanced immune response on subsequently encountering the same antigen

meningitis Inflammation or infection of the meninges

mesophile A microorganism having an optimum growth temperature between 25°C and 40°C; such an organism is said to be mesophilic

mesosome A prokaryotic cell organelle (an infolding of the cytoplasmic membrane) possibly involved in cellular respiration

messenger RNA (mRNA) The type of RNA that contains the exact same genetic information as a single gene on a DNA molecule

MHC Major histocompatibility complex

MHC-I The class of MHC antigens (-A, -B and -C) that present peptides to CD8+ T cells

MHC-II The class of MHC antigens (-DP, -DQ and -DR) that present peptides to CD4+ T cells

microbial antagonism The killing, injury or inhibition of one microbe by the substances produced by another

microbial homeostasis The natural stability of the resident microflora of a site

microbicidal agent A chemical or drug that kills microorganisms; a microbicide

micrometre A unit of length, equal to one-millionth of a metre

minimum infective dose The minimum number of microorganisms required to cause an infection

mitosis A process of cell reproduction consisting of a sequence of modifications of the nucleus that result in the formation of two daughter cells with exactly the same chromosome and DNA content as that of the original cell

monoclonal antibodies Antibodies produced by hybridomas. Such antibodies are of exceptional purity and specificity

monocyte A relatively large mononuclear leucocyte; monocytes present in the blood differentiate into tissue-resident macrophages

monokine Soluble protein mediator released by activated monocytes and macrophages; monokines represent one category of cytokines

monotrichous Possessing only one flagellum

motile Possessing the ability to move

mRNA Messenger RNA

mucocutaneous Affects both skin and mucous membranes

mucosa-associated lymphoid tissue (MALT) Non-encapsulated dispersed aggregates of lymphoid cells positioned to protect the main passages by which microorganisms gain entry to the body (alimentary, respiratory and urinogenital tracts)

muramyl dipeptide A constituent of mycobacteria that is a potentially useful adjuvant for human vaccines

mutant A phenotype in which a mutation is manifested

mutation An inheritable change in the character of a gene; a change in the sequence of base pairs in a DNA molecule

mutualism A symbiotic relationship in which both parties derive benefit

mycelium (pl. mycelia) A fungal colony; composed of a mass of intertwined hyphae

mycology The branch of science concerned with the study of fungi

mycosis (pl. mycoses) A fungal disease

myelitis Inflammation or infection of the spinal cord

myocarditis Inflammation of the myocardium (the muscular walls of the heart)

nanometre A unit of length, equal to one-billionth of a metre

natural killer (NK) cell A type of cytotoxic human blood lymphocyte that kills cells (e.g. virus-infected cells, tumour cells) expressing low levels of MHC molecules

necrosis Death of tissues or cells

negative selection Depletion of thymocytes bearing TCRs that bind strongly to MHC + self peptides

neoplasia Literally 'new growth' of cells, but usually applied to benign or malignant cancers

nephritis Inflammation of the kidneys

neurotoxin A bacterial toxin that attacks the nervous system

neutrophil A type of granulocyte found in blood; its granules contain neutral substances that attract neither acidic nor basic dyes; also called a polymorphonuclear cell (PMN)

niche The function or role of an organism in a habitat. Species with identical niches will, therefore, be in competition

nitric oxide A major cytotoxic product of phagocytic cells, responsible for killing microorganisms

NK Natural killer; a type of lymphocyte

nosocomial infection Infection acquired while hospitalized

N-region addition The insertion of small numbers of non-templated nucleotides at junctions between BCR and TCR V(D)J segments

nuclear membrane The membrane that surrounds the chromosomes and nucleoplasm of a eukaryotic cell

nucleic acid Macromolecule consisting of linear chains of nucleotides (e.g. DNA, mRNA, tRNA, rRNA)

nucleolus A dense portion of the nucleus, where ribosomal RNA (rRNA) is produced

nucleoplasm That portion of a cell protoplasm that lies within the nucleus

nucleotide The basic unit or building block of nucleic acids; each nucleotide consists of a purine or pyrimidine combined with a pentose (ribose or deoxyribose) and a phosphate group

nucleus (pl. **nuclei**) That portion of a eukaryotic cell that contains the nucleoplasm, chromosomes and nucleoli

obligate aerobe An organism that requires 20% oxygen (the amount found in atmospheric air) to survive

obligate anaerobe An organism that cannot survive in oxygen

occlusal Surface on the top of the tooth

oedema Swelling due to an accumulation of watery fluid in cells, tissues or body cavities

oligonucleotide A compound made up of a small number of nucleotides, used to probe for complementary sequences within a gene

oncogene Gene expressed in malignant cells, the product of which may cause abnormal growth regulation

oncogenic Capable of causing cancer

oophoritis Inflammation or infection on an ovary

opportunist A microbe with the potential to cause disease when an opportunity arises (e.g. in HIV infection when resistance is low) but which does not do so under ordinary circumstances; also called an opportunistic pathogen

opportunistic infection Infection that only occurs in immunosuppressed or immunodeficient patients

opsonin A substance (such as an antibody or complement component) that enhances phagocytosis

opsonization Coating of particles with antibody or complement products to permit binding to Fc or C-receptors on phagocytes

osteomyelitis Inflammation of bone caused usually by infection

passive immunization Transfer of preformed antibodies to a non-immune individual, e.g. placental transfer of IgG antibodies to the fetus

PCR Polymerase chain reaction

perforin Molecule released by cytotoxic T cells and NK cells which polymerizes on target cell membranes, forming transmembrane channels

pericoronitis Infection around the crown of an erupting tooth

periodontopathogen An organism implicated in the aetiology of periodontal disease

peripheral tolerance Induction of specific non-responsiveness in anti-self T cells which have survived negative selection in the thymus

Peyer's patches Aggregations of lymphoid tissue in the lower ileum

phagocyte A cell that can engulf particles and digest them in cytoplasmic vacuoles

phenotype The properties shown by a body or cell that are due to expression of its genotype

pili Syn. Fimbriae; a specialized pilus called the sex pilus can form a link between recipient and donor cells during bacterial conjugation (mainly in Gram-negative bacteria)

pleiotropy Having several different activities. Used especially in describing cytokines

polyclonal activation Induction of a state of activation in a high proportion of lymphocytes (as opposed to the very low proportion activated by a given antigen)

polymerase chain reaction (PCR) A method of producing multiple copies of DNA using polymerase enzymes; this amplification process can be used to detect a microbe present in low cell numbers

polymorphonuclear leucocyte A phagocytic cell whose nucleus is composed of two or more lobes

positive selection The process of allowing those thymocytes whose TCRs bind with low affinity to MHC molecules + self peptides to survive

pre-B cells Cells that are committed to the B-cell lineage but have not yet expressed mature BCRs

primary lymphoid organs The sites of lymphocyte development: bone marrow and thymus

primary response The immune response that occurs on first exposure to a given antigen

prion Proteinaceous infectious particle that is the agent of slowly progressive chronic diseases such as variant Creutzfeldt–Jakob disease (v-CJD); smallest known infectious agent

prodromal phase The period between infection and the appearance of the symptoms

programmed cell death Self-destruction of cells that do not receive special signals for survival

prophylaxis Prevention of a disease or a process that can lead to a disease

proteosome Organelle responsible for processing of cytoplasmic proteins into peptides for antigen presentation

protoplasm The semifluid matter within living cells; cytoplasm and nucleoplasm are examples

protozoa (sing. **protozoan**) Unicellular eukaryotes found in water and soil; some are pathogens (e.g. *Entamoeba oralis*, found in the mouth)

purine A molecule found in certain nucleotides and, therefore, in nucleic acids; adenine and guanine are purines found in both DNA and RNA

pus A fluid product of inflammation, containing leucocytes, tissue debris and dead and dying bacteria

pyelonephritis Inflammation of certain areas of the kidneys, most often the result of bacterial infection

pyogenic Pus-producing; causing the production of pus

pyrimidine A molecule found in certain nucleotides and, therefore, in nucleic acids; thymine and cytosine are pyrimidines found in DNA; cytosine and uracil are pyrimidines found in RNA

pyrogen An agent that causes a rise in body temperature; such an agent is said to be pyrogenic

reactive oxygen intermediaries Cytotoxic products of phagocytes responsible for killing microorganisms

recombinant DNA technology The artificial manipulation of segments of DNA from one organism into the DNA of another organism, to allow cloning of the gene and synthesis of the specific gene product

recombinant vaccine A vaccine produced by recombinant DNA technology

redundancy Having the same activity as several other molecules. Used especially in describing cytokines

reservoir of infection Living or non-living material in or on which a pathogen multiplies and/or develops

resident microflora Members of the indigenous microflora that are more or less permanent

restriction enzyme Enzyme that breaks DNA at a specific nucleotide sequence

retrovirus A virus that transcribes its RNA into DNA and back again; this is accomplished by the presence of the enzyme reverse transcriptase

reverse transcriptase An enzyme that converts RNA into DNA

ribonucleic acid (RNA) A macromolecule of which there are three main types: messenger RNA (mRNA), ribosomal RNA (rRNA), and transfer RNA (tRNA); found in all cells, but only in certain viruses (RNA viruses)

ribosomal RNA (rRNA) The type of RNA molecule found in ribosomes

ribosome Organelle which is the site of protein synthesis in both prokaryotic and eukaryotic cells

RNA polymerase The enzyme necessary for transcription (see transcription)

rRNA Ribosomal RNA

saprophyte An organism that lives on dead or decaying organic matter; such an organism is said to be saprophytic

secondary disease A disease that follows the initial disease

secondary lymphoid organs Lymph nodes, spleen and mucosa-associated lymphoid tissue, the sites where lymphocytes encounter and respond to antigen

secondary response The immune response that occurs when memory T or B cells encounter antigen for a second or subsequent time

selective medium Culture medium that allows a certain organism or group of organisms to grow while inhibiting growth of all other organisms

septicaemia A disease consisting of chills, fever, prostration; the presence of large quantities of bacteria and/or their toxins in the blood

sequestered antigen Self antigen which is normally hidden from the immune system and does not induce neonatal tolerance. Following tissue damage these antigens may be released and stimulate an autoimmune response

sequestrum A necrotic piece of bone

serological procedure Immunodiagnostic test procedure performed using serum

serology Branch of science concerned with serum and serologic procedures

sex pilus A specialized pilus through which one bacterial cell (the donor cell) transfers genetic material to another bacterial cell (the recipient cell) during conjugation

sialadenitis Infection of the salivary glands

sialagogue Substance that encourages saliva production

sialolith Stone in the salivary gland

signal 1 An activation signal delivered through the BCR or TCR which alone is not sufficient for B-cell or T-cell activation

signal 2 A second activation signal required for lymphoid cell activation; for T cells this is mediated by binding of CD28 to B7 on an APC, for B cells CD40 must bind to CD40L on T helper cells

sinus A tissue tract or space lined with epithelium from which pus or fluids drain

Sjögren's syndrome A syndrome with dry mouth (xerostomia), dry eyes and rheumatoid arthritis

slime layer A non-organized, non-attached layer of glycocalyx surrounding a bacterial cell

SLPI Salivary leucocyte protease inhibitor (a proline-rich protein found in saliva that inhibits viruses such as HIV)

species A specific member of a given genus (e.g. *Porphyromonas gingivalis* is a species in the genus *Porphyromonas*). The name of a particular species consists of two parts — the generic name (the first name) and the specific epithet (the second name); singular species is abbreviated 'sp.', while plural species is abbreviated 'spp.'

specific epithet The second part (second name) in the name of a species

spirochaete Spiral-shaped bacterium (e.g. *Treponema denticola*)

spleen Secondary lymphoid organ important in the induction of immune responses to antigens present in the blood

sporadic disease A disease that occurs occasionally, usually affecting one person; neither endemic nor epidemic

sporicidal agent A chemical agent that kills spores; a sporicide

sporulation Production of one or more spores

stationary phase Bacterial growth phase during which organisms are dying at the same rate at which new organisms are being produced; the third phase in a bacterial growth curve

sterile Free of all living microorganisms, including spores

sterilization The destruction of all microorganisms, including spores

streptokinase A kinase produced by streptococci

subgingival Below the gingival (gum) margin; e.g. pertaining to a sample taken from the gingival crevice or periodontal pocket

substrate The substance that is acted upon or changed by an enzyme

subunit vaccine Vaccine that employs only immunogenic subunits of a pathogen, rather than the whole organism

superantigen Molecule that stimulates a subset of T cells by binding to TCR Vβ and MHC-II

superinfection An overgrowth of one or more particular organisms; often organisms that are resistant to an antimicrobial agent that the patient is receiving

surrogate light chains Polypeptides which together with the constant region of IgM produce a primitive receptor on the surface of pre-B cells

symbiosis The living together or close association of two dissimilar organisms

syncytium Multinucleate giant cell formed by fusion of several cells

synergism As used in this book, the correlated action of two or more microorganisms so that the combined action is greater than that of each acting separately (e.g. when two microbes accomplish more than either could do alone)

synthetic peptide vaccine Vaccine which employs only peptide epitopes of a pathogen

systemic infection See generalized infection

taxonomy The systematic classification of living things

T cell T lymphocyte

T-cell receptor (TCR) Heterodimers (αβ or γδ) on the surface of T cells which recognize and bind antigenic peptides presented by MHC molecules on APCs

T cytotoxic cells A subset of T cells that recognize antigenic peptides presented by MHC-I molecules and can kill the peptide-bearing cell

teichoic acid Polymer found in the cell walls of Gram-positive bacteria

terminal deoxynucleotidyl transferase An enzyme that causes the addition of nucleotides to the junctions between BCR and TCR V(D)J segments

tetanolysin Another neurotoxin produced by tetanus bacillus

tetanospasmin Another neurotoxin produced by *Clostridium tetani*; causes tetanus

TGF Transforming growth factor

T$_H$0 A newly activated T helper cell which secretes a wide range of lymphokines

T$_H$1 A T helper cell which produces IL-2, IFNγ and LT and induces macrophage activation

T$_H$2 A T helper cell which produces IL-4, IL-5 and IL-10 and induces B-cell activation

T helper cell T-cell subset required for activating the effector functions of macrophages, B cells, NK cells and other T cells

thermophile An organism that thrives at a temperature of 50°C or higher; such an organism is said to be thermophilic

thrombus A blood clot within a vessel

thymic selection Deletion of potentially self-reactive thymocytes and retention of thymocytes able to recognize foreign peptides presented by MHC molecules

thymocyte Precursor of mature T cells

thymus Organ in the mediastinal cavity anterior to and above the heart. Primary lymphoid organ for T-lymphocyte development

T lymphocyte Subset of lymphocytes that recognizes antigenic peptides in the context of MHC-I or -II molecules. See T cytotoxic cell, T helper cell, T suppressor cell

TNF Tumour necrosis factor

tolerance Specific non-reactivity to an antigen

tonsils Secondary lymphoid tissue in the pharynx

toxaemia The presence of toxins in the blood, especially during septicaemia

toxigenicity The capacity to produce toxin — a measure of virulence; a microorganism capable of producing a toxin is said to be toxigenic

toxin As used in this book, a poisonous substance produced by a microorganism

toxoid A toxin that has been modified artificially to destroy its toxicity but retain its antigenicity; toxoids are used as vaccines (e.g. tetanus toxoid)

transcription Transfer of the genetic code from one type of nucleic acid to another; usually, the synthesis of a mRNA molecule from a DNA template

transduction Transfer of genetic material (and its phenotypic expression) from one bacterial cell to another via bacteriophages

transfection Introduction of a segment of DNA into the genes of another organism

transfer RNA (tRNA) The type of RNA molecule that is capable of combining with (and thus activating) a specific amino acid; involved in protein synthesis (translation); the anticodon on a tRNA molecule recognizes the codon on an mRNA molecule

transformation In microbial genetics, transfer of genetic information between bacteria via uptake of naked DNA; bacteria capable of taking up naked DNA are said to be 'competent'

transforming growth factor beta (TGFβ) Cytokine with generally suppressive activity against cytokine-secreting cells

transient microflora Temporary members of the indigenous microflora that are 'in transit' (e.g. *E. coli* in the oral cavity)

translation The process by which mRNA, tRNA and ribosomes effect the production of proteins from amino acids; protein synthesis

transporter associated with antigen processing (TAP) Molecule responsible for transporting peptides from proteosome to endoplasmic reticulum for association with MHC-I

T regulator cell T-cell subset that suppresses immune reactions by producing mainly TGFβ and/or IL-10

T suppressor cell T-cell subset that negatively regulates immune responses, usually by interfering with T helper cell function

tuberculocidal agent A chemical or drug that kills *Mycobacterium tuberculosis*, the agent of tuberculosis

tumour necrosis factor (TNF) Cytokine that can damage tumour cells; TNFα and TNFβ (also known as lymphotoxin) are important mediators of inflammation and have other immune regulatory functions

universal precautions Safety precautions taken by health-care workers to protect themselves from cross-infection, where all patients are treated as if they were carrying an infection

urethritis Inflammation or infection of the urethra

urticaria A vascular reaction of the skin often caused by an allergic reaction

vaccination Stimulation of a specific immune response against a pathogen in order to provide protection against natural exposure to that pathogen

vacuole Membrane-bound storage space in the cell

vector An invertebrate animal (e.g. mite, mosquito) capable of transmitting pathogens among vertebrates

vegetation Blood clot on the heart lining or endocardium

V genes Genes encoding the variable region of antibodies, BCRs and TCRs

virion A complete, infectious viral particle

virucidal agent A chemical or drug that kills viruses; a virucide

virulence A measure of pathogenicity; invasiveness and toxigenicity contribute to virulence

virus Acellular microorganism that is smaller than a bacterium; an intracellular parasite

V region The part of an antibody, BCR or TCR responsible for binding to a specific epitope

xerostomia Dryness of the mouth, usually due to impairment of salivary gland function

zoonosis (pl. zoonoses) An infectious disease or infestation transmissible from animals to humans

Index

Numbers in **bold** refer to tables and illustrations